EXERCISE, CALORIES, FAT, AND CANCER

ADVANCES IN EXPERIMENTAL MEDICINE AND BIOLOGY

Recent Volumes in this Series

A Continuation Order Plan is available for this series. A continuation order will bring delivery of each new volume immediately upon publication. Volumes are billed only upon actual shipment. For further information please contact the publisher.

EXERCISE, CALORIES, FAT, AND CANCER

Edited by

Maryce M. Jacobs

American Institute for Cancer Research
Washington, D.C.

PLENUM PRESS • NEW YORK AND LONDON

Library of Congress Cataloging in Publication Data

Exercise, calories, fat, and cancer / edited by Maryce M. Jacobs.
    p.   cm. — (Advances in experimental medicine and biology; v. 322)
    "Based on the American Institute for Cancer Research conference on exercise, calories, fat, and cancer, held September 4-5, 1991, in Pentagon City, Virginia" — T.p. verso.
    Includes bibliographical references and index.
    ISBN 978-1-4684-7955-3   ISBN 978-1-4684-7953-9 (eBook)
    DOI 10.1007/978-1-4684-7953-9
    1. Cancer — Nutrition aspects — Congresses. 2. Fat — Physiological effect — Congresses. 3. Exercise — Physiological aspects — Congresses. 4. Low-calorie diet — Physiological aspects — Congresses. 5. Carcinogenesis — Congresses. 6. Cancer — Animal models — Congresses. I. Jacobs, Maryce M. II. American Institute for Cancer Research. III. Series.
    [DNLM: 1. Caloric Intake — physiology — congresses. 2. Dietary Fats — adverse effects — congresses. 3. Exercise — physiology — congresses. 4. Neoplasms — etiology — congresses. 5. Neoplasms, Experimental — chemically induced — congresses. W1 AD559 v. 322 / QZ 202 E954 1991]
RC267.45.E94   1992
616.99'4071 — dc20
DNLM/DLC   92-49867
for Library of Congress   CIP

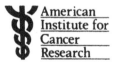

American
Institute for
Cancer
Research

Based on the proceedings of an American Institute for Cancer Research conference on Exercise, Calories, Fat, and Cancer, held September 4-5, 1991, in Pentagon City, Virginia

ISBN 978-1-4684-7955-3

© 1992 Plenum Press, New York
Softcover reprint of the hardcover 1st edition 1992
A Division of Plenum Publishing Corporation
233 Spring Street, New York, N.Y. 10013

Preface

The American Institute for Cancer Research (AICR) sponsored its second annual conference on nutrition and cancer. The theme was "Exercise, Calories, Fat, and Cancer" and the conference was held September 4-5, 1991 at the Ritz Carlton Hotel in Pentagon City, Virginia. This proceedings volume contains chapters from the platform presentations and abstracts from each poster presentation. Relationships among physical activity, calorie consumption, energy expenditure, dietary fat, and cancer are described in the context of epidemiologic, animal, and *in vitro* studies.

Dietary recommendations to lower cancer risk are based on expanding evidence relating nutrition and cancer. Identification of the precise dietary contribution to disease is complicated by the concurrent genetic and environmental contributions, in addition to the inherent difficulties in gathering and interpreting epidemiologic data. Individual variations in cancer risk are the result of differences in genetic and environmental factors including sources and amounts of calories consumed, metabolism, and energy expenditure. Human and animal studies describing independent and combined influences of exercise, calorie restriction, and dietary fat on carcinogenesis are reported in this volume.

Exercise: Data from epidemiologic studies on alumni of Harvard and the University of Pennsylvania associate physical activity with some cancers. The appearance of cancer at certain sites is inversely related to the frequency, duration, and intensity of physical activity. Moderate and high levels of activity correlate with lower colon cancer risk. The protective effects on colon cancer of energy expenditure, diet, decreased transit time, and possibly of increased prostaglandins, testosterone, and anti-oxidants are discussed. Prostate cancer risk is also lower in alumni with high energy expenditure. In the Harvard/University of Pennsylvania study increased physical activity does not appear to influence breast cancer risk.

Another chapter presents data from questionnaires sent to over 5000 female graduates, half of whom participated in organized athletic activity when in college. The rates of reproductive system cancers (uterus, ovary, cervix, and vagina) and of breast cancer are significantly lower in the former athletes than in the non-athletes. Factors that are considered to contribute to the decreased cancer rates in former athletes are discussed. These include late menarche, early menopause, restriction in dietary fat, leanness with increased formation of non-estrogenic metabolites from estradiol, and fatness with increased conversion of estrogen to potent estrogenic metabolites.

Data from studies in laboratory animals are presented that support and expand on human study data relating physical activity to cancer rates. Contrasting responses to voluntary and forced exercise are reported in several chapters. Based on a review of many studies in animals, *voluntary exercise* appears to consistently reduce the incidence and/or number of tumors in breast, colon, liver, and pancreatic tissue and conteracts the promoting effect of a high-fat diet. In contrast, *forced exercise* yields inconsistent results causing inhibition, no change, or stimulation of neoplasia. Additional studies in animals show that *voluntary* exercise during the post-initiation phase inhibits chemically and virally induced mammary tumor development and inhibits growth of transplantable metastasizing mammary tumors.

The variations in the effects of exercise on the carcinogenic response are related to differences in intensity and type (e.g. motorized cages, swimming, and treadmill running) of exercise. Other variables appear to be sex, energy expenditure, body weight, body composition, endocrine status, stress, and food consumption, especially dietary fat intake. Increases in prolactin secretion and in immune function with exercise reported in epidemiologic and experimental animal studies also have been related to the protective effect of exercise against some cancers. All together, data from human and animal studies suggest there might be an exercise threshold. That is, a specific type, intensity, and duration of exercise might be identified that affords optimal protection against cancer.

Calories and Fat: Several chapters consider mechanisms by which fat and calories influence carcinogenesis either independently or together. Lifetime studies in selected rat and mouse strains to determine the effects of reduced calorie intake on multiple physiologic, biochemical and pathological endpoints are in progress at the National Center for Toxicological Research. These studies have indicated that a restriction in total calorie intake by 40% of *ad libitum* controls lengthens lifespan, delays the onset of many degenerative diseases, including cancer, reduces lipid metabolism and the accumulation of free radicals, increases superoxide dismutase, and alters drug and xenobiotic metabolic systems. Reduced susceptibility to chemical carcinogens with calorie restriction has been related to reductions in cytochrome P450 activity and in DNA adduct formation.

Modifications of a variety of specific cellular events in an attempt to explain how calorie consumption and dietary fat might affect carcinogenesis are addressed. The influence of calorie restriction, fiber, and fat on cell proliferation, hence carcinogenesis, is one example. Excessive cell proliferation is associated with mutation, a critical process in carcinogenesis. Factors that alter cellular proliferation may have the potential to alter carcinogenesis. Data are presented from rodent studies. Restriction in calories up to 40% inhibits cell labeling, and cell proliferation, in many tissues with the most profound inhibition in the duct cells of the mammary gland.

Attempts to distinguish and prioritize differential effects of calorie restriction and energy expenditure on carcinogenesis are an underlying theme throughout the proceedings. Over seventy years ago a rise in human cancer rates was linked to excess calorie intake and early on in mice an inhibition of tumor growth was linked to under-feeding. Because of varied life-styles, human data do not conclusively establish whether it is the dietary fat or calorie intake that correlates directly with cancer incidence. Controlled dietary studies in animals designed to make this distinction indicate that the incidence of neoplasms is clearly related to calorie restriction. Further, the degree of calorie restriction required to lower the incidence of neoplasms still provides calories sufficient to maintain adult body weight, albeit a weight lower than in controls fed *ad libitum*. Calorie restriction reduces the incidence of spontaneous, transplanted, and induced tumors. Energy restriction also reduces tumor multiplicity and tumor burden. Mice fed restricted calories and high fat have fewer tumors than mice fed higher calories *ad libitum* and low fat. The enhancing effect of dietary fat can be obliterated by calorie restriction. The molecular mechanisms by which calorie restriction confers a protective effect are being investigated. The studies target multiple hormone activities, metabolism of carbohydrate, fat, and protein, as well as over-all energy expenditure. Recommendations of a life-style to reduce cancer risk include consuming appropriate levels of fruits, vegetables, and whole-grain cereals, less sugar and fats, especially polyunsaturated fats, restricted calories, and maintaining weight control with these eating patterns and exercise.

The site-specific inhibition of growth of a transplantable colon tumor (CT-26) by dietary marine oils and data comparing the effects of different amounts and types of lipids on the growth of chemically induced and transplantable tumors are described. The dietary marine oils (eicosapentaenoic and docosahexaenoic n-3 polyunsaturated oils) impair the growth of CT-26 implants in the bowel and lung, but not in the subcutis of the back; and implants in the back grow at the same rate in animals fed low or high levels of saturated or polyunsaturated n-6 or n-3. There are local areas of tumor necrosis in marine oil-inhibited colon tumor implants and not in n-6 polyunsaturated and saturated lipid-promoted tumors.

A review of the data from animal models is presented that supports and expands observations on fat effects in humans. Many studies attempt to elucidate the mechansims by which dietary fat influences the onset and development of cancer in mammary and other tissues. Primary observations are that an increase in dietary fat enchances mammary tumorigenesis, and the magnitude of the enhancement depends on the type of fat and duration of feeding. Fat can promote mammary tumor development in highly susceptible and genetically resistant rat strains and may act as a cocarcinogen. Contrary to frequent reports, data are presented showing increased quantities of unsaturated fats of vegetable origin can enhance mammary tumorigenesis more than high levels of saturated fats of animal origin. Feeding high fat during initiation does not profoundly or consistently affect turmorigenesis; while feeding high fat during promotion enhances tumor development. The possibility that there may be a threshold level of dietary fat and linoleic acid, whereby a further increase of either does not further increase mammary tumor development, is proposed. Studies on the effects of monounsaturated fatty acids from tropical oils, fish oils rich in omega-3 fatty acids, and *trans* versus *cis* fatty acids on chemically induced, spontaneous, and transplantable, mammary tumors are elucidated. *In vitro* studies suggest maximal growth stimulation of normal and neoplastic mammary cell growth requires linoleic acid and hormones such as insulin, progesterone, estrogen, and prolactin. How arachidonate and its metabolites stimulate tumor growth and confirmation of the role of leukotrienes in tumorigenesis are discussed. The observation that large reductions in fat consumption and only very small reductions in energy consumption can substantially reduce mammary tumorigenesis supports the notion that calories may be the predominant determinant of mammary tumorigenesis.

In several chapters the authors address the involvement of immune system components, membrane structure and function, of endocrine activities, and of energy metabolism in tumor cell growth. Studies with dehydroepiandrosterone (DHEA), an androgenic steroid, effects on azaserine-induced pre-neoplastic pancreatic foci, and tumor formation are presented. DHEA-fed animals eat less, gain less weight, have lower body fat, elevated energy and fat metabolism, and increased number and size of pre-neoplastic foci in pancreas compared with pair-fed controls. The focus of several studies is to learn how steroids affect fat metabolism with the idea that an optimal nutritional state, with respect to the amount and type of fat, can be determined.

Epidemiologic studies in the United States and other countries to identify factors that correlate with breast cancer risk are described in several chapters. The increase in breast cancer in Japanese women who adapt to the higher fat Western diet is cited. The observation that the magnitude of the increased cancer risk may be obscured by inaccuracies in mortality data, and in fat consumption estimates, is discussed. Another epidemiologic study shows a low incidence of breast cancer in southern Italy where the consumption of olive oil is high. Olive oil is rich in oleic acid, and omega-9 fatty acid, that does not affect mammary tumor promotion in rats as markedly as omega-6 PUFAs. Human and animal data suggest an apparent threshold for the fat effect. It is proposed that total fat calories at or below 20% do not affect carcinogenesis, whereas total fat calories at or above 30% promote carcinogenesis. The optimal diet proposed to lower human breast cancer risk contains 25% total fat calories and 25 grams of fiber per day.

Data and difficulties encountered in dietary intervention studies to lower breast cancer risk are reviewed. The studies discussed are the Women's Health Trial (a low-fat intervention study), the Nutrition Adjuvant Study, the Women's Intervention Study (WINS), the Swedish and Finnish Breast Cancer Studies, a Canadian Study and a proposed American Cancer Society Study. Epidemiologic data on the influence of exercise and of dietary saturated and unsaturated fat, phytoestrogen, alchol, fiber, and protein intake on breast concer are discussed. Confounding factors in interpreting human study data include inaccuracies in diet assessments, under-reporting of food intake, lack of measurements of compliance, poor long-term adherence to low-fat diets, combined effects of low fat, low energy, and decreased body weight, and discrepancies in adjusting energy intakes.

Many studies were reported in platform and poster presentations at the American Institute for Cancer Research Conference on "Exercise, Calories, Fat, and Cancer." Considerably more research is needed to identify theresholds in exercise, calorie restriction, and dietary fat consumption that might afford optimal protection against cancers at different sites. Throughout these proceedings difficulties in distinguishing and quantifying direct effects of exercise, energy metabolism, and dietary fat on cancer risk and the carcinogenic process are emphasized. Inconsistencies appear in the data from both human and animal studies regarding relationships between amounts and types of physical activity, dietary fat and calories, or energy utilization and carcinogenesis. Individual variations in genetics, physiology, age, and sex in addition to variations in study protocols contribute to the diversity of research findings. Continued research is targeted to resolve these problems and clarify the influence of exercise, calories, and fat on carcinogenesis.

The Editor

Maryce M. Jacobs, Ph.D. is presently Vice President for Research at the American Institute for Cancer Research in Washington D.C.. She received her Ph.D. in Biological Chemistry from the University of California at Los Angeles in 1970. Prior to her present position, Dr. Jacobs was a Biochemical Toxicologist for five years for The MITRE Corporation in McLean, VA, six years at the Eppley Institute for Cancer Research in Omaha, NE as Associate Professor and Industrial Contract Coordinator, and six years at M.D. Anderson Hospital and Tumor Institute in Houston, TX. While at M.D. Anderson, Dr. Jacobs also served as Cochairman of the Biochemistry Area of the University of Texas Graduate School of Biomedical Sciences for two years.

Dr. Jacobs' primary research interest is inhibition of chemical carcinogenesis with dietary factors, particularly selenium. She is a leader in this area having published some of the earliest studies on selenium inhibition of colon carcinogens, as well as of liver and lung carcinogens. Dr. Jacobs has also reported her research findings on antimutagenic, anticlastogenic, and antiangiogenic properties of selenium. In addition, she has described acute, subchronic, and chronic toxicity parameters of selenium in rodents.

Dr. Jacobs is a member of several prestigious organizations among which include the American Association for Cancer Research, the American Academy of Clinical Toxicology, the American Association for Advancement of Science, the American Chemical Society, American Men and Women in Science, and the Society of Toxicology. In addition, Dr. Jacobs has served as Vice President of the National Capital Area Chapter of the Society of Toxicology.

Contributors

Nile L. Albright, Department of Surgery, New England Deaconess Hospital, Boston, Massachusetts 02181

Tenley E. Albright, Department of Surgery, New England Baptist Hospital, Boston, Massachusetts 02181

William T. Allaben, National Center for Toxicological Research, Jefferson, Arkansas 72079

Roswell K. Boutwell, McArdle Laboratory for Cancer Research, University of Wisconsin Medical School, Madison, Wisconsin 53706

Elizabeth Boylan, Department of Biology, Queens College, City University of New York, Flushing, New York 11367

Selwyn A. Broitman, Departments of Microbiology and Pathology, Boston University School of Medicine, Boston, Massachusetts 02118

Francis Cannizzo, Jr., Departments of Microbiology and Pathology, Boston University School of Medicine, Boston, Massachusetts 02118

Ming Chou, National Center for Toxicological Research, Jefferson, Arkansas 72079

David B. Clayson, Toxicology Research Division, Bureau of Chemical Safety, Food Directorate, Health Protection Branch, National Health and Welfare, Ottawa, Ontario K1A OL2, Canada

Leonard A. Cohen, Division of Nutrition and Endocrinology, American Health Foundation, Valhalla, New York 10595

Thomas L. Dao, Professor of Surgery Emeritus, Roswell Park Memorial Institute, 666 Elm Street, Buffalo, New York 14263

Peter H. Duffy, National Center for Toxicological Research, Jefferson, Arkansas 72079

Johanna T. Dwyer, Frances Stern Nutrition Center, New England Medical Center Hospitals, 750 Washington Street, Boston, Massachusetts 02111

Marcy Epstein, Division of Nutrition and Endocrinology, American Health Foundation, Valhalla, New York 10595

Gabriel Fernandes, Department of Medicine, University of Texas Health Science Center, 7703 Floyd Curl Drive, San Antonio, Texas 78284

Ritchie J. Feuers, National Center for Toxicological Research, Jefferson, Arkansas 72079

Rose E. Frisch, Center for Population Studies, and Department of Population Sciences, Harvard School of Public Health, 9 Bow Street, Cambridge, Massachusetts 02138

Theresa C. Giles, Department of Pharmacology and Toxicology, Dartmouth Medical School, Hanover, New Hampshire 03756

Ronald W. Hart, National Center for Toxicological Research, Jefferson, Arkansas 72079

D. Mark Hegsted, New England Regional Primate Research Center, Harvard Medical School, Southboro, Massachusetts 02181

Russell Hilf, Biochemistry Department, University of Rochester, School of Medicine and Dentistry, Box 607, 601 Elmwood Avenue, Rochester, New York 14642

Penny Jee, Toxicology Research Division, Bureau of Chemical Safety, Food Directorate, Health Protection Branch, National Health and Welfare, Ottawa, Ontario K1A OL2, Canada

David Kritchevsky, The Wistar Institute, 3601 Spruce Street, Philadelphia, Pennsylvania 19104

Julian E. A. Leakey, National Center for Toxicological Research, Jefferson, Arkansas 72079

I-Min Lee, Department of Epidemiology, Harvard School of Public Health, Boston, Massachusetts 02181

Eric Lok, Toxicology Research Division, Bureau of Chemical Safety, Food Directorate, Health Protection Branch, National Health and Welfare, Ottawa, Ontario K1A OL2, Canada

Loren D. Meeker, Department of Mathematics, University of New Hampshire, Durham, New Hampshire 03824

Roger Mongeau, Nutrition Research Division, Bureau of Nutritional Sciences, Food Directorate, Health Protection Branch, National Health and Welfare, Ottawa, Ontario K1A OL2, Canada

Eduardo A. Nera, Toxicology Research Division, Bureau of Chemical Safety, Food Directorate, Health Protection Branch, National Health and Welfare, Ottawa, Ontario K1A OL2, Canada

Ralph S. Paffenbarger, Jr., Division of Epidemiology, Stanford University School of Medicine, Stanford, California 94305 and the Department of Epidemiology, Harvard School of Public Health, Boston, Massachusetts 02181

Walisundera M. N. Ratnayake, Nutrition Research Division, Bureau of Nutritional Sciences, Food Directorate, Health Protection Branch, National Health and Welfare, Ottawa, Ontario K1A OL2, Canada

B. D. Roebuck, Department of Pharmacology and Toxicology, Dartmouth Medical School, Hanover, New Hampshire 03756

Adrianne E. Rogers, Department of Pathology, Boston University School of Medicine and The Mallory Institute of Pathology, Boston City Hospital, 80 East Concord Street, Boston, Massachusetts 02118

Anne M. Ronan, Department of Animal and Nutritional Sciences, University of New Hampshire, Durham, New Hampshire 03824

David P. Rose, American Health Foundation, Division of Nutrition and Endocrinology, Valhalla, New York 10595

Isaac Schiff, Department of Gynecology, Massachusetts General Hospital, Boston, Massachusetts 02181

Fraser W. Scott, Nutrition Research Division, Bureau of Nutritional Sciences, Food Directorate, Health Protection Branch, National Health and Welfare, Ottawa, Ontario K1A OL2, Canada

Anthony R. Tagliaferro, Department of Animal and Nutritional Sciences, University of New Hampshire, Durham, New Hampshire 03824

Emanuela Taioli, American Health Foundation, Division of Epidemiology, 320 East 43rd Street, New York, New York 10017

Henry J. Thompson, Laboratory of Nutrition Research, AMC Cancer Research Center, Denver, Colorado 80214

Jaya T. Venkatraman, Department of Medicine, University of Texas Health Science Center, 7703 Floyd Curl Drive, San Antonio, Texas 78284

Clifford W. Welsch, Department of Pharmacology and Toxicology, Michigan State University, East Lansing, Michigan 48824

Alvin L. Wing, Department of Epidemiology, Harvard School of Public Health, Boston, Massachusetts 02181

Jelia Witschi, Department of Nutrition, Harvard School of Public Health, Boston, Massachusetts 02181

Ernst L. Wynder, American Health Foundation, Division of Epidemiology, 320 East 43rd Street, New York, New York 10017

Grace Wyshak, Center for Population Studies, and Department of Biostatistics, Harvard School of Public Health, Department of Medicine, Harvard Medical School, Boston, Massachusetts 02181

Edith Zang, Division of Nutrition and Endocrinology, American Health Foundation, Valhalla, New York 10595

Contents

Chapter 11
Enhancement of Pancreatic Carcinogenesis by Dehydroepiandrosterone 119
Anthony R. Tagliaferro, B. D. Roebuck, Anne M. Ronan and
Loren D. Meeker

Chapter 12
Caloric Restriction and Experimental Carcinogenesis 131
David Kritchevsky

Chapter 13
Breast Cancer — The Optimal Diet 143
Ernst L. Wynder, Emanuela Taioli and David P. Rose

Chapter 16
Dietary Fat, Calories, and Mammary Gland Tumorigenesis 203
   Clifford W. Welsch

Chapter 17
Dietary Fat and Breast Cancer: A Search for Mechanisms 223
   Thomas L. Dao and Russell Hilf

Chapter 18
Selected Recent Studies of Exercise, Energy Metabolism, Body Weight, and Blood Lipids Relevant to Interpretation and Design of Studies of Exercise and Cancer

Adrianne E. Rogers

Chapter 1

Exercise, Calories, and Fat: Future Challenges

D. MARK HEGSTED
Keynote speaker

I. Introduction

Developments in nutrition in the last 10 to 15 years have been remarkable. Less than 15 years ago the McGovern Committee published the Dietary Goals for the United States.[1] They were vigorously opposed—by the Food and Nutrition Board of the National Academy, the American Medical Association and practically everyone else. They were followed by the Dietary Guidelines for Americans[2] which were attacked in a similar fashion. Today these recommendations are, for all practical purposes, national nutrition policy. Although all of the issues are still discussed and researched, I see little evidence that the recommendations will be changed. I find it particularly interesting that the recommendations of the Diet and Health Committee of the Food and Nutrition Board[3] are quantitatively similar to those in the Dietary Goals.

One of the major objections raised originally, and continually, was that the primary basis for the recommendations came from epidemiologic data. Most of medicine is taught as an experimental science. Epidemiology is said to provide hypotheses for study but can provide no "proof" of anything. There is no doubt that the experimental method is powerful when appropriate experiments can be designed but only when good design and control are possible. I seriously doubt that many of the hypotheses relating diet to chronic disease can be adequately tested by field trials. In any event, I think we should remember that some of the greatest intellectual achievements—scientific achievements—have been developed by observation and deduction, such as evolution, the geologic history and structure of the earth and many others. Science is not limited to subjects which can be approached experimentally.

We face some serious challenges, however, in attempting to expand the evidence relating disease to nutrition and in the application of such knowledge.

D. Mark Hegsted • New England Regional Primate Research Center, Harvard Medical School, Southboro, Massachusetts

Exercise, Calories, Fat, and Cancer, Edited by M.M. Jacobs
Plenum Press, New York, 1992

II. Body Weight and Disease Risk

I would call your attention to the recent paper[4] that evaluated the effect of changes in body weight in the Framingham Study. Large fluctuations in body weight were found to be a serious health risk and may exceed the risk of moderate obesity itself. It has long been apparent that most weight-reduction schemes do not work in the long run. While I don't suppose that the success of any of the many approaches that have been tried are accurately known, a failure rate of 95% may be reasonable. It does not appear that we have been very successful in controlling obesity and the question can be asked whether the emphasis on avoidance of obesity over many years has been a net benefit or a loss.

I don't want to over-do it but we know there is excessive concern about obesity. Anorexia and bulemia are apparently increasing. I suppose that women's fashions have had a greater impact than nutritionists or the medical community on what women consider an appropriate body weight but I believe there are both health and psychologic hazards in over-emphasizing problems when no effective treatment is available. Now, with major programs to control blood pressure and serum cholesterol, if we all had our blood pressure and serum lipid levels tattooed on our foreheads, most of us might be under the same kind of pressure as those who are over-weight.

Ernst Wynder has said that "We want people to die young as late as possible." I think we might add to that, that we also want people to be reasonably happy while they extend their lives. Whether we are talking about exercise, calories or fat, too severe recommendations will not only fail but may have unfortunate effects.

III. Calories and Energy Expenditure

About calories. The nutrition bibles tell us that there are only two variables that really count—calorie intake and energy expenditure. How many times have we heard that 10 extra calories a day for umpteen years equals so many pounds of fat? I weigh about 5 pounds more now than I did over 50 years ago. I have probably consumed about 36.5 million calories and I have gained about 2000 pounds. I don't believe for a minute that the two essentially voluntary activities—intake and exercise—are harmonized to that degree. I am sure that we have dozens of internal controls over body composition and what happens to the calories we eat.[5]

The trouble with studies of energy metabolism is that we have no adequate measure of efficiency. We know that if we measure the amount of gas our car consumes and the heat produced that they would be equal. But these measures are meaningless unless we measure how many miles we get. The body differs, of course, in that if we step too hard on the gas, some energy will be converted to fat. But there is no reason to believe that the efficiency of the body is the same at all times or with all sources of fuel or that all people have the same efficiency. It is not how many calories we eat or burn that is over-riding but what happens to those calories.

Why is it that rats fed identical amounts of food do not grow at the same rate or develop the same body composition? Animal breeders have known for many years that you can easily selectively breed for efficiency and body composition. This is not simply a matter of energy intake and physical activity. I believe the biochemists when they tell us the maximal number of ATPs or high-energy bonds one can get from a calorie of fat or sugar. I see no reason to believe, however, that we are always at maximal efficiency, if ever. There are many ways that energy can be wasted in the body or the efficiency of ATP utilization modified.[5] When we learn what controls the yield of useful energy when foodstuffs are oxidized, we may begin to understand this problem.

I think we[6] showed clearly some years ago that, in young rats, calories from fat promote the deposition of body fat. It is of particular interest that in those animals, high-fat diets increased body fat even when the total energy intake was not sufficient to allow maximal growth. That is, even in partially starved animals, the energy from fat and carbohydrate was not equally available for all purposes. The energy from fat favored fat deposition rather than lean body mass. The conversion of dietary fat to body fat must be very efficient, probably about 90% efficient; the conversion of carbohydrate to fat cannot be more than about 40% efficient. But what controls the amount of fat or other material deposited in different body compartments?

We and others have also shown that animals fed low-protein diets waste energy.[7,8] The number of calories required to maintain weight in baby monkeys fed a low-protein diet is 10 to 15% greater than in those fed an adequate amount of protein. These are extreme situations but clear evidence that the efficiency with which animals utilize energy can vary and that the source of energy is important.

It is not that calories are not important. Obviously they are. But the simplified message we put out that a calorie is a calorie, equivalent under all conditions and regardless of their source or who eats them, is, I am sure, wrong.

IV. Food Composition Estimation and Evaluation

Regardless of how good or bad the epidemiologic data are, I suppose we would all prefer to have nice, clear-cut field trials demonstrating that lowering serum cholesterol does reduce heart attacks, that low-fat or high-fiber diets prevent cancer, etc. As I have already indicated, I am not convinced that many of the major problems related to the chronic diseases and nutrition can be answered in controlled trials where diet is modified and the end result evaluated.

One obvious reason, of course, is that these diseases are, in fact, chronic, the eventual outcome of insults over long periods of time which, in some cases, may be a lifetime. Just how long it takes is not very clear. Most of our diets probably impose a moderate risk but it may take a very severe dietary restriction to reverse the pathology or it may not be completely reversible.

As I see it, the evidence increases that few people can accurately report what they eat and I will predict that all of our methods of estimating food consumption will be under severe and increasing criticism in the future. We now appear to have for the first time an entirely independent estimate of total energy intake—the use of double-labeled water—which can be applied in the field. The results are discouraging. The British have always believed that the best means of getting accurate estimates of food intake was by having the subjects weigh their food for a week or so. In this country, a food record has been preferred since it is obviously less intrusive. I think it will be clear within a few years that neither is adequate.

The paper of Livingstone et al.[9] is rather remarkable. Some 31 subjects participated and completed a 7-day weighed-food record on two different occasions. A comparison of the calculated energy intake on these two occasions appeared to show that the second trial confirmed the first. There was a correlation coefficient of 0.79, which is better agreement than most people have found in comparisons of either the same or different dietary methods. Yet when the energy expenditure was estimated by the double-labeled water method, the average reported energy intake was about 15% too low and three subjects underestimated intake by 50 percent. A review[10] of the few comparisons now available (i.e., comparison of the reported energy intake from various kinds of dietary methods and energy expenditure by double-labeled water) indicates that in most instances the dietary data yield substantial underestimates of actual intake. A recent abstract from the English group[11] is not more encouraging. Estimates of energy intake by different methods and different dietitians yielded mean energy intakes of 64 to 84% of the energy expenditure. Few individuals appear to be capable of estimating energy intake within 10%. They say that "personal factors" strongly influence "cooperation" but when different methods of estimating intake are compared, it is not necesarily the same people who seriously underestimate intake. In these studies they rarely find signficant overestimation of energy intake indicating that there is a serious bias in the data as well as random error.

It is not necessary to dwell on the difficulties of estimating what we eat; we are all aware of them. It is not that the data we collect are meaningless, but I am sure that we are going to have to do some hard thinking about what such data mean and the conclusions we can draw from it.

With regard to field trials, it seems likely that when people know what they are expected to eat, they will report intakes that err on the side of the prescribed diet. Few participants want to demonstrate that they do not follow the diet if they continue in the trial so the bias is likely to be in that direction. There will always be slippage over time with a tendency for consumption to return to usual levels. Thus, all field trials will err on the side of no-effect, whether or not the hypothesis being tested is true or not. Negative field trials can probably never clearly demonstrate that diet is not effective but will be very discouraging when they yield a negative result, especially when they are as costly as they are.

Having emphasized how bad dietary data can be, I should say that I find it remarkable that so many studies have found that high levels of consumption of carotene or food sources of carotenoids protect against cancer.[12,13] It is perfectly clear that quantitative estimates of carotene consumption are very difficult to obtain. On the day you eat your carrots or spinach, carotene intake is very high, but it is very low on the days you don't eat such foods. It is likely that the protective effects are due to the anti-oxidant properties of carotenoids and perhaps other materials in such foods. It would seem to me that the only reasonable explanation for the findings is that the protective effect must be large—much greater, in fact, than the data indicate. It must be sufficient to overcome all the inadequacies of the data collected, the variations in genetic susceptibility, etc., all of which tend to yield negative findings.

V. Genetics, Diet, and Disease

It seems that about half of the research effort in biology these days is devoted to the search for genes, their structure and function. How useful such data will be in relation to most chronic diseases is unclear to me. I suppose that most of these diseases will involve several genes and identification of related genes will indicate increased risk but not certainty of disease. I worry that identification of individual "risk" may lead to too much emphasis upon the individual rather than upon the community. I believe it is clear that dietary instruction at the individual level, even when risk is rather high, usually fails. Effective dietary modification must involve at least the family. We will be truly effective when we modify the diet of the community.

In the U. S. about one in nine women will develop breast cancer. It is certain that if all women ate exactly the same diet—say the average American diet, whatever that is—they would not all get breast cancer. Similarly, we could all eat the same diet but we would not all have the same levels of serum lipids or be equally susceptible to heart attacks. In all metabolic trials very large differences in the serum cholesterol levels, not related to diet, have been observed. We[14,15] found that in a group of men who had been screened to remove real hypercholesterolemics or those with exceptionally low cholesterol levels, that the individual serum cholesterol levels varied about 100 mg/dl when they were all fed the same diet. The maximum change in the average serum cholesterol that we could achieve by manipulation of dietary fat and cholesterol was also about l00 mg/dl. These differences in dietary fat composition we examined were much greater than will ever be observed in most communities.

Hence, it is certain that most of the variation in serum cholesterol levels observed within any reasonably homogeneous community is due to differences, presumably genetic, in the way people respond to diet rather than to differences in what they eat. It is not surprising, therefore, that in most communities little or no relationship between estimated fatty acid or cholesterol intakes to serum cholesterol can be shown. We know that serum cholesterol can be modified by dietary fat and cholesterol. Negative findings within communities cannot disprove a dietary effect.

Whether we are dealing with fat and heart disease, salt and hypertension, fat or fiber and cancer, calcium and osteoporosis, or any other problem, it is certain that individuals vary in susceptibility. An environmental or dietary effect on the disease must represent a modification, to greater or lesser degree, of the genetic susceptibility. I think one serious weakness in the epidemiologic data is that we don't know how to deal with these variations in susceptibility, which obviously tend to obscure the evidence of dietary effects even when they are important. Perhaps in the future we will have additional indicators of risk due to genetic factors that can be taken into account.

Many, of course, have commented on the weaknesses of international comparisons relating diet to disease. They are fairly obvious but I suspect that, relatively speaking, the dietary data are not much worse than what we collect by other methods. Although the range of genetic susceptibility is large, migrant studies indicate that the over-all susceptibility of populations is probably not greatly different. Furthermore, in many populations we are dealing with long-term effects, diets which vary over a wide range of composition but have not varied a great deal over time, and with large sample sizes. I have more faith in many of these comparisons of populations than I do of studies within communities.

VI. Diets and Dietary Guidelines

Changing diets requires time. Many kinds of activities are important in educating the American public about desirable food habits and how to achieve them. I am reasonably optimistic about what we have achieved so far and the prognosis for the future. I suspect, however, that the food industries may very well determine what happens. We are eating more prepared and semi-prepared foods. I expect few people will be willing to spend more time in the kitchen and our diet will increasingly depend upon what the food industries make available. Many, if not most, Americans will eat a decent diet if it is not much more expensive and tastes as good as what they usually eat. Much of the food industry is trying to develop such products.

I would say a word in defense of the food industries. Nobody approves fraudulent advertising. On the other hand, an appropriate diet is composed of many foods and the consumer must select from a vast array of products. The contribution that individual foods make toward a good diet may not be large but the sum of many modest changes becomes important. Much of what the consumer knows comes from advertising. Advertising should be factual but the limitations on advertising should not be so severe that the consumer is deprived of the information required to make appropriate food selections.

Obviously, any list of problems reflects the interests of whoever makes the list as is clear here. But, to go back to the beginning, if I were to re-write the Dietary Guidelines now, I would probably include a serving or two of fish weekly and place more emphasis upon the vegetable sources of carotenoids. However, we made reasonable estimates of how Americans ought to be modified 10-15 years ago and I see no serious challenge to those recommendations. No doubt Dietary Guidelines can be and will be improved, but we are on the right track.

Acknowledgment

Supported in part by NIH grant No. RR00168 from the Division of Research Resources.

References

1. The Senate Select Committee on Nutrition and Human Needs, "Dietary Goals for the United States," 2nd Ed. U.S. Government Printing Office, Washington, D.C. (1977).
2. U.S. Department of Agriculture/U.S. Department of Health and Human Services, "Nutrition and Your Health: Dietary Guidelines for Americans," Home and Garden Bulletin No. 228. U.S. Government Printing Office, Washington, D.C. (1980).
3. Food and Nutrition Board, National Research Council, "Diet and Health: Implications for reducing risk of chronic disease," National Academy Press, Washington, D.C. (1989).
4. L. Lissner, P.M. Odell, R.B. D'Agustino, J. Stokes III, B.E. Kreger, A.J. Belanger, and K.D. Brownell, Variability of body weight and health outcomes in the Framingham population, *N Eng J Med*. 324:1839 (1991).
5. D.M. Hegsted, Energy needs and energy utilization, *Nutr Rev*. 32:32 (1974).
6. K. Donato and D.M. Hegsted, Efficiency of energy utilization of various sources of energy for growth, *Proc Natl Acad Sci USA*. 82:4866 (1985).
7. K.W. Samonds and D.M. Hegsted, Protein deficiency and energy restriction in young Cebus monkeys, *Proc Natl Acad Sci USA*. 75:1600 (1978).
8. L.M. Ausman, D.L. Gallina and D.M. Hegsted, Protein-calorie malnutrition in squirrel monkeys: adaptive response to caloric deficiency, *Am J Clin Nutr*. 50:1190 (1989).
9. M.B.E. Livingstone, A.M. Prentice, J.J. Strain, W.A. Coward, A.E. Black, M.E. Barker, P.G. McKenna, and R.G. Whitehead, Accuracy of weighed dietary records in studies of diet and health, *Br Med J*. 300:708 (1990).
10. D.A. Schoeller, How accurate is self-reported dietary energy intake?, *Nutr Rev*. 48:373 (1990).
11. A.E. Black, S.A. Jebb, S.A. Bingham, Validation of energy and protein intakes assessed by diet history and weighed records against energy expenditure and 24 h nitrogen excretion, *Proc Nutr Soc Abstacts of Communications*, Sept 6-7 (1991).
12. W.C. Willett and B. MacMahon, Diet and cancer — An overview, *N Eng J Med*. 310:633 (1984).
13. R.G. Ziegler, A review of epidemiologic evidence that carotenoids reduce risk of cancer, *J Nutr*. 119:115 (1989).
14. D.M. Hegsted, R.B. McGandy, M.L. Myers and F.J. Stare, Quantitative effects of dietary fat on serum cholesterol in man, *Am J Clin Nutr*. 17:281 (1965).
15. R.B. McGandy, D.M. Hegsted, F.J. Stare, Dietary fats, carbohydrates and atherosclerotic vascular disease, *N Eng J Med*. 277:417 & 469 (1967).

Chapter 2

The Influence of Physical Activity on the Incidence of Site-Specific Cancers in College Alumni

RALPH S. PAFFENBARGER, JR.,
I-MIN LEE and ALVIN L. WING

I. Introduction

The past dozen years have seen wide acceptance of epidemiologic evidence that adequate physical activity promotes physical fitness and counters tendencies toward development of coronary heart disease, a chief cause of early debilitation and premature death. But the evidence that physical activity influences cancer incidence is less clear, perhaps because cancer is a variety of diseases differing in underlying cause, age of onset, organ of involvement, induction period, and clinical course. Since exercise is a natural function of the body, its health benefits are thought to be achieved through its effects on all body systems, and accordingly it deserves serious study in relation to any effect it may have on prevention or delay in cancer occurrence.

Data from a large population of college alumni that were studied primarily for hypertensive-metabolic-atherosclerotic disease have been reviewed further for incidence of cancer in relation to levels of leisure-time, recreational activity. This report is intended to offer a brief overview of salient epidemiologic observations on these alumni in relation to findings on exercise and cancer incidence.

Archives of 40-75 years ago from the University of Pennsylvania and Harvard College have provided physical, psychologic, and sociocultural data recorded many years before the onset of site-specific cancers, and as prospective observations have afforded opportunity to examine etiologically oriented hypotheses relatively free of recall or interviewer bias.[1-3] These records from 1916-1950, plus mail questionnaires returned in 1962 or 1966, in 1977, and in 1988, together with death certificate data from 1916-1985, have permitted explorations

---

Ralph S. Paffenbarger, Jr. ● Division of Epidemiology, Stanford University School of Medicine, Stanford, California and the Department of Epidemiology, Harvard School of Public Health, Boston, Massachusetts; I-Min Lee and Alvin L. Wing ● Department of Epidemiology, Harvard School of Public Health, Boston, Massachusetts

Exercise, Calories, Fat, and Cancer, Edited by M.M. Jacobs
Plenum Press, New York, 1992

of physical activity and other personal characteristics for relation to the incidence of site-specific cancers.

II. College Sports and Site-Specific Cancers

In a first set of observations, college entrance physical examinations for 51,977 men from Harvard and the University of Pennsylvania, and for 4706 women from the latter university, provided data on more than 1.8 million person-years of follow-up during which 3375 cancer cases (1675 fatal and 1700 nonfatal) occurred through 1978.[4]

Physical activity as measured here refers to whether or not students had participated in intramural (house) or varsity (inter-collegiate) sports play. In their early college experience, about half the students had engaged in sports for five or more hours per week. Table 1 lists site-specific cancers and relative risks (RR) of developing these cancers in the interval from college entrance through 1978, by presence vs. absence of sports play at the breakpoint of five hours per week. For example, the relative risk (RR) of developing stomach cancer was 5% higher among students who played sports five or more hours per week than among students who played less or not at all (not significant). More active students were less likely to develop rectal cancer (RR=0.46) and more likely to develop prostate cancer (RR=1.66) than their age-comparable, less active classmates during follow-up (28-62 years) after college entrance.   Other relationships between sports play and specific cancer incidence were essentially null. Potential confounding characteristics were not considered, and although five or more hours of college sports suggests interest in a physically active way of life, this level of activity may or may not have persisted into the middle and advanced years.

Table 1.   Relative Risks (RR)[a] of Developing Selected Cancers (Nonfatal or Fatal) among 56,683 Harvard and University of Pennsylvania Alumni, 1916-1950 through 1978, by College Sports Play Pattern

Cancer	Total cases in 1,800,000 person-years	Sports play ≤5 hr/wk ~900,000 person-years		P
		Cases	RR of cancer	
Stomach	41	22	1.05	0.898
Colon	201	114	0.91	0.604
Rectum	53	24	0.46	0.038
Colorectum	254	138	0.80	0.168
Pancreas	86	48	0.86	0.554
Lung	194	116	1.22	0.286
Breast	46	16	0.96	0.920
Prostate	154	104	1.66	0.028
Testes	45	25	1.20	0.628
Kidney	53	29	0.95	0.888
Urinary bladder	58	25	0.72	0.304
Melanoma	59	30	1.05	0.876
Brain	54	32	1.51	0.238
Hodgkin's disease	52	29	0.73	0.336
Non-Hodgkin's lymphoma	86	40	0.67	0.134
All leukemias	81	42	0.84	0.588

[a] Computed by a proportional hazards model adjusting for differences in age and sex.[33]

Determination of rectal cancer occurrence from official death certification is suspected as unreliable, and although little relationship exists between higher levels of college sports play and the incidence of colon cancer in middle and later years (RR=0.91). Such a relationship for combined colon and rectal cancer (RR=0.80) was in the direction of a protective effect.

The relative risk of breast cancer (RR=0.96), a cancer suspected of being less common among women whose habits include greater participation in sports[5] was unassociated with activity as measured here. But again, potential confounding variables, such as body weight-for-height and catamenial and reproductive events were not taken into account. And, college sports play may be a poor long-term indicator of physical activity in midlife.

III. Alumni Physical Activity and Site-Specific Cancers

In a next set of observations, life-style habits were examined with emphasis on leisure-time physical activity in the middle and later years of life, after college, among 16,936 Harvard alumni. This group represented a subset of the total population who had reported on their exercise, social, and health status in 1962 or 1966 and were followed for site-specific cancer mortality through 1988.[4,6-9]

Alumni were classified by their exercise habits as reported through postal questionnaires. They indicated how many city blocks they walked daily, how many stairs they climbed up daily, and the types, frequencies, and durations of their sports or recreational participation in hours per week. Walking one mile rated 100 kilocalories (kcal); climbing and descending five stories (100 stairs), 40 kcal; and sports and recreation were classified in an index by standards of intensity as light, mixed, and moderately vigorous rated at 5, 7.5, and 10 kcal per minute. From these reported data, a physical activity index was computed per week. The index was regarded as an estimate or indicator rather than absolute total of energy output, largely in leisure time. When divided into ranges of less than 500, 500 to 1999, and 2000 or more kcal per week, index increments represented 15, 45, and 39% of the person-years, respectively.

Table 2 shows total and cause-specific death rates for the Harvard alumni along this gradient of energy expenditure. A total of 3939 (23%) of the men died between the ages of 35 and 94 years in the over 371,000 person-years of follow-up ending in 1988. Underlying causes of death totaled 43% from cardiovascular disease, 31% from cancer, 14% from other natural causes, and 12% from trauma. Death rates were adjusted for differences in age, cigarette smoking, and body weight-for-height—all strong predictors of death from many causes, including many cancers.

A decline in death rates with increasing activity was seen for all causes, all cardiovascular diseases, coronary heart disease, and chronic obstructive respiratory disease. But when examined for all cancer, and separately as site-specific cancers, energy output of leisure time among college alumni had little distinctive influence on death rates from any of these cancers. Death rates from colon cancer trended toward an inverse relationship with the physical activity index, just as they had in the larger experience with different method and time of assessment of energy expenditure, namely sports play during college time. Further, higher levels of physical activity measured as walking, climbing stairs, and participation in more vigorous activities in contemporary time trended toward a direct association with prostate cancer, just as five or more hours of sports play in college related to increased incidence of such cancer (both nonfatal and fatal) in a longer period of follow-up.

As defined and quantified in college, and on a single assessment in the early 1960s, physical activity showed little definite effect on the incidence of cancer occurrence. The types or amounts of exercise considered thus far are known to induce cardiovascular fitness (e.g., increased VO_2, max, reduced heart rate, and lowered blood pressure level), and

Table 2. Cause-Specific Death Rates per 10,000 Person-Years[a] among 16,936 Harvard Alumni, 1962 through 1988, by Physical Activity Index

Cause	Total deaths in 371,000 person-years	Physical activity index, kcal/week			P for trend
		<500	500-1999	2000+	
All causes	3939	116.8	108.8	97.4	<0.001
All natural causes	3475	103.4	96.3	85.3	<0.001
All cardiovascular diseases	1690	54.0	47.5	38.8	<0.001
Coronary heart diseases	1144	36.2	31.8	26.9	<0.001
Stroke	283	10.1	7.3	6.6	0.021
All respiratory diseases	216	8.1	5.8	4.7	0.006
All cancers	1213	32.0	32.9	32.6	0.336
Lung	224	5.5	6.1	6.2	0.413[b]
Colon	125	3.5	3.7	2.9	0.156
Rectum	24	0.3	0.5	1.0	0.048[b]
Colorectum	149	3.8	4.2	3.8	0.396
Pancreas	83	1.8	2.4	2.2	0.423[b]
Prostate	162	3.8	3.7	5.2	0.051[b]
All unnatural causes	464	13.4	12.5	12.0	0.150

[a] Computed by a proportional hazards model adjusting for differences in age, cigarette smoking, and body-mass index.[33]
[b] Opposite to all-cause trend.

metabolic fitness (e.g., improved lipoprotein profile and increased insulin sensitivity).[10] But they may be too imprecise, above the threshold level, or of the wrong type necessary to show an influence on risks of cancer occurrence.

IV. Long-Term Physical Activity and Colon Cancer

Since measurement of physical activity at a single point in time may not adequately reflect activity over the long term, we undertook study of 17,148 Harvard alumni followed prospectively for up to 26 years for the development of colon cancer (nonfatal and fatal), physical activity levels being assessed in both 1962 or 1966 and in 1977. A total of 225 cases developed in over 231,000 person-years of follow-up.[6]

In this set of observations a MET score was assigned to every sport, based on generally accepted values.[11,12] (One MET is defined as the energy expended while sitting quietly, and is equivalent to 3.5 ml of oxygen per kilogram of body weight per minute in the average adult.) To estimate the energy expended in each sport, its MET score was multiplied by body weight in kilograms and hours of play per week. Total energy expenditure was estimated from summing the resultant kcal per week from walking, stair-climbing, and sports play.

Alumni were then grouped into three activity levels by energy expenditure in kcal per week: "inactive" (less than 1000), "moderately active" (1000 to 2499), and "highly active" (2500 or more) as of 1962 or 1966. Person-years were counted beginning three years from the return of questionnaires in these years until questionnaires were returned in 1977, until death, or until clinical onset of colon cancer in the interim. In 1977, activity levels were recomputed from questionnaire responses of that year; person-years were counted from 1980 through 1985 for fatal cancers, and from 1980 through 1988 for nonfatal colon cancers.

As seen in Table 3, alumni classified as being moderately active had a 12% lower risk of developing colon cancer as compared with those less active, while alumni classified as highly active had a 15% lower risk. These reductions in risk are not statistically significant, nor is the trend of decreasing hazard rates with increased levels of inactivity.

In a separate analysis (Table 4), activity levels in 1962 or 1966 and in 1977 were assessed jointly to measure the effect of change or lack of change in relation to colon cancer incidence through 1985 for fatal outcomes, and through 1988 for nonfatal outcomes. There were 110 new colon cancer cases in 72,000 person-years of observation from 1980 through 1988. Using the experience of alumni who were physically inactive at both questionnaire assessments as standard, alumni who were moderately or highly active at both assessments experienced half the risk of colon cancer in the follow-up period. Men who had increased their physical activity between assessments tended to be at lower risk than the standard group (although the difference is not significant) while men who had decreased their activity were at similar risk to that for men who were inactive at both assessments (again not significant).

Table 3. Relative Risks (RR)[a] of Developing Colon Cancer (Nonfatal or Fatal) among 17,148 Harvard Alumni, by Physical Activity Levels Assessed in 1962 or 1966 with Follow-Up from 1965 or 1969 through 1977, and in 1977 with Follow-Up from 1980 through 1988

Physical activity level[b]	No. of cases in 231,000 person-years	RR of colon cancer[c]	90% confidence interval
Inactive	88	1.00	—
Moderately active	77	0.88	0.68–1.14
Highly active	60	0.85	0.64–1.12

[a] Computed by a Poisson regression model adjusting for differences in age.[34]
[b] Inactive = energy expenditure <1000 kcal/wk on walking, stair climbing, and sports playing; moderately active = 1000–2499 kcal/wk; highly active = 2500 or more kcal/wk.
[c] P for trend = 0.31.

Table 4. Relative Risks (RR)[a] of Developing Colon Cancer (Nonfatal or Fatal) among 17,148 Harvard Alumni, by Physical Activity Levels Assessed both in 1962 or 1966 and in 1977 with Follow-Up from 1980 through 1988

Physical activity level[b]	No. of cases in 72,000 person-years	RR of colon cancer	90% confidence interval
Inactive	24	1.00	—
Moderately active	11	0.52	0.28–0.94
Highly active	10	0.50	0.27–0.93
Increased	34	0.87	0.56–1.35
Decreased	31	1.02	0.65–1.60

[a] Computed by a Poisson regression model adjusting for differences in age.[34]
[b] Inactive = energy expenditure <1000 kcal/wk in walking, stair climbing, and sports playing; moderately active = 1000–2499 kcal/wk; highly active = 2500 or more kcal/wk; increased = upward change between categories; decreased = downward change between categories.

We conclude that higher levels of physical activity may provide some protection against the development of colon cancer. We can suggest two possible explanations for the finding that only men who were moderately or highly active in both 1962 or 1966 and 1977 were at lower risk of colon cancer. Either persistently higher levels of energy expenditure are necessary for protection, or measuring physical activity at two or more points in time increases the precision of measurement.

There are several mechanisms by which increased activity could protect against the development of colon cancer. Shortening intestinal transit may protect against this cancer by reducing contact time between colonic mucosa and such potential carcinogens as bile acids and their metabolites. And higher levels of energy expenditure may decrease transit time, especially in the ascending colon and proximal two-thirds of the transverse colon. A second mechanism may be via increased levels of certain prostaglandins, e.g., prostaglandin F2α, which is increased in men who exercise strenuously, and which in animals strongly inhibits growth of chemically induced colon cancer. A third mechanism may be through increased production of anti-oxidant enzymes, which may induce a protective effect on colon cancer.

There are a variety of potential limitations to these observations, e.g., selection bias, confounding by diet or other variables, and the imprecision of relying on death certification for case ascertainment. To offset such problems, we had excluded all cases from study that had onset of cancer within three years of reporting physical activity levels, thus reducing selection bias toward low-level activity as a result of disease. Diet could have confounded the relationship between physical activity and colon cancer. Nevertheless, if decreased transit time were the primary mechanism of exercise-induced protection, then diet would be an intermediary in the causal pathway, since potential carcinogens may be diet-derived. Misclassification of diagnoses on death certificates generally results from the over-reporting of colon and the under-reporting of rectal cancers. If, in fact, physical activity protects against colon and not against rectum, cancer findings consistent with much recent work,[13-27] this would result in an underestimate of the protective effect of energy expenditure on colon cancer.

V. High Levels of Physical Activity and Prostate Cancer

High testosterone levels have long been suspected as playing a role in the development of prostate cancer.[28-32] Since physical activity may induce lower circulating levels of testosterone, an active and fit way of life may indeed prevent or delay the clinical expression of prostate cancer. Using the same methods and population of Harvard alumni studied for predictors of colon cancer, we searched for any relationship between physical activity patterns in the 1960s and 1970s and risk of developing prostate cancer through the 1980s. A total of 419 clinically recognized cases of prostate cancer developed in men aged 30-79 during 228,000 person-years of follow-up.[7]

As in the study of colon cancer, we found that moderately and highly active alumni had the same risk of developing prostate cancer as their inactive counterparts when but a single assessment of physical activity was made (Table 5). These findings held for both older and younger alumni.

When activity levels were assessed jointly in 1962 or 1966 and in 1977, and at different breakpoints of physical activity (1000 and 4000 kcal per week), the findings are somewhat different for older alumni. Table 6 depicts risks of developing prostate cancer among 5048 alumni aged 70 or older and shows that the very highly active (expending 4000 or more kcal per week) had a significantly lower incidence rate as compared with moderately active and inactive men (RR=0.53). However, when incidence rates were examined by 1000 kcal per week increments of energy output, no evidence of a dose-response relationship was seen.

Table 5. Relative Risks (RR)[a] of Developing Prostate Cancer (Nonfatal or Fatal) among 17,719 Harvard Alumni, by Physical Activity Levels Assessed in 1962 or 1966 with Follow-Up from 1965 or 1969 through 1977, and in 1977 with Follow-Up from 1980 through 1988

Physical activity level[b]	No. of cases in 228,000 person-years	RR of prostate cancer[c]	95% confidence interval
Inactive	153	1.00	—
Moderately active	146	0.97	0.77–1.21
Highly active	120	0.99	0.78–1.26

[a] Computed by a Poisson regression model adjusting for differences in age.[34]
[b] Inactive = energy expenditure <1000 kcal/wk in walking, stair climbing, and sports playing; moderately active = 1000–2499 kcal/wk; highly active = 2500 or more kcal/wk.
[c] P for trend = 0.94.

Table 6. Relative Risks (RR)[a] of Developing Prostate Cancer (Nonfatal or Fatal) among 5048 Harvard Alumni Aged 70 Years or Older by Physical Activity Levels Assessed in 1962 or 1966 with Follow-up from 1965 or 1969 through 1977, and in 1977 with Follow-up from 1980 through 1988

Physical activity level (kcal/wk)	No. of cases in 31,000 person-years	RR of prostate cancer[b]	95% confidence interval
<1000	75	1.00	—
1000–3999	106	1.08	0.80–1.45
≥4000	13	0.53	0.29–0.95

[a] Computed by a Poisson regression model adjusting for differences in age.[34]
[b] P for trend = 0.17.

Although these findings suggest that men who are highly active in terms of total energy expended each week in leisure time may be at lower risk of developing prostate cancer than their inactive classmates, the present observations are too meager to provide much assurance of this.

VI. Physical Activity and Breast Cancer Incidence

In prospective observations of life-style habits that might predict risk of various chronic diseases in middle-aged women, we studied physical activity patterns and incidence rates of breast cancer among 2370 University of Pennsylvania alumnae aged 40-50 years in 1962. In 15 years of follow-up, 73 breast cancers (nonfatal or fatal) were identified. We constructed a physical activity index from reported walking, stair-climbing, and recreational sports, as was done for Harvard alumni (see Section III). In over 25,000 person-years of follow-up, alumnae who expended 1000 or more kcal per week were only slightly less likely to develop breast cancer than less active alumnae (RR=0.88). This risk estimate, adjusted for differences in age, body-mass index, and history of maternal cancer was not significant (95% confidence interval, 0.54-1.43). This small experience, not adjusted for many potential confounding characteristics (e.g., factors of womanhood), fails to lend support to the idea that active and fit women are at lower lifetime risk of breast cancer.[5]

VII. Conclusion

Where energy expenditure of occupational and leisure time may have only limited direct value in reducing the incidence or delaying the onset of the composite of human cancers, various types and amounts of exercise influence: physiologic and biochemical events, choice and results of diet, autoimmune mechanisms, and body-fat depositions—all of which are thought to be related to cancer occurrence. Accordingly, continued attention to the type, timing, frequency, intensity, and constancy of physical energy expenditure, for its influence on cancer incidence and progression, is warranted and should be encouraged.

Acknowledgment

Supported by research grants (R01 CA 44854) from the National Cancer Institute and (R01 HL 34174) from the National Heart, Lung and Blood Institute.

Report number XLVII in a series on chronic disease in former college students.

References

1. R.S. Paffenbarger, Jr., P.A. Wolf, J. Notkin, and M.C. Thorne, Chronic disease in former college students: I. Early precursors of fatal coronary heart disease, *Am J Epidemiol.* 83:314 (1966).
2. R.S. Paffenbarger, Jr., J. Notkin, D.E. Krueger, P.A. Wolf, M.C. Thorne, E.J. LeBauer, and J.L. Williams, Chronic disease in former college students: II. Methods of study and observations on mortality from coronary heart disease, *Am J Public Health.* 56:962 (1966).
3. A.S. Whittemore, R.S. Paffenbarger, Jr., K. Anderson, and J. Lee, Chronic disease in former college students: XXVII. Early precursors of site-specific cancers in college men and women, *J Natl Cancer Inst.* 74:43 (1985).
4. R.S. Paffenbarger, Jr., R.T. Hyde, and A.L. Wing, Physical activity and incidence of cancer in diverse populations: A preliminary report, *Am J Clin Nutr.* 45:312 (1987).
5. R.E. Frisch, G. Wyshak, N.L. Albright, T.E. Albright, I. Schiff, K.P. Jones, J. Witschi, E. Shiang, E. Koff, and M. Marguglio, Lower prevalence of breast cancer and cancers of the reproductive system among former college athletes compared to non-athletes, *Br J Cancer.* 52:885 (1985).
6. I.-M. Lee, R.S. Paffenbarger, Jr., and C.-c. Hsieh, Chronic disease in former college students: XLIV. Physical activity and risk of colorectal cancer among college alumni, *J Natl Cancer Inst.* 83:1324 (1991).
7. I.-M. Lee, R.S. Paffenbarger, Jr., and C.-c. Hsieh, Chronic disease in former college students: XLVI. Physical activity and risk of prostatic cancer among college alumni, *Am J Epidemiol.* 135:169 (1992).
8. R.S. Paffenbarger, Jr., R.T. Hyde, A.L. Wing, and C.H. Steinmetz, Chronic disease in former college students: XXV. A natural history of athleticism and cardiovascular health, *J Amer Med Assoc.* 252:491 (1984).
9. R.S. Paffenbarger, Jr., R.T. Hyde, A.L. Wing, and C.-c. Hsieh, Chronic disease in former college students: XXX. Physical activity, all-cause mortality, and longevity of college alumni, *N Engl J Med.* 314:605 (1986); 315:399 (1986).
10. C. Bouchard, R.J. Shephard, T. Stephens, J.R. Sutton, and B.D. McPherson, (eds), "Exercise, Fitness, and Health," Human Kinetics Books, Champaign, (1990).
11. C.J. Caspersen, B.P.M. Bloemberg, W.H.M. Saris, R.K. Merritt, and D. Kromhout, The prevalence of selected physical activities and their relation with coronary heart disease risk factors in elderly men: the Zutphen study, 1985, *Am J Epidemiol.* 133:1078 (1991).

12. B.E. Ainsworth, D.R. Jacobs, Jr., and A.S. Leon, Compendium of physical activities: classification of energy costs of human physical activities, *Med Sci Sports Exerc.* 1992 (In press).

13. D.H. Garabrant, J.M. Peters, T.M. Mack, and L. Bernstein, Job activity and colon cancer risk, *Am J Epidemiol.* 119:1005 (1984).

14. J.E. Vena, S. Graham, M. Zielezny, M.K. Swanson, R.E. Barnes, and J. Nolan, Lifetime occupational exercise and colon cancer, *Am J Epidemiol.* 122:357 (1985).

15. M. Gerhardsson, S.E. Norell, H. Kiviranta, N.L. Pedersen, and A. Ahlbom, Sedentary jobs and colon cancer, *Am J Epidemiol.* 123:775 (1986).

16. J.E. Vena, S. Graham, M. Zielezny, J. Brasure, and M.K. Swanson, Occupational exercise and risk of cancer, *Am J Clin Nutr.* 45:318 (1987).

17. A. H. Wu, A. Paganini-Hill, R.K. Ross, and B.E. Henderson, Alcohol, physical activity, and other risk factors for colorectal cancer: A prospective study, *Br J Cancer.* 55:687 (1987).

18. M.L. Slattery, M.C. Schumacher, K.R. Smith, D.W. West, and N. Abd-Elghany, Physical activity, diet, and risk of colon cancer in Utah, *Am J Epidemiol.* 128:989 (1988).

19. M. Gerhardsson, B. Floderus, and S. E. Norell, Physical activity and colon cancer risk, *Int J Epidemiol.* 17:743 (1988).

20. R.K. Severson, A.M.Y. Nomura, J.S. Grove, and G.N. Stemmermann, A prospective analysis of physical activity and cancer, *Am J Epidemiol.* 130: 522 (1989).

21. R.C. Brownson, S.H. Zahm, J.C. Chang, and A. Blair, Occupational risk of colon cancer. An analysis by anatomic subsite, *Am J Epidemiol.* 130:675 (1989).

22. D. Albanes, A. Blair, and P.R. Taylor, Physical activity and risk of cancer in the NHANES I population, *Am J Public Health.* 79:744 (1989).

23. M. Fredriksson, N.O. Bengtsson, L. Hardell, and O. Axelson, Colon cancer, physical activity, and occupational exposures. A case-control study, *Cancer.* 63:1838 (1989).

24. R.K. Peters, D.Y. Garabrant, M.C. Yu, and T.M. Mack, A case-control study of occupational and dietary factors in colorectal cancer in young men by subsite, *Cancer Res.* 49:5459 (1989).

25. R. Ballard-Barbash, A. Schatzkin, D. Albanes, M.H. Schiffman, B.E. Kreger, W.B. Kannel, K.M. Anderson, and W.E. Helsel, Physical activity and risk of large bowel cancer in the Framingham Study, *Cancer Res.* 50:3610 (1990).

26. M. Gerhardsson de Verdier, G. Steineck, U. Hagman, A. Rieger, and S.E. Norell, Physical activity and colon cancer: A case-referent study in Stockholm, *Int J Cancer.* 46:985 (1990).

27. A.S. Whittemore, A.H. Wu-Williams, M. Lee, Z. Shu, R.P. Gallagher, J. Deng-ao, Z. Lun, W. Xianghui, C. Kun, D. Jung, C.-Z. Teh, L. Chengde, X.J. Yao, R.S. Paffenbarger, Jr., and B.E. Henderson, Diet, physical activity, and colorectal cancer among Chinese in North America and China, *J Natl Cancer Inst.* 82:915 (1990).

28. C. Huggins, and C.V. Hodges, Studies on prostatic cancer. I. The effect of castration, of estrogen and of androgen injection on serum phosphatases in metastatic carcinoma of the prostate, *Cancer Res.* 1:293 (1941).

29. D.G. Zaridze, and P. Boyle, Cancer of the prostate: epidemiology and aetiology, *Br J Urol.* 59:493 (1987).

30. R. Ghanadian, C.M. Puah, and E.P.N. O'Donoghue, Serum testosterone and dihydrotestosterone in carcinoma of the prostate, *Br J Cancer.* 39:696 (1979).

31. M.A. Jackson, J. Kovi, M.Y. Heshmat, T.A. Ogunmuyiwa, G. W. Jones, A.O. Williams, E.C. Christian, E.O. Nkposong, M.S. Rao, A.G. Jackson, and B.S. Ahluwalia, Characterization of prostatic carcinoma among blacks: a comparison between a low-incidence area, Ibadan, Nigeria, and a high-incidence area, Washington, DC, *The Prostate.* 1:185 (1981).

32. B. Ahluwalia, M.A. Jackson, G.W. Jones, A.O. Williams, M.S. Rao, and S. Rajguru, Blood hormone profiles in prostate cancer patients in high-risk and low-risk populations, *Cancer.* 48:2267 (1981).

33. D.R. Cox, Regression models and life tables, *J Roy Soc Stat.* 34:187 (1972).

34. E.L. Frome, The analysis of rates using Poisson regression models, *Biometrics.* 39:665 (1983).

Chapter 3

Effects of Voluntary Exercise and/or Food Restriction on Pancreatic Tumorigenesis in Male Rats

THERESA C. GILES and B. D. ROEBUCK

I. Introduction

Pancreatic cancer is the fifth leading cause of death due to cancer in the United States,[1] yet thus far the only strong etiological association with this disease is cigarette smoking.[2] Hence, research into preventative strategies not only provides practical applications to public health recommendations, but may elucidate carcinogenesis mechanisms.

Various epidemiologic studies have demonstrated a consistent association between increased activity levels and a decreased rate of death due to cancer whether for increased occupational activity[3-5] or recreational exercise,[6] for former participation in college athletics,[7,8] or for general increases in physical activity.[9,10] Furthermore, several studies report an inverse relationship between exercise and mortality regardless of cigarette smoking status.[10,11]

These epidemiologic data provide a basis for the animal-exercise model in the study of cancer prevention, while consistent findings between the two, such as the suggestion that exercise may reduce cancer risk by decreasing obesity,[6,12] affirm potential applications of the animal model to humans. In rat cancer models both dietary fat and/or the availability of energy appear to act as promoters in the post-initiation phase of carcinogenesis,[13-16] thus suggesting a link between obesity and increased cancer risk. It remains unclear whether dietary fat acts directly as a promoter or whether it simply increases the caloric density of the diet, nevertheless, decreases in energy intake[15] or increases in energy expenditure can inhibit cancer development.[16-18]

Findings among animal studies indicate that the type or amount of exercise may influence cancer development; treadmill studies have demonstrated enhancement,[19,20] while voluntary exercise appears to inhibit,[18] but protection from tumor development is not necessarily proportional to amount of exercise performed.[16,17] Perhaps treadmill exercise represents stressful or intensive forms of activity, while voluntary wheel running mimics

---

Theresa C. Giles and B. D. Roebuck ● Department of Pharmacology and Toxicology, Dartmouth Medical School, Hanover, New Hampshire

Exercise, Calories, Fat, and Cancer, Edited by M.M. Jacobs
Plenum Press, New York, 1992

17

recreational forms of exercise. This is consistent with epidemiologic findings that "heavy" exercise tended to increase the risk of death from cancer of the lung, colon, and pancreas relative to moderate exercise.[11] Treadmill running as employed by Thompson et al.,[19,20] which produced enhancement of carcinogenesis, constituted considerably less total, but more intensive, exercise than voluntary wheel running.[16-17]

Thus, it appears important to explore methodologies of voluntary wheel running in order to improve the model. One potential problem with current methods is the individual animal variability in running performance. Female rats show a greater propensity to run voluntarily than do male rats, yet females are more resistant to the pancreatic carcinogen, azaserine.[17] A recent study by Russell et al.[21] demonstrated increased voluntary exercise activity in male rats by introducing a relatively mild (10%) dietary restriction. Food intake was adjusted upward or downward at intervals in order to keep running within a set criteria. In the current experiment we attempted to duplicate this reported exercise protocol as applied to our well-characterized rat-azaserine model of pancreatic cancer.[22]

II. Materials and Methods

A. Animals, Diets, and Treatments

Thirty-five, 7-day-old male Lewis rats with lactating dams were purchased from Charles River Breeding Laboratories, Wilmington, MA. The three litters of pups were housed with their dams in a controlled environment of 25°C, 50% relative humidity, and a 12-hour light-dark cycle. The dams were provided with purified AIN-76A[23,24] diet (but without the anti-oxidant ethoxyquin) and deionized water ad libitum. At 15, 20, and 24 days of age each pup was injected intraperitoneally with 30 mg of azaserine (Calbiochem-Behring Corp., La Jolla, CA), dissolved in 0.9% NaCl solution, per kg body weight, yielding a total dose of 90 mg azaserine/kg body weight. The pups were weaned at 24 days of age, and at 28 days of age were assigned to one of four experimental groups: 1) sedentary/ad libitum fed (n=10), 2) exercise/ad libitum fed (n=10), 3) sedentary/food restricted (n=8), and 4) exercise/food restricted (n=7) (Figure 1). Rats assigned to the two sedentary groups were transferred to suspended wire mesh cages, while rats assigned to the exercise groups were transferred to wire-bottomed housing units attached to running wheels (type H8002, Lab Products, Inc., Maywood, NJ). The wheels are 34.5 cm in diameter and 11.5 cm wide. Upon assignment to the groups, all rats were fed a powdered, purified 20% unsaturated fat diet ad libitum for 2 weeks. The composition of the diet was: 34.5% sucrose, 23.5% casein, 20.0% corn oil, 10.3% corn starch, 5.86% cellulose, 4.11% AIN mineral mix, 1.17% AIN vitamin mix, 0.35% methionine, and 0.23% choline bitartrate, yielding a caloric density of 4.54 kcal/g. At 6 weeks of age, food restriction was instituted for groups 3 and 4: a pre-weighed allotment of food was given to these rats approximately halfway through the light phase of their light-dark cycle. Groups 1 and 2 continued to receive food ad libitum. Food consumption was measured for one 24-hour period once each week, and the body weights of the rats were measured weekly for the duration of the experiment.

B. Exercise Monitoring

Odometers were attached to the running wheels to record the number of revolutions generated daily by each rat (one revolution is equivalent to 1.08 m.) Based on the protocol of Russell et al.,[21] in which a 10% food restriction resulted in a consistent voluntary running pattern of 6000-10,000 m/day, we initiated a 10% dietary restriction (that is, 90% of ad libitum intakes by weight) for groups 2 and 4 in order to enhance the running (<2000 m/day) previously observed in ad libitum-fed rats. The mean food intake of the sedentary/ad libitum-fed group for two consecutive days was used as a baseline from which the initial

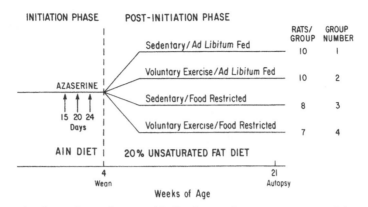

Figure 1. Schematic of experimental protocol indicating carcinogen treatment, and the post-initiation treatment protocols.

10% restriction was calculated for the two restricted groups. Accordingly, the food-restricted groups 3 and 4 received 12 g of food/day at the commencement of restriction. Running was monitored daily in order to achieve the target goal of 6,000-10,000 m/day of mean group running by the exercise/food-restricted group (group 4). After 3 days of restriction, the running was below the goal and thus the food allotment was decreased to 11 g/day. At this intake level, the running goal was achieved for several days; however, the degree of food restriction relative to group 1 (sedentary/*ad libitum*) rats had become increasingly severe as group 1 increased both in size and in food intake. At this point an attempt to decrease the degree of food restriction while maintaining the extensive running, was made by gradually increasing the food allotment over the next 3 weeks until the animals were once again receiving a 10% restriction in food intake compared to group 1. This scheme resulted in dramatic decreases in running activity corresponding to the increases in food allotment, until at 10 weeks of age the running activity of the food-restricted group was again equivalent to that of the exercise/*ad libitum*-fed rats (group 2). Therefore, again we decreased the food allotment by 1 g every 3 days, until the animals were receiving 12 g food. This level of food intake was equivalent to a 33% restriction compared to the concurrent sedentary/*ad libitum* (group 1) intakes, yet running did not resume but rather continued to decline. In a final effort to stimulate extensive running, the restricted rats were fed *ad libitum* for 7 days followed by a 20% food restriction for 4 days. However, this resulted in only a modest increase in running, such that the distances run by the restricted group were only one-and-one-half times that of the nonrestricted group. At 14 weeks of age, all rats were returned to *ad libitum* feeding for the duration of the experiment, although both groups of exercise rats were still allowed access to the running wheels.

C. Autopsy and Histopathology

At 21 weeks of age, the rats were anesthetized with ether and killed by guillotine. The entire pancreas, liver, kidneys, and perirenal and epididymal fat pads were excised and weighed. The entire pancreas was fixed in Bouin's fixative. The pancreatic tissue was processed for histologic study by routine methods, and the paraffin-embedded sections were stained with hematoxylin and eosin for examination by light microscopy. Azaserine-induced lesions of atypical acinar cells, henceforth called foci, were identified and classified as acidophilic or basophilic in general accord with the criteria of Rao *et al.*[25] and Roebuck *et al.*[26] Quantitative stereologic measurements of pancreatic foci were accomplished by previously published procedures.[26,27] From the observed number and area of the focal transections the mean number and size of the foci per cubic cm of pancreas were determined by the quantitative stereologic methods of Pugh et al.[27] as applied to the pancreas.[26]

D. Statistics

Data from the four treatment groups were analyzed by Two-Way Analysis of Variance (ANOVA), by access to exercise, and by dietary restriction. There were no interactions between the two factors for any of the variables. The amount of exercise performed by the two exercise groups was compared by Student's t-test. Significant p values for each variable are reported in Tables 1 and 2. All statistical analyses of foci data are based upon the calculated volumetric data (Table 3), i.e., number of foci per cubic centimeter, mean focal diameter, and the volume percent of the pancreas that is occupied by foci. The volume percent is a measurement analogous to tumor burden. Extent of exercise, organ weight, and tumor burden were evaluated by the Pearson r correlation.

III. Results

Figure 2 illustrates the post-weaning growth curves for the four groups. At 4 weeks of age, the mean body weights for the four groups were identical. All rats gained weight at approximately the same rate during the first 2 weeks of the protocol when the average

Table 1. Pancreas, Fat Pad, and Body Weights (g)[a]

Group	n	Pancreas wt	Pancreas wt/100g Body wt	Body wt 12 wks	Body wt 21 wks	Fat pad wt Perirenal	Fat pad wt Epididymal
1 sed/ad lib	10	1.21 ± 0.03	0.256 ± .007	354 ± 6	474 ± 10	21.63 ± 0.77	10.31 ± 0.76
2 ex/ad lib	10	1.28 ± 0.06	0.279 ± .009	354 ± 6	457 ± 10	19.13 ± 1.05	9.26 ± 0.65
3 sed/restr	8	1.13 ± 0.04	0.245 ± .004	296 ± 2	462 ± 9	22.01 ± 0.96	8.95 ± 0.84
4 ex/restr	7	1.15 ± 0.02	0.262 ± .004	280 ± 2	441 ± 5	17.82 ± 0.71	8.13 ± 0.40
Restriction		p=0.03	——	p=0.0000	——	——	——
Exercise		——	p=0.013	——	——	p=0.001	——

[a]Values were analyzed by Two-Way ANOVA, by restriction, and by exercise. There were no significant interactions. All significant p values are shown. Data are shown as mean ± SEM.

Table 2. Exercise and Food Intake Values[a]

Group	Exercise (m/day)	Food intake (g/day) Restr. period	Food intake (g/day) Post-restr.	Food intake (g/day) Total
1 sed/ad lib	——	16.74 ± 0.25	17.00 ± 0.33	16.85 ± 0.27
2 ex/ad lib	1012 ± 92	16.28 ± 0.28	17.08 ± 0.43	16.61 ± 0.25
3 sed/restr	——	13.18 ± 0.04	19.92 ± 0.54	15.96 ± 0.24
4 ex/restr	2272 ± 206	12.98 ± 0.03	18.26 ± 0.50	15.15 ± 0.22
Restriction		p=0.0000	p=0.0001	p=0.0001
Exercise		——	——	p=0.048
t test	p<0.001			

[a]Food intake values were analyzed by Two-Way ANOVA, by restriction, and by exercise. There were no significant interactions. Data are shown as mean ± SEM. All significant p values are shown. Exercise values were analyzed by Student's t test.

food intake for the four groups was similar and prior to the initiation of food restriction (Figure 3). Access to exercise appears to have an immediate effect on food consumption as noted by the lower intakes of the two exercise groups during the first week of exercise (Figure 3). The food intake of the two *ad libitum*-fed groups ranged from an initial intake of approximately 8 g/day to approximately 19 g/day at 10 weeks of age when intake was at its highest; these rats continued to gain weight throughout the study even though intake subsided slightly during the second half of the experiment. The overall pattern of food consumption for the two *ad libitum*-fed groups was similar. Food restriction, implemented from 6 to 13 weeks of age, resulted in slower weight gain for the food-restricted groups, such that at 12 weeks of age there was a significant effect of food restriction on body weight (Figure 2 and Table 1). Although the magnitude of restriction was identical for the two food-restricted groups, the sedentary/food-restricted rats (group 3) gained weight at a slightly faster rate than the exercise/food-restricted rats (group 4) during the restriction period,

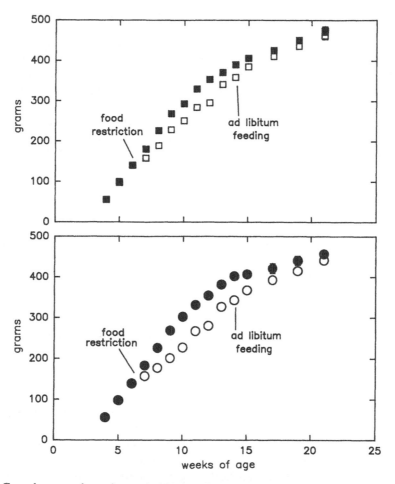

Figure 2. Growth curves for sedentary/*ad libitum* (■), exercise/*ad libitum* (●), sedentary/restricted (□), and exercise/restricted (O) rats. *Ad libitum* feeding is indicated by filled symbols and open symbols indicate restricted groups. Food restriction and return to *ad libitum* feeding for groups 3 and 4 are indicated by arrows. Except where indicated SEM bars are smaller than the symbol.

suggesting that exercise caused an additional energy deficit in this group. After restriction was abandoned, the difference between the body weights of the *ad libitum*-fed groups and the restricted groups steadily decreased as the previously restricted rats increased their consumption to quantities greater than those of the *ad libitum*-fed rats (Figures 2 and 3). During the food-restriction period (weeks 6 to 14), the mean intake of the restricted rats was lower than that of the *ad libitum*-fed rats, and post-restriction their intake was higher (Table 2). The mean food consumption of the total experiment was affected by both the restriction and exercise factors such that there was a significant effect of each (Table 2). At autopsy, the pancreas and both perirenal and epididymal fat pad weights were measured. Food restriction produced a significant decrease in pancreas weights (Table 1). When the ratios of pancreas wt/100 g body weight were compared among groups, exercise increased these values such that a significant effect was found (Table 1). For the exercise groups, the fat pads were small and the perirenal fat pads were significantly smaller compared to the sedentary groups (Table 1). These findings suggest that restriction directly interfered with pancreatic growth, while exercise primarily affected other aspects of body composition such as fat pad deposition (Table 1).

The voluntary running behavior of the two exercised groups is plotted in Figure 4. The mean running of the exercise/*ad libitum*-fed rats (group 2) varied from approximately 0.8 to 2.9 km/day from 4 weeks of age to 12 weeks of age, with a peak of activity at 7 to 8 weeks of age. At 13 weeks of age the running decreased to less than 1 km/day. This exercise activity represents a previously observed pattern of voluntary running in *ad libitum*-fed rats, including the peak of activity.[16-18] With food restriction at week 6, the exercise/food-restricted rats (group 4) demonstrated a dramatic increase in running activity in comparison to the initial 2 weeks of running by this group, and in comparison to the corresponding running by the *ad libitum*-fed rats (group 2). At 7 to 8 weeks, activity reached a plateau of approximately 8 to 10.8 km/day (Figure 4). This plateau corresponded with an approximate food restriction of 30% compared to *ad libitum* intakes. In an attempt to reverse the restriction regimen of group 4 which had become increasingly severe as the rats gained in weight, we gradually increased the food allotment. At approximately 9 weeks of age the running began to decrease and by 10 weeks of age had approached the low level of the exercise/*ad libitum* group. Between weeks 11 and 12 another period of restriction was begun in an attempt to re-induce extensive running, however, the desired response was not obtained, and the rats were permanently returned to an *ad libitum*-fed diet at 14 weeks of age. The running pattern continued to decrease gradually in both groups of rats until at 21 weeks of age, the animals were running less than 0.5 km/day (Figure 4). In spite of only a short extensive exercise period for the restricted rats (group 4), the mean total running of this group was significantly greater than that of the exercise/*ad libitum* rats (group 2) (Table 2).

Table 3 contains the observed and calculated quantitative stereologic data and statistical analysis of the azaserine-induced acidophilic foci in pancreatic sections in the four groups. As established in previous experiments, azaserine induces two phenotypically different populations of foci, acidophilic and basophilic.[25,26] The acidophilic foci are typically larger and more numerous, thus accounting for approximately 97% of the focal burden at 4 months post-initiation. This population also appears to be a better predictor of the occurrence of adenomas and carcinomas in long-term experiments.[22,26] Thus, only data from acidophilic foci are reported. The number of acidophilic foci per cubic cm of pancreas was decreased in groups 2, 3, and 4 in comparison to the sedentary/*ad libitum*-fed rats (group 1). Restriction without exercise showed the largest decrease (33% compared to control), yet neither restriction nor exercise showed a statistically significant effect. The mean focal diameter was notably lower only in the exercise/restricted group; these findings are in contrast to previous studies in this laboratory where exercise significantly decreased the mean focal diameter of measured foci, but had a lesser effect on foci number.[17] The volume percent,

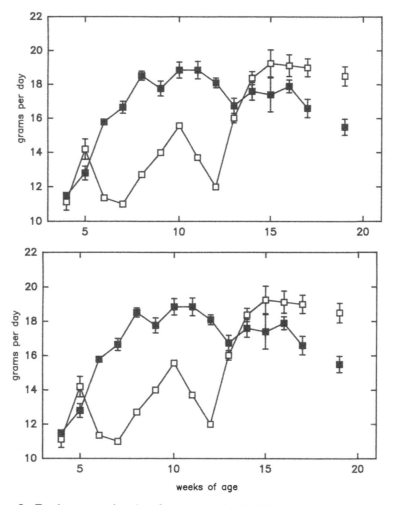

Figure 3. Food consumption data for groups 1-4. See Figure 2 for symbol legends.

or focal burden, of acidophilic foci was decreased from the sedentary/*ad libitum*-fed rats (group 1) by 37%, 43%, and 56% in groups 2, 3, and 4, respectively. A significant effect of dietary restriction (p=0.0183) was noted for this variable by Two-Way ANOVA, but an effect of exercise just missed statistical significance (p=0.0540).

IV. Discussion

The data in this experiment indicate that voluntary exercise may slow the development of putative pre-neoplastic foci in rats exposed to a pancreatic carcinogen. Food restriction, which has been shown to significantly decrease tumor focal development in other studies,[13-16] exhibited a significant effect on pancreatic tumor burden despite the fact that restriction was abandoned halfway through the experiment. Exercise was sufficient to inhibit focal development in both exercise groups, but the greatest overall decrease in volume percent of the pancreas occupied by foci was found in the rats that were food restricted and had access to the exercise wheels (Table 3). So although exercise did not yield a statistically significant effect, it lowered the tumor burden to an extent similar to that of dietary restriction: when

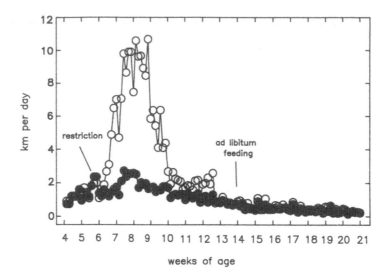

Figure 4. Daily activity patterns for exercise/*ad libitum* (●) and exercise/restricted (○) rats.

Table 3. Acidophilic Foci Data[a]

Group	n	No. foci observed	No. foci/ cm^2	Mean focal area (mm^{2}x100)	No. foci/ cm^3	Mean focal diameter (μm)	Volume %
1 sed/*ad lib*	10	65.8 ±6.26	35.31 ±3.36	10.89 ±1.10	1017.96 ±84.57	343.86 ±19.21	4.061 ±0.622
2 ex/*ad lib*	10	53.7 ±6.92	26.18 ±3.19	9.48 ±0.77	751.70 ±88.45	348.18 ±10.48	2.546 ±0.399
3 sed/restr	8	40.63 ±6.80	22.70 ±3.90	9.65 ±1.49	680.24 ±116.62	333.91 ±17.05	2.299 ±0.530
4 ex/restr	7	52.0 ±7.02	22.25 ±2.61	7.90 ±0.49	731.26 ±79.60	302.58 ±9.93	1.783 ±0.274
Restriction					—	—	p=0.0183
Exercise					—	—	p=0.0540

[a]All values were analyzed by Two-Way ANOVA, by restriction, and by exercise. There were no significant interactions. All significant p values are shown. Data are shown as mean ± SEM.

exercise was combined with restriction, it inhibited the volume percent of pancreas occupied by foci by greater than 50%.

The extent of cumulative exercise was compared to tumor burden (Pearson *r* correlation analysis), and in agreement with previous studies[16,17] was not statistically significant. We interpret this to indicate that exposure to exercise can delay or inhibit carcinogenesis, but that the inhibition is not directly proportional to amount of work performed. In fact, Cohen *et al.*[16] demonstrated an inverse relationship between voluntary exercise and mammary carcinogenesis, in that the rats which exercised the least were afforded the greatest protection from tumor development.

It is unknown whether the inhibitory effects exerted by exercise and/or food restriction are direct or indirect, but previous work in this laboratory suggests that inhibition is not directly related to intense running activity, but rather to some indirect effect caused by exercise.[17] In this study the effect of exercise on perirenal fat pad weights suggests that the exercised rats were leaner than their sedentary counterparts regardless of food intake (Table 1). Additionally, perirenal fat pad weight was significantly correlated with volume percent foci (r=0.56, p<0.01), by Pearson r correlation analysis, suggesting a relationship between body composition and inhibition of focal development. Furthermore, while exercise was not directly correlated with volume percent data, it was significantly correlated with perirenal fat pad weight (r=–0.50, p<0.01), suggesting that exercise may exert an indirect effect on development of foci by reducing fat deposition. Food consumption was significantly correlated with fat pad weight (r=0.56, p<0.01) as well as with volume percent foci data (r=0.61, p<0.01) and therefore restriction and exercise may work via similar mechanisms in reducing focal development.

Of additional importance in this study was our inability to duplicate the outcome of the Russell protocol,[21] which held promise for "boosting" the amount of "voluntary" exercise activity in our pancreatic cancer model, and thus enhancing the effect due to exercise. Dietary restriction has been demonstrated to inhibit carcinogenesis in pancreas[13,14] as well as in other cancer models[15,16] and thus introduces a confounding variable when used as a means of enhancing exercise activity. Indeed whether the additional decrease in volume percent foci in the exercise/restricted group was due to the greater extent of exercise exhibited by these rats or due to the combination of (extensive) exercise and dietary restriction is uncertain. Furthermore, we did not find that a 10% dietary restriction was sufficient to induce or sustain elevated running. Instead, only severe decreases in the food allotment produced the desired effect. While our experiment was designed to differentiate between the effects of restriction and exercise, we felt that a severe restriction would further complicate interpretation of the results and thus abandoned the restriction regimen. Therefore, we were unable to achieve the effect reported by Russell et al.[21] on voluntary running by introducing a 10% dietary restriction with 3-day interval adjustments on weanling male rats.

Both access to exercise and dietary restriction were effective in decreasing the tumor burder of azaserine-induced pancreatic foci. These variables may elicit similar metabolic mechanisms, perhaps such as effecting decreases in body fat deposition. This work supports other data suggestive of voluntary exercise either as an important alternative to caloric restriction, or as a way to lessen the severity of dietary restriction needed to inhibit carcinogenesis.[15-18]

V. Summary

Studies were undertaken to evaluate the effects of caloric restriction on voluntary exercise in a rat model of pancreatic cancer. Suckling male Lewis rats were initiated with 3 doses (30 mg/kg body weight) of the pancreatic carcinogen azaserine. At 28 days of age they were weaned to one of four experimental protocols; namely, sedentary/ad libitum fed, voluntary exercise/ad libitum fed, sedentary/food restricted, and voluntary exercise/food restricted. Voluntary exercise was provided by free access to running wheels fitted with odometers. Food restriction was intended to be mild, at less than 10% reduction of ad libitum intake. Putative pre-neoplastic pancreatic foci were identified microscopically at 4 months post-azaserine treatment. As previously shown, food restriction led to increased wheel activity, but the increased activity could not be maintained beyond the first half of the post-initiation treatment phase. Additionally, the extensive wheel running occured only when available food was restricted by greater than 10%. Exercise *per se* had a lesser effect compared to food restriction on pancreatic tumorigenesis.

Acknowledgments

This work was supported by Grant 88A29 from the American Institute for Cancer Research, Washington, D.C. The authors thank Robert Holthus for technical assistance with the rats, Denise MacMillan for assistance with the analyses of the pancreatic foci, and Karen Baumgartner for statistical analysis.

References

1. E. Silverberg and J.A. Lubera, Cancer statistics, 1989, *CA-Cancer J Clin.* 39:3 (1989).
2. T.M. Mack, Pancreas, *in*: "Cancer Epidemiology and Prevention," D. Schottenfeld and J. Fraumeni, eds., W.B. Sanders Company, Philadelphia (1982).
3. D.H. Garabrant, J.M. Peters, T.M. Mack, and L. Bernstein, Job activity and colon cancer risk, *Am J Epidem.* 119:1005 (1984).
4. M. Gerhardsson, S.E. Norell, H. Kiviranta, N.L. Pedersen, and A. Ahlbom, Sedentary jobs and colon cancer, *Am J Epidem.* 123:775 (1986).
5. J.E. Vena, S. Graham, M. Zielezny, J. Brasure, and M.K. Swanson, Occupational exercise and risk of cancer, *Am J Clin Nutr.* 45:318 (1987).
6. E.R. Eichner, Exercise, lymphokines, calories, and cancer, *The Physician and Sportsmedicine.* 15:109 (1987).
7. R.E. Frisch, G. Wyshak, N.L. Albright, T.E. Albright, I. Schiff, J. Witschi, and M. Marguglio, Lower lifetime occurence of breast cancer and cancers of the reproductive system among former college athletes, *Am J Clin Nutr.* 45:328 (1987).
8. M.M. Gauthier, Can exercise reduce the risk of cancer?, *The Physician and Sportsmedicine.* 14: 171 (1986).
9. R. Ballard-Barbash, A. Schatzkin, D. Albanes, M.H. Schiffman, B.E. Kreger, W.B. Kannel, K.M. Anderson, and W.E. Helsel, Physical activity and risk of large bowel cancer in the Framingham study, *Cancer Res.* 50:3610 (1990).
10. R.S. Paffenbarger Jr., R.T. Hyde, A.L. Wing, and C. Hsieh, Physical activity, all-cause mortality, and longevity of college alumni, *N Engl J Med.* 314:605 (1986).
11. L. Garfinkel, and S.D. Stellman, Mortality by relative weight and exercise, *Cancer.* 62:1844 (1988).
12. J.O. Holloszy, E.K. Smith, M. Vining, and S. Adams, Effect of voluntary exercise on longevity of rats, *J Appl Physiol.* 59:826 (1985).
13. B.D. Roebuck, J.D. Yager, and D.S. Longnecker, Dietary modulation of azaserine-induced pancreatic carcinogenesis in the rat, *Cancer Res.* 41:888 (1981).
14. B.D. Roebuck, J.D. Yager, D.S. Longnecker, and S.A. Wilpone, Promotion by unsaturated fat of azaserine-induced pancreatic carcinogenesis in the rat, *Cancer Res.* 41:3961 (1981).
15. D.M. Klurfeld, C.B. Welch, M.J. Davis, and D. Kritchevsky, Determination of degree of energy restriction necessary to reduce DMBA-induced mammary tumorigenesis in rats during the promotion phase, *J Nutr.* 119:286 (1989).
16. L.A. Cohen, K. Choi, and C. Wang, Influence of dietary fat, caloric restriction, and voluntary exercise on *N*-nitrosomethylurea-induced mammary tumorigenesis in rats, *Cancer Res.* 48:4276 (1988).
17. B.D. Roebuck, J. McCaffrey, and K. Baumgartner, Protective effects of voluntary exercise during the postinitiation phase of pancreatic carcinogenesis in the rat, *Cancer Res.* 50:6811 (1990).
18. B.S. Reddy, S. Sugie and A. Lowenfels, Effect of voluntary exercise on azoxymethane-induced colon carcinogenesis in male F344 rats, *Cancer Res.* 48:7079 (1988).
19. H.J. Thompson, A.M. Ronan, K.A. Ritacco, A.R. Tagliaferro, and L.D. Meeker, Effect of exercise on the induction of mammary carcinogenesis, *Cancer Res* 48:2720 (1988).

20. H.J. Thompson, A.M. Ronan, K.A. Ritacco, and A.R. Tagliaferro, Effect of type and amount of dietary fat on the enhancement of rat mammary tumorigenesis of exercise, *Cancer Res.* 49:1904 (1989).

21. J.C. Russell, W.F. Epling, D. Pierce, R.M. Amy, and D.P. Boer, Induction of voluntary prolonged running by rats, *J Appl Physiol.* 63:2549 (1987).

22. B.D. Roebuck, K.J. Baumgartner, and D.S. Longnecker, Growth of pancreatic foci and development of pancreatic cancer with a single dose of azaserine in the rat, *Carcinogenesis.* 8:1831 (1987).

23. G. Bieri, Report of the American Institute of Nutrition *ad hoc* Committee on standards of nutritional studies, *J Nutr.* 107:1340 (1977).

24. G. Bieri, Second report of the *ad hoc* committee on standards for nutritional studies, *J Nutr.* 110:1726 (1980).

25. M.S. Rao, M.P. Upton, V. Subbarao, and D.G. Scarpelli, Two populations of cells with differing proliferative capacities in atypical acinar cell foci induced by 4-hydroxy-aminoquinoline-1-oxide in the rat pancreas, *Lab Invest.* 46:527 (1982).

26. B.D. Roebuck, K.J. Baumgartner, and C.D. Thron, Characterization of two populations of pancreatic atypical acinar cell foci induced by azaserine in the rat, *Lab Invest.* 50:141 (1984).

27. T.D. Pugh, J.H. King, H. Koen, D. Nychka, J. Chover, G. Wahba, Y. He, and S. Goldfarb, Reliable stereological method for estimating the number of microscopic hepatocellular foci from their transections, *Cancer Res.* 43:1261 (1983).

Chapter 4

Former Athletes Have a Lower Lifetime Occurrence of Breast Cancer and Cancers of the Reproductive System

ROSE E. FRISCH, GRACE WYSHAK, NILE L. ALBRIGHT,
TENLEY E. ALBRIGHT, ISAAC SCHIFF and JELIA WITSCHI

I. Introduction

We have found that women who were athletes in college had a significantly lower prevalence (lifetime occurrence) rate of cancers of the reproductive system (uterus, ovary, cervix, and vagina) and breast cancer than did the non-athletes.[1] In accord with these findings, the former athletes also have a significantly lower prevalence of benign tumors of these tissues.[2]

The study comparing the cancer risk of former college athletes and non-athletes was suggested by the findings that strenuous exercise delays menarche[3-5] and that women dancers and athletes, including college athletes, have a high incidence of oligomenorrhea and secondary amenorrhea.[3,5-7] Also, women with weight loss in the range of 10 to 15% of normal weight-for-height, which is equivalent to a loss of a third of body fat, become amenorrheic.[8] Both these underweight women[9] and lean athletes,[10-12] have altered hypothalamic regulation of gonadotropin secretion and, consequently, low levels of estrogen. These findings raised the question, are there differences in the long-term reproductive and general health of women who had been college athletes compared to college non-athletes?

Rose E. Frisch • Center for Population Studies, and Department of Population Sciences, Harvard School of Public Health, 9 Bow Street, Cambridge, Massachusetts; Grace Wyshak • Center for Population Studies, and Department of Biostatistics, Harvard School of Public Health, Department of Medicine, Harvard Medical School, Boston, Massachusetts; Nile L. Albright • Department of Surgery, New England Deaconess Hospital, Boston, Massachusetts; Tenley E. Albright • Department of Surgery, New England Baptist Hospital, Boston, Massachusetts; Isaac Schiff • Department of Gynecology, Massachusetts General Hospital, Boston, Massachusetts; Jelia Witschi • Department of Nutrition, Harvard School of Public Health, Boston, Massachusetts

Exercise, Calories, Fat, and Cancer, Edited by M.M. Jacobs
Plenum Press, New York, 1992

II. Subjects and Methods

The subjects were 5,398 living alumnae who responded to a detailed questionnaire sent in 1981 to 7,559 alumnae listed as currently alive by the alumnae offices of eight colleges and two universities. Of the 5,398 respondents, 2,622 were former athletes and 2,776 were former non-athletes. These women resided throughout the United States and abroad. The response rate was 71.4%; 71.9% for the athletes and 70.1% for the non-athletes. The relatively low rate of non-deliverable questionnaires, 3.6% (272), indicated the alumnae offices kept their listing of living alumnae up-to-date. Alumnae classes dated from 1925 to 1981.

Details of the procedures for obtaining rosters of athletes and non-athletes and of the 14-page questionnaire have been previously reported.[1]

The criteria for an athlete were: women who had been on at least one varsity team, house team, or other intramural team for one or more years, and/or had achieved other athletic distinction, such as awarding of a college letter. Team sports included basketball, crew, dance, fencing, field hockey, gymnastics, lacrosse, soccer, softball, squash, swimming, tennis, track, and volleyball. Team training had to be regular, i.e., at least two practice sessions a week during the college year or longer. Non-team athletes (1.0%) were included if they trained regularly, for example, running at least 2 miles a day for 5 days a week.

Almost two-thirds (64.2%) of the athletes were on more than one college team; the mean number of teams was 2.6 ± 0.03. Of the college athletes, 83.5% were on a team 2 or more years; 39% were on a team for all 4 years.

A. Pre-College Athletic Training

Questions on pre-college athletic training included age at beginning of regular athletic training, number and type(s) of team(s), whether year-round or not, length of break, and whether pre-college training was more or less rigorous than college training.

Of the former college athletes, 82% had also been on an athletic team in high school or earlier, compared to 25% of their non-athletic classmates.

B. Current Exercise

Questions on current exercise included type, number of hours per day and per week, and whether year-round or not.

C. Medical and Reproductive History

In addition to the questions on athletics, the 14-page questionnaire requested detailed medical history, reproductive history from menarche through the menopause, including births and pregnancy outcome, smoking history, current health problems, height, weight, weight changes, and current diet.

The questions on cancer or malignant tumors were: age the cancer was diagnosed, type or site, biopsy history, (age occurred, inpatient/outpatient, diagnosis), type(s) of treatment(s) of the cancer, history of hospitalizations (reason, age occurred, treatment), and family history of cancer in female blood relatives.

Our cover letter stated long-term health as the purpose of the study; the letter did not state that we were going to compare athletes and non-athletes.

D. Statistical Methods

All rates are either age-specific or age-adjusted.[1] Relative risk is reported as non-athletes/athletes throughout the paper.

Multiple logistic regression analyses were done to determine the effects of possible confounding factors on the risk of reproductive cancers and breast cancer. These factors included: age, number of pregnancies, family history of cancer, being an athlete or non-athlete, leanness, age of menarche, ever smoked, use of oral contraceptives, and use of hormones for menopausal symptoms.

Age of natural menopause was estimated by probit analysis. Natural menopause was defined as 12 consecutive months (or more) without cycles after age 40. Body composition of respondents of all ages was estimated by the equations of Cohn et al.,[13] and Ellis et al.[14] (Appended).

III. Results

A. Cancers of the Reproductive System

Figure 1 and Table 1 show that the prevalence (lifetime occurrence) rate of reproductive system cancers (uterus, ovary, cervix, and vagina) is consistently lower for the athletes than for the non-athletes.

The relative risk (RR) adjusted by multiple logistic regression is 2.53, 95% confidence limits (CL) (1.17, 5.47) (Table 2). Other significant risk factors for cancers of the reproductive system are: age, use of hormones for menopausal symptoms, RR=2.26, 95% CL (1.02, 5.01), and smoking (ever/never) RR=3.47, 95% CL (1.38, 8.70).

The age-adjusted rates (by the direct method) for cancers of the reproductive tract are 3.7 per thousand for the athletes compared to 9.5 per thousand for the non-athletes. The age adjusted RR is 2.62, with 95% CL (1.24 to 5.54) (Table 2).

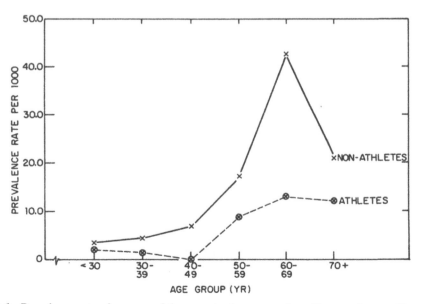

Figure 1. Prevalence rate of cancers of the reproductive system for athletes and non-athletes by age group. (Reprinted from the *British Journal of Cancer* with permission.)

B. Breast Cancer

Figure 2 and Table 1 show that the prevalence rate of breast cancer is consistently lower for the athletes than for the non-athletes.

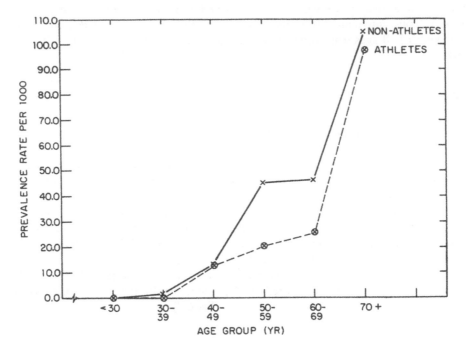

Figure 2. Prevalence rate of breast cancer for athletes and non-athletes by age group. (Reprinted from the *British Journal of Cancer* with permission.)

Table 1. Age-Specific Prevalence (Lifetime Occurrence) Rates of Cancers of the Reproductive System and Breast Cancer of Athletes and Non-Athletes

	Athletes (N=2,622)				Non-athletes (N=2,776)			
	Reproductive system cancers[a]		Breast cancer		Reproductive system cancers[b]		Breast cancer	
Age (years)	No.	Rate/ 1000	No.	Rate/ 1000	No.	Rate/ 1000	No.	Rate/ 1000
< 30	2	2.0	0	0.0	2	3.6	0	0.0
30–39	1	1.5	0	0.0	5	4.6	2	1.8
40–49	0	0.0	5	13.0	3	6.7	6	13.3
50–59	3	8.8	7	20.6	6	17.1	16	45.6
60–69	2	13.0	4	26.0	10	42.6	11	46.8
70+	1	12.2	8	97.6	2	21.0	10	105.3
Total	9	3.4	24	9.2	28	10.1	45	16.2

[a] The 9 cancers were: cervix 4, uterus 4, and ovary 1.
[b] The 28 cancers were: cervix 10, uterus 11, ovary 5, vagina 1, and choriocarcinoma 1.

The relative risk for non-athletes/athletes adjusted by multiple logistic regression is RR=1.86, 95% CL (1.00, 3.47) (Table 2). Other significant risk factors for breast cancer in the logistic model are: age, history of cancer in the family, RR=2.04, 95% CL (1.20, 3.38), and age of menarche (14 years and over vs. under 12 years), RR=0.37, 95% CL (0.14, 0.95). Nulliparity was not significant and age of first live birth did not differ between those with or without breast cancer.

The age-adjusted rates for breast cancer are 10.1 per 1,000 for the athletes and 15.6 per 1,000 for non-athletes; the age-adjusted RR=1.54, 95% CL (0.96, 2.48) (Table 2). The age-adjusted rates for breast cancer for subjects who had ever been pregnant are 13.7 per 1,000 for the athletes and 22.2 per 1,000 for the non-athletes (Table 2). No subject under age 30 had a breast cancer.

The age-specific rates for breast cancer of the non-athletes showed the pre- and post-menopausal pattern similar to other well-nourished Western populations.[15] The athletes, however, have a less steep rise in the perimenopausal period (Figure 2).

C. Family History of Cancer, and Other Characteristics of the Alumnae

The characteristics of the athletes and non-athletes are set forth in Table 3. The family history of cancer of athletes did not differ from that of non-athletes. Athletes were significantly taller than non-athletes and slightly heavier, but leaner, in all age groups. (Their leanness may be underestimated since an athlete's weight may consist of more lean mass than that of a non-athlete of the same weight.[5,16,17]) Athletes had a later age of menarche and an earlier age of natural menopause than non-athletes (Table 3). Pregnancy histories are similar between the two groups. A lower percentage of athletes used oral contraceptives and estrogens for the menopause than did non-athletes (Table 3).

Table 2. Relative Risk (Non-Athletes/Athletes) Adjusted by Multiple Logistic Regression (line 1), and Adjusted for Age Only, (line 2), and Age-adjusted Rates per 1,000, for Cancers of the Reproductive System and Breast Cancer of Athletes and Non-Athletes

Type of cancer	Relative risk (95% confidence limits)	Age-adjusted rates per thousand[a]	
		Athletes	Non-athletes
Reproductive system cancers	2.53 (1.17, 5.47)	3.7 ± 1.2	9.5 ± 1.8
	2.62 (1.24, 5.54)		
Breast cancer	1.86 (1.00, 3.47)	10.1 ± 2.0	15.6 ± 2.2
	1.54 (0.96, 2.48)		
Breast cancer, ever pregnant	2.02 (1.03, 3.94)	13.7 ± 2.9	22.2 ± 3.5
	1.64 (0.98, 2.67)		

[a] Age strata: Under 30, 30-39, 40-49, 50-59, 60-69, 70 years and over. Rates are adjusted by the direct method. The standard population is the population of the athletes and non-athletes combined.

Table 3.   Characteristics of Athletes and Non-Athletes: Values Are Age-Adjusted Rates ± SE% or Means ± SEM[a]

Characteristic	Athletes	Non-athletes
Family history of cancer[b](%)	49.8 ± 1.0	51.7 ± 1.0
Cancer in mother (%)	18.1 ± 0.8	17.9 ± 0.7
Breast cancer in mother (%)	6.9 ± 0.5	7.5 ± 0.5
Breast cancer in sister(s) (%)	1.2 ± 0.2	1.2 ± 0.2
Height (cm)	166.8 ± 0.1	165.3 ± 0.1[c]
Weight (kg)	60.0 ± 0.2	59.2 ± 0.2[c]
Percent fat (estimated)	32.9 ± 0.1	34.0 ± 0.1[c]
Age of menarche (year) (by year and month)	13.0 ± 0.0	12.7 ± 0.0[c]
Age of menarche (year) (by year)	13.1 ± 0.0	12.9 ± 0.0[c]
Age of natural menopause (year)	51.3 ± 0.2	52.0 ± 0.3[d]
Ever pregnant (%)	61.9 ± 0.8	61.1 ± 0.8
Ever pregnant: no. of pregnancies	2.8 ± 0.0	2.7 ± 0.0
No. live births	2.2 ± 0.0	2.1 ± 0.0
Age at first birth (years)	27.1 ± 0.1	27.4 ± 0.1
Ever use OCs [e](<60 years) (%)	59.4 ± 1.0	65.1 ± 0.9[c]
Ever use estrogens for menopause (≥40 years) (%)	16.2 ± 1.1	20.4 ± 1.1[f]
Hysterectomies (%)	6.5 ± 0.5	7.8 ± 0.4[d]
Pre-college training (%)	82.4 ± 0.8	24.9 ± 0.8[c]
Ever smoked (%)	46.8 ± 0.9	48.7 ± 0.9
Now exercising regularly (%)	73.5 ± 0.9	57.0 ± 1.0[c]
Now restricting diet (%)	42.0 ± 1.0	46.2 ± 1.0[d]
Now on low-fat diet (%)	20.8 ± 0.8	21.3 ± 0.8

[a]   Values in the table are rounded to the nearest tenth.
[b]   Female blood relatives.
[c] $p \leq 0.001$.
[d] $p \leq 0.05$.
[e]   Oral contraceptives.
[f] $p \leq 0.01$.

A much higher percentage of athletes (82.4%) were on teams in secondary school or earlier than were non-athletes (24.9%) in all age groups. About 74% of the athletes reported they now were exercising regularly year round, compared to 57% of the non-athletes.

IV. Discussion

A remarkable result was that the subjects who had participated in organized athletic activity while in college had a lower lifetime occurrence rate of cancers of the reproductive system and breast cancer than their non-athletic classmates.

"The time course of carcinogenesis commonly extends over 20 years or more."[18] What might be the reasons for the difference in prevalence rates of these cancers between athletes and non-athletes? Genetic factors are unlikely, since the family histories of cancer of the athletes and non-athletes are similar. Strong evidence against selection or reporting biases is the fact that the prevalence rates for both reproductive and breast cancers of the non-athletes are in accord with the national data.[19] The prevalence rate of reproductive cancers for non-athletic alumnae 60-69 years is 4.2%; this rate is similar to the cumulative incidence rate for United States white women of all classes, ages 0-74 years, 5.8%, and to the comparable Connecticut rate, 4.9%.[19] (The rate of non-athletic alumnae ages 70 years and over, 2.1%, includes only two women.)

The prevalence rate of breast cancer for the non-athletic alumnae 70 years and over, 10.5%, is comparable to the cumulative incidence rate for white women 0-74 years in the United States, 8.2%, and the comparable Connecticut rate, 8.5%.[19] A slightly higher cumulative incidence rate is expected for college women compared to the general population.[18]

The later menarche of the athletes in all age groups is in accord with other studies of athletes.[5] Their earlier age of menopause compared to non-athletes would also be expected because they are less fat. Both early menarche[8,20] and late menopause[20] are related to greater fatness. Pertinent to our results, a higher risk of cancer of the breast,[20-24] and cancer of the endometrium[25,26] are associated with early menarche,[24] later menopause and greater relative fatness.[26]

Since the characteristics of the former athletes are associated with a lower risk of sex hormone-sensitive cancers, it is very improbable that our results are due to a greater cancer mortality in every age group of the athletes compared to the non-athletes. Also, we have found that, in accord with the cancer data, the former athletes have a significantly lower prevalence of benign tumors of the reproductive system and benign breast disease.[2]

The present-day small, but significant, difference in relative leanness between athletes and non-athletes may have existed long term, and been larger at earlier ages, since 82.4% of the athletes were on teams in secondary school or earlier, compared to only 24.9% of the non-athletes. Apter and Vihko[24] report that early maturers (who were fatter than late maturers), had higher serum concentrations of estradiol than the leaner, later maturing girls both before and after menarche, in relation to chronological age.

Fatness is associated with an increased extraglandular conversion of androgen to estrogen[12,25-27] and the metabolism of estrogen to more potent forms,[27,28] which have been observed in association with breast cancer.[29,30] Conversely, leanness is associated with an increased metabolism of estradiol (E_2) to the non-estrogenic metabolite, 2-hydroxyestrone, a catechol estrogen. When body fat was quantified by magnetic resonance imaging, athletes had one-third less fat than the non-athletes, although their body weights did not differ significantly,[16] and the relative leanness of the athletes was significantly correlated with an increase in the 2-hydroxylated, non-potent form of estrogen.[31]

Diets low in fat and saturated fat have also been shown to shift the pattern of estrogen metabolism toward the non-potent 2-hydroxylated catechol estrogens.[32] There is evidence that athletes with early training eat less fat than those trained at later ages.[5,33] Many studies show a relation between total intake of fat and risk of cancer.[18,34,35] About equal percentages of non-athletes and athletes reported they were restricting fat in their diet at present. The important difference for cancer risk, however, may be that many of the former athletes restricted themselves to low-fat diets for four or five decades,[18] compared to more recent restrictions of diet by the non-athletes.

Excess body weight is associated with a diminished capacity of serum sex-hormone-binding globulin and an elevated percentage of serum estradiol in the free state.[27] The latter may be related to increased risk of breast cancer[36] and cancer of the endometrium.[27]

Bernstein *et al.*[37] suggest that early, moderate physical activity may reduce the risk of breast cancer by reducing the frequency of ovulatory cycles in adolescence. These authors found that young, post-menarcheal girls participating in moderate physical activity had an increase of anovulatory menstrual cycles. After adjustment for age at menarche, and years since menarche, there was a significant dose-related trend in the risk of anovulatory menstrual cycles associated with increasing levels of physical activity.

Cohen *et al.*, in this volume and a 1988 report,[38] suggested that energy restriction and voluntary moderate exercise reduced tumor yields in induced mammary tumorigenesis in female rats. Voluntary exercise reduced tumor yields and delayed time of tumor appearance in high fat diet, exercising animals to levels similar to those found in low-fat, *ad libitum*, sedentary animals.

The former athletes have a slightly shorter interval (about 0.5 year) from menarche to age of first birth (Table 3) which may contribute to a lower risk of breast cancer.[39,40] There does not seem to be a breast cancer risk related to use of oral contraceptives,[21] although there is now controversy about increased risk from long-term use before age 25.[41,42] In our study none of the breast cancer cases reported were diagnosed before age 30. The majority of cases were reported by women age 50 years and over; oral contraceptives were not available to these women when they were under 25 years. In accord with other studies, we found an increased risk of cancers of the reproductive system with use of estrogens for menopausal symptoms,[43] and that smoking was a risk factor.[44]

These data indicate that long-term exercise, which was not Olympic or marathon level, but moderate and regular, reduces the risk of sex-hormone-sensitive cancers later in life. Recent data showing moderate exercise also reduces the risk of non-reproductive system cancers suggest that other factors, such as changes in immunosurveillance[45] may, in addition to body composition changes, be involved.

Whatever the mechanisms, the observed reduction in cancer risk associated with physical exercise has potential for public health: the data indicate that young girls should begin regular, moderate exercise before menarche, thus entraining a lifestyle that can lower the risk of cancer in the menopausal years.

Acknowledgments

We thank: the alumnae and the Alumnae Associations and the Athletic Offices of: Barnard, Bryn Mawr, Mount Holyoke, Radcliffe, Smith, Springfield, Vassar, and Wellesley Colleges and the Universities of Southern California and Wisconsin, for their generous cooperation; and Meg Tyler for preparation of the manuscript. This research was done under the auspices of the Advanced Medical Research Foundation, Boston.

References

1. R.E. Frisch, G. Wyshak, N.L. Albright, T.E. Albright, I. Schiff, K.P. Jones, J. Witschi, E. Shiang, E. Loff, and M. Marguglio, Lower prevalence of breast cancer and cancers of the reproductive system among former college athletes compared to non-athletes, *Br J Cancer*. 52:885 (1985).
2. G. Wyshak, R.E. Frisch, N.L. Albright, T.E. Albright, and I. Schiff, Lower prevalence of benign diseases of the breast and benign tumours of the reproductive system among former college athletes compared to non-athletes, *Br J Cancer*. 54:841 (1986).
3. R.E. Frisch, G. Wyshak, and L. Vincent, Delayed menarche and amenorrhea in ballet dancers, *N Engl J Med*. 303:17 (1980).
4. M.P. Warren, The effects of exercise on pubertal progression and reproductive function in girls, *J Clin Endocrinol Metab*. 51:1150 (1980).

5. R.E. Frisch, A. von Gotz-Welbergen, J.W. McArthur, T. Albright, J.Witschi, B. Bullen, J. Birnholz, R.B. Reed, and H. Hermann, Delayed menarche and amenorrhea of college athletes in relation to age of onset of training, *J Am Med Assoc.* 246:1559 (1981).

6. E. Dale, D.H. Gerlach, and A.L. Wilhite, Menstrual dysfunction in distance runners, *Obstet Gynecol.* 54:47 (1979).

7. B. Schwartz, D.C. Cumming, E. Riordan, M. Selye, S.S.C. Yen, and R.W. Rebar, Exercise-associated amenorrhea: a distinct entity?, *Am J Obstet Gynecol.* 141:662 (1981).

8. R.E. Frisch and J.W. McArthur, Menstrual cycles: fatness as a determinant of minimum weight for height necessary for their maintenance or onset, *Science* 185:949 (1974).

9. R.A. Vigersky, A.E. Andersen, R.H. Thompson, D.L. Loriaux, Hypothalamic dysfunction in secondary amenorrhea associated with simple weight loss, *N Engl J Med.* 297:1141 (1977).

10. J.D. Veldhuis, W.S. Evans, L.M. Demers, M.O. Thorner, D. Wakat, and A.D. Rogel, Altered neuroendocrine regulation of gonadotropin secretion in women distance runners, *J Clin Endocrin Metab.* 61:557 (1985).

11. D.C. Cumming, M.M. Vickovic, S.R. Wall, and M.B. Fluker, Defects in pulsatile LH release in normally menstruating runners, *J Clin Endocrin Metab.* 60:810 (1985).

12. R.J. Hershcopf and H.L. Bradlow, Obesity, diet, endogenous estrogens, and the risk of hormone-sensitive cancer, *Am J Clin Nutr.* Suppl. 45:283 (1987).

13. S.H. Cohn, S. Vartsky, A. Yasumura, A. Sawitsky, I. Zanzi, A. Vaswani, and K.J. Ellis, Compartmental body composition based on total-body nitrogen, potassium, and calcium, *Am J Physiol.* 239 (*Endocrinol Metab.* 2): E 524 (1980).

14. K.J. Ellis, K.K. Shukla, S.H. Cohn, and R.N. Pierson, Jr., A predictor for total body potassium in man based on height, weight, sex, and age: applications in metabolic disorders, *J Lab Clin Med.* 83(5):716 (1974).

15. F. De Waard, Premenopausal and postmenopausal breast cancer: one disease or two?, *J Nat Cancer Inst.* 63:549 (1979).

16. E.L. Gerard, R.C. Snow, D.N. Kennedy, R.E. Frisch, A.R. Guimarals, R.L. Barbieri, A.G. Sorenson, T.K. Egglin, and B.R. Rosen, Overall body fat and regional fat distribution in young woman: Quantification with MR Imaging, *Am J Roentgen.* 157:99 (1991).

17. A.R. Behnke, B.G. Feen, and W.C. Welham, The specific gravity of healthy men: body weight/volume as an index of obesity, *J Am Med Assoc.* 118:495 (1942).

18. National Research Council, "Diet, Nutrition, and Cancer," National Academy Press, Washington, (1982).

19. J.L. Young, Jr., C.L. Percy, and A.J. Asire, Surveillance, epidemiology and end results, incidence and mortality data, 1973-1977, *Natl Cancer Inst Monogr.* 57:202 (1981).

20. B. Sherman, R. Wallace, J. Bean, and L. Schlabaugh, Relationship of body weight to menarcheal and menopausal age: implications for breast cancer risk, *J Clin Endocrinol Metab.* 52:488 (1981).

21. A.B. Miller and R.D. Bulbrook, The epidemiology and etiology of breast cancer, *N Engl J Med.* 303:1246 (1980).

22. M.C. Pike, B.E. Henderson, and J.T. Casagrande, *in*: "Banbury Report 8, Hormones and Breast Cancer," M.C. Pike, P.K. Siiteri, and C.W. Welsch, eds., Cold Spring Harbor Laboratory, Banbury, (1981).

23. F. De Waard, *in*: "Banbury Report 8: Hormones and Breast Cancer," M.C. Pike, P.K. Siiteri, and C.W. Welsch, eds., Cold Spring Harbor Laboratory, Banbury, (1981).

24. D. Apter and R. Vihko, Early menarche, a risk factor for breast cancer, indicates early onset of ovulatory cycles, *J Clin Endocrinol Metab.* 57:82 (1983).

25. J.M. Grodin, P.K. Siiteri, and P.C. MacDonald, Source of estrogen production in postmenopausal women, *J Clin Endocrinol Metab.* 36:207 (1973).

26. S.P. Forney, L. Milewich, G.T. Chen, J.L. Garlock, B.E. Schwartz, C.D. Edman, and P.C. MacDonald, Aromatization of androstenedione to estrone by human adipose tissue in vitro. Correlation with adipose tissue mass, age, and endometrial neoplasia, *J Clin Endocrinol Metab.* 53:192 (1981).

27. P.K. Siiteri, Extraglandular estrogen formation and serum binding of estradiol: relationship to cancer, *J Endocrinol.* 89:119 (1981).

28. J. Fishman, R.M. Boyar, and L. Hellman, Influence of body weight on estradiol metabolism in young women, *J Clin Endocrinol Metab.* 41:989 (1975).

29. J. Schneider, D. Kinne, A. Fracchia, V. Pierce, K.E. Anderson, H.L. Bradlow, and J. Fishman, Abnormal oxidative metabolism of estradiol in women with breast cancer, *Proc Natl Acad Sci.* 79:3047 (1982).

30. H.L. Bradlow, C.P. Martucci, and J. Fishman, Evidence for a cancer risk related increase in estradiol 16 α-hydroxylation, *The Endocrine Society Program and Abstracts*, Abstract 162 (1983).

31. R.E. Frisch, R. Snow, E.L. Gerard, L. Johnson, D. Kennedy, R. Barbieri, and B.R. Rosen, Magnetic Resonance Imaging of body fat of athletes compared to controls, and the oxidative metabolism of estradiol, *Metabolism.* 41:191 (1992).

32. C. Longcope, S. Gorbach, B. Goldin, M. Woods, J. Dwyer, A. Morrilla, and J. Warram, The effect of a low fat diet on estrogen metabolism, *J Clin Sudocrind Metab.* 64:1246 (1987).

33. R.E. Frisch, Amenorrhea, vegetarianism, and/or low fat, *Lancet.* i:1024 (1984).

34. P. Hill, L. Garbaczewski, P. Helman, J. Huskinsson, E. Sporangisa, and E.L. Wynder, Diet, lifestyle, and menstrual activity, *Am J Clin Nutr.* 33:1192 (1980).

35. D.W. Cramer, W.R. Welch, G.B. Hutchison, W. Willett, and R.E. Scully, Dietary animal fat in relation to ovarian cancer risk, *Obstet Gynecol.* 63:833 (1984).

36. J.W. Moore, G.M.G. Clark, R.D. Bulbrook, J.L. Hayward, J.J. Mora, L. Hammond, and P.K. Siiteri, Serum concentrations of total and non-protein bound estradiol in patients with breast cancer and in normal controls, *Int J Cancer* 29:17 (1982).

37. L. Bernstein, R.K. Ross, R.A. Lobo, R. Hanisch, M.D. Krailo, and B.E. Henderson, The effects of moderate physical activity on menstrual cycle patterns in adolescence: Implications for breast cancer prevention, *Br J Cancer.* 55:681 (1987).

38. L.A. Cohen, K. Choi, and C-X Wang, Influence of dietary-fat, caloric restriction, and voluntary exercise on N-Nitrosomethylurea-induced mammary tumorigenesis in rats, *Cancer Research.* 48:4276 (1988).

39. B. MacMahon, P. Cole, and J. Brown, Etiology of human breast cancer: a review, *J Nat Cancer Inst.* 50:21 (1973).

40. J. Cairns, Mutation, selection and the natural history of cancer, *Nature.* 255:197 (1975).

41. M.C. Pike, M.D. Krailo, B.E. Henderson, and A. Duke, Breast cancer in young women and use of oral contraceptives: possible modifying effect of formulation and age at use, *Lancet* ii:926 (1973).

42. R. Gambrell, Jr., Oral contraceptives and breast cancer, *Lancet.* ii:1201 (1983).

43. H. Jick, R.N. Watkins, J.R. Hunter, B.J. Dina, S. Madsen, K.J. Rothman, and A.M. Walker, Replacement estrogens and endometrial cancer, *N Engl J Med.* 300:218 (1979).

44. W. Winkelstein, Jr., E.J. Shillitoe, R. Brand, and K.K. Johnson, Further comments on cancer of the uterine cervix, smoking, and herpes virus infection, *Am J Epidemiol.* 119:1 (1984).

45. L.T. MacKinnon, T.W. Chick, A. vanAs, and T.B. Tomasi, Effects of prolonged intense exercise on natural killer cells, (Abstract #59) *Med Sci Sports Exerc.* 19 (Suppl.):S 10 (1987).

Appendix

Predictions of Body Composition by Equations

of Cohn *et al.*[13] and Ellis *et al.*[14]

Predicted potassium, $K_p = aW^{\frac{1}{2}} Ht^2$;

W = weight (kg);

Ht = height (meters);

a (for females) = 4.58 –0.010 age (years).

Lean body mass (LBM) (for females) = K_p x 0.442 kg.

Fat (kg) = Body weight (kg) - LBM (kg).

%Fat = Fat/body weight

Chapter 5

Voluntary Exercise and Experimental Mammary Cancer

LEONARD A. COHEN, ELIZABETH BOYLAN,
MARCY EPSTEIN and EDITH ZANG

> Plato quoting Socrates: *"And is not bodily habit spoiled by rest and illness, but preserved for a long time by motion and exercise?"* Theaetetus: *"True"*[1]

I. Introduction

Both epidemiologic and experimental studies suggest that physical activity may protect against several forms of cancer. Regarding experimental mammary cancer, exercise has been shown to enhance or inhibit tumorigenesis depending on the type of activity employed. Voluntary exercise, consistently inhibited while forced exercise either enhanced or inhibited depending on experimental conditions. The present study explored the protective role of voluntary activity on two different kinds of chemically induced mammary tumors, [N-nitrosomethylurea(NMU) and 7,12-dimethylbenz(a)anthracene (DMBA)], a virally induced mouse mammary tumor (MMTV) and a transplantable metastasizing mammary tumor (R13672). Its purpose was to determine whether the protective effect of energy expenditure was a species-, strain-, carcinogen-, diet-, or stage-specific phenomenon, or whether it was a general phenomenon affecting all aspects of mammary carcinogenesis. The results of these studies indicate that voluntary exercise inhibits the development of both the NMU- and DMBA-induced mammary tumors and the MMTV-induced mouse mammary tumor under high-fat (HF) 20-23% wt/wt) conditions. The results in the R13762 model study were less clear. Under HF conditions, voluntary exercise exerted a statistically insignificant enhancement of pulmonary metastases in retired breeders, but had the opposite effect in medium-fat (MF, 11.5% wt/wt) conditions. When only the most active half of the HF animals were compared to sedentary controls, a statistically significant enhancement of pulmonary metastases was found. These studies indicate that, with regard to primary prevention,

Leonard A. Cohen, Marcy Epstein and Edith Zang • Division of Nutrition and Endocrinology, American Health Foundation, Valhalla, New York; Elizabeth Boylan • Department of Biology, Queens College, City University of New York, Flushing New York

Exercise, Calories, Fat, and Cancer, Edited by M.M. Jacobs
Plenum Press, New York, 1992

voluntary activity during the post-initiation phase inhibits mammary tumor development whether chemically or virally induced. With regard to secondary prevention, under HF conditions, activity may enhance both the volume and number of lung metastasis, while the converse may occur under MF conditions, indicating that interactions between dietary fat (energy intake) and activity (energy expenditure) may play an important role in determining the effects of physical activity on the metastatic process. Remaining to be clarified are the effects of the degree and amount of exercise, the effects of activity on the initiation and progression phases of carcinogenesis, the nature of the interaction between fat intake, activity and mammary carcinogenesis, and, lastly, the underlying cellular mechanisms responsible for the protective effects of physical exercise.

Early Studies

As the above quote illustrates, the notion that physical exercise confers health benefits has been a theme common to both ancient and modern cultures. However, the intuitive certainty with which Theaetetus answered Socrates's question 2,000 years ago remains to be borne out experimentally today.

As Drs. Paffenbarger and Frisch have shown (see Chapters 2 and 4, this volume) there is epidemiologic evidence to suggest that inactive individuals are at increased risk of cancer, particularly cancer of the colon and reproductive tract and breast. Laboratory animal model studies indicating an inverse association between forced activity and the development of a variety of tumor types go back to the early reports of Sivertsen and Hastings[2] and Milone[3] in the 1920s. However, systematic analysis of this phenomenon didn't begin until the 1940s with the work of Rusch and Kline.[4] Since then, a number of reports have appeared on the effects of forced exercise with somewhat inconsistent results[4-13] (Table 1).

Table 1. Forced Activity and Experimental Neoplasia

Author	Date	Model	Type of exercise	Result
Rusch & Kline Cancer Res. 4:116-18	1944	Fibrosarcoma (implant)	Rotating drum	Inhibition
Hoffman *et al.* Cancer Res. 22:597-99	1962	Walker carcinoma (implant)	Swimming & treadmill	Inhibition
Moore & Tittle Surgery 73:329-332	1973	DMBA mammary tumor	Treadmill	Inhibition
Norton *et al.* J. App. Physiol. 46:654-657	1979	3MC-induced sarcoma	Tenotony of synergist	No change
Deuster *et al.* Med. Sci. Sports Exer. 17:385-392	1985	Walker carcinoma (implant)	Treadmill	Inhibition
Bennink *et al.* Fed. Proc. 45:1087	1986	DMBA mammary tumor	Treadmill	Inhibition
Yedinak *et al.* Fed. Proc. 46:436	1987	DMBA mammary tumor	Treadmill	Inhibition
Thompson *et al.* Cancer Res. 48:2720-23	1988	DMBA mammary tumor	Treadmill	Stimulation
Thompson *et al.* Cancer Res. 49:1904-08	1989	DMBA mammary tumor	Treadmill	Stimulation
Baracos Can J. Physiol & Pharmacol. 67:864-70	1989	Morris hepatoma 7777 (implant)	Swimming	Inhibition

These studies involved forced exercise, such as running in a motorized cage, swimming, or treadmill running. In some cases, the exercise was extremely strenuous, with animals running on a treadmill for as long as 16 hours a day.[4,5] In addition, in most cases, exercise took place during daylight, despite the fact that the rat is a nocturnal animal. Since stress can influence tumor development,[5] it serves as a potential confounding variable in any experiment involving involuntary exercise. As a consequence, it is difficult to sort out the effects of stress from the effects of activity. To overcome this problem, a number of investigators have turned to voluntary exercise using a wheel cage unit that allows ingress to and egress from an activity wheel equipped with an odometer to record activity over time. As of the present, voluntary activity has consistently been shown to reduce the incidence and/or number of primary tumors or neoplastic foci in breast, colon, liver, and pancreatic tumor models[14-19] (Table 2).

II. The NMU Model

With regard to mammary cancer, we have previously shown that voluntary exercise counteracts the promoting effect of a high-fat diet in the N-nitrosomethylurea (NMU)-induced mammary tumor model.[15] Tumor incidence was reduced almost to the level of a low-fat diet (Table 3). Interestingly, the rats that exercised least exhibited the greatest tumor suppression (Figure 1). The activity profile (Figure 2), typical of rodents,[20-27] indicated an early interest in the wheel followed by a gradual diminution of interest. Nonetheless, all animals avidly used the activity wheel. While quantitative measures of exercise intensity, such as VO_2max, were not assessed, observation indicated that the animals walked rapidly rather than ran and showed no signs of fatigue or exhaustion. Body composition analysis (Table 4) indicated that animals fed diets containing different amounts of fat gained weight similarly and had similar amounts of body fat. Active animals exhibited a significant decrease in total body fat but an increase in body weight gain (Figure 3) and food

Table 2. Voluntary Activity and Experimental Neoplasia

Author	Date	Model	Carcinogen	Result
Andrianopoulaus et al. Anticancer Res. 7:849-52	1987	Colon	DMH	Inhibition
Cohen et al. Cancer Res. 48:4276-83	1988	Mammary	NMU	Inhibition
Reddy et al. Cancer Res. 48:7079-81	1988	Colon	AOM	Inhibition
Krieger et al. 72nd Annual Mtg. Fed Proc. #3304	1988	Liver	AFB_1	Inhibition
Benjamin et al. 72nd Annual Mtg. Fed Proc. #5202	1988	Mammary	DMBA	Inhibition
Roebuck et al. Cancer Res. 50:6811-16	1990	Pancreas	Azaserine	Inhibition

Table 3. Mammary Tumor Incidence

Group	Treatment	% of fat	No. of rats	Non-palpable[a] adenocarcinoma No.	Incidence(%)	Palpable[b] adenocarcinoma No.	Incidence(%)	Total[c] adenocarcinoma No.	Incidence(%)
1	Sedentary	5	36	13	36	12[d]	33[d]	21	58
2	Sedentary	10	36	18	50	21	58	28	78
3	Sedentary	20	36	16	45	25	70	28	78
4	Active	20	30	12	40	14	47	19	63

[a] Number of animals with one or more non-palpable adenocarcinomas.
[b] Number of animals with one or more palpable adenocarcinomas.
[c] Number of animals with one or more palpable and/or non-palpable tumors.
[d] Test for overall negative trend: Group 3 > Group 2 > Group 1 ($p<0.05$) (Bartholomew's test). Group 3 vs. Group 1 ($p<0.05$); Group 2 vs. Group 1 ($p<0.05$); Group 3 vs. Group 4 ($p<0.05$) by Fisher's exact test (palpable adenocarcinoma).

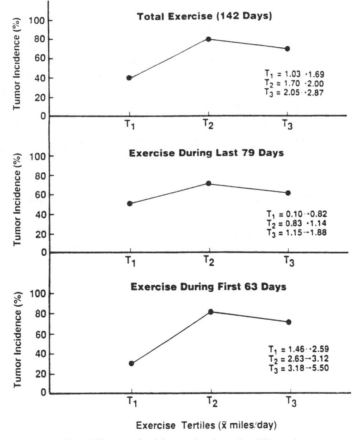

Final Tumor Incidence by Level of Exercise

Figure 1. Tumor incidence plotted as a function of the amount of activity. The ranges of the exercise tertiles for total exercise (top), early exercise (middle) and late exercise (bottom) are denoted above. Each exercise tertile consisted of 10 animals (total N=30). Data from Reference 15.

Table 4. Body Composition as a Percentage of the Total

| Group | No. of animals | Percentage of Total | | | | Body weight (g) |
		Fat	Protein	Moisture	Ash	
1	6	19.4 ± 3.6[a](21)[b]	17.7 ± 1.5(17)	56.8 ± 2.8(56)	4.4 ± 1.4(4.6)	192.8 ± 6.3(195)
2	6	19.0 ± 2.0 (17)	18.3 ± 0.8(18)	56.7 ± 1.5(56)	4.3 ± 0.9(4.6)	191.7 ± 7.7(195)
3	5	20.7 ± (20)	17.8 ± 0.3(18)	53.3 ± 4.3(50)	4.0 ± 0.3(3.8)	197.2 ± 8.9(201)
4	8	16.0 ± 4.7 (14)	18.6 ± 1.6(18)	58.0 ± 4.4(59)	4.1 ± 0.9(3.7)	212.0 ± 16.5(209)

[a] Mean ± SD.
[b] Median.
[c] Statistical analysis was by the Student t test (two-tailed comparison). The percentage of fat: Group 3 vs. Group 4, $p < 0.05$ ($p < 0.03$, one-tailed test). The percentage of moisture: Group 3 vs. Group 4, $p < 0.06$, $p < 0.035$, one-tailed). All other pairwise comparisons were not significant.

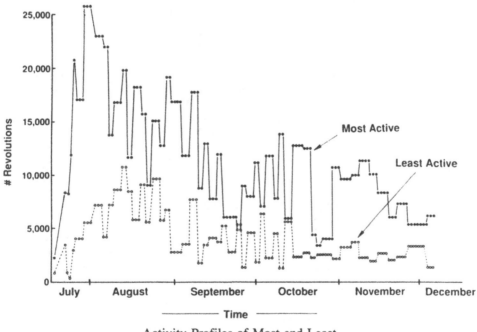

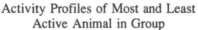

Activity Profiles of Most and Least
Active Animal in Group

Figure 2. Plot of activity vs. time for F-344 rat depicting the activity profile for the most and least active animals in the active group. Note that early interest in wheel running subsided over time. All animals exhibited a similar chronological pattern of activity. Data from Reference 15. One complete revolution of the wheel is equivalent to 3.53 ft; 1496 revolutions equal 1 mile.

consumption.[15] This latter result is in keeping with other reports [21,24,25] indicating that female rats, in contrast to males, compensate for increased energy expenditure by increasing food intake. Female rats also tend to be more active than males: female F344 rats, for example, are 10 times more active than their male counterparts.[16]

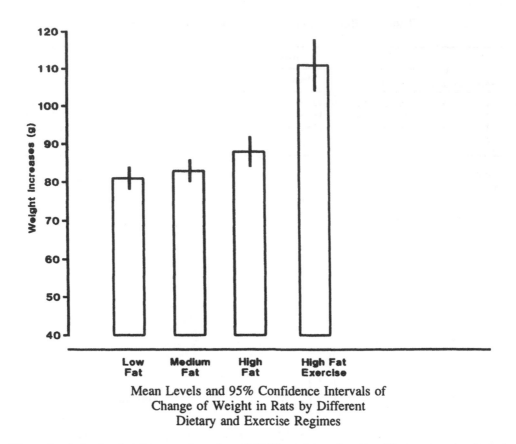

Mean Levels and 95% Confidence Intervals of
Change of Weight in Rats by Different
Dietary and Exercise Regimes

Figure 3. Animal weight increase from day of NMU administration (day 55 of age) to day 210 of age (termination). Differences between groups 1 (low-fat-sedentary), 2 (medium-fat-sedentary), and 3 (high-fat-sedentary), NS. Group 4 (high-fat-active) significantly elevated compared to groups 1-3 (p=<0.05). Data from Reference 47.

Various mechanisms have been proposed to explain the health effects of exercise[28-41] (Table 5). One which we investigated involves mediation, via the hypothalamo-pituitary axis, by the polypeptide hormone prolactin. Prolactin is a known promoter of both the DMBA and MNU mammary tumor[42] and may promote human breast cancer development.[43] Hence, one way in which activity could serve as an anti-promoter is to block prolactin secretion by the anterior pituitary. We, therefore, measured circulating prolactin using both immuno- and bioassay [44-46] methods at termination of the experiment.[47] As seen in Figures 4 and 5, activity had no significant effects on either form of prolactin. This does not necessarily mean that prolactin changes are irrelevant to the activity effect[48] but does suggest that voluntary activity does not exert major long-term effects on prolactin secretion by the anterior pituitary.

While the inhibitory effect of voluntary activity has been demonstrated convincingly in the NMU model, it remained to be determined whether the same effect could be demonstrated in other breast cancer models. To this end, we embarked on a series of comparative studies using three different models of human breast cancer (Table 6): the DMBA-induced mammary tumor, the MMTV mouse mammary tumor, and the R13762 transplantable metastasizing mammary tumor.

Table 5. Activity and Cancer Prevention: Hypothetical Mechanisms

System	References
1) Altered endocrine profile	28-32
2) Altered prostaglandin metabolism	33
3) Increased endorphin production	28, 34
4) Enhanced immune function	35-38
5) Altered adiposity/fat distribution	39
6) Enhanced free-radical/antioxidant functions	40
7) Stimulation of colonic peristalsis	41

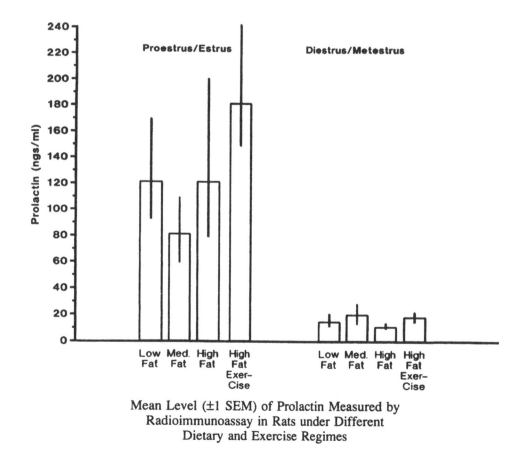

Mean Level (±1 SEM) of Prolactin Measured by
Radioimmunoassay in Rats under Different
Dietary and Exercise Regimes

Figure 4. Circulating prolactin levels measured at termination. Prolactin measured by bioassay as described in Reference 46. Groups 1-4 as described in legend to Figure 3.

Table 6. Mammary Tumor Models: Voluntary Activity and Breast Cancer

Model	Agent or procedure	Mode of action	Outcome	Species	Stage in carcinogenesis
Chemically induced	NMU	Direct-acting	Primary	Rat	Promotion
	DMBA	Host-activated	Primary	Rat	Promotion
Virally induced	MMTV	RNA-retrovirus	Primary	Mouse	Promotion
Transplantable (R-13762)	Subcutaneous implant	Metastasis to lung and liver	Primary and metastasis	Rat (retired breeder)	Progression

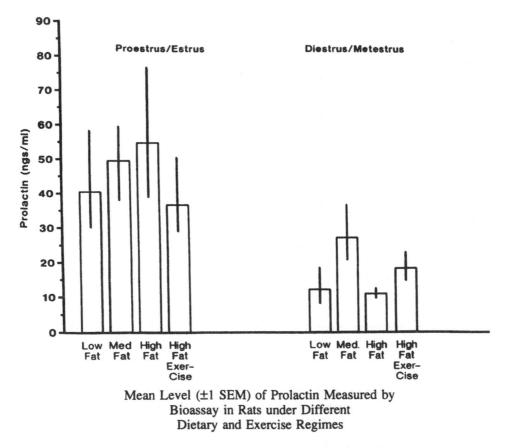

Mean Level (±1 SEM) of Prolactin Measured by
Bioassay in Rats under Different
Dietary and Exercise Regimes

Figure 5. Circulating prolactin levels measured at termination. Prolactin measured by immunoassay as described in Reference 46. Groups 1-4 as described in legend to Figure 3.

III. The DMBA Model

This experiment was designed to test not only whether voluntary activity suppressed the tumor-promoting effect of a high-fat diet, but whether the effect was dependent on the dose of initiating carcinogen. In general, it has been observed that at high carcinogen doses, the effects of promoters (and anti-promoters) are attenuated and, conversely, at low doses these effects are more pronounced. Since humans are exposed to low doses of carcinogens, this implies that promoters and anti-promoters play a major role in human carcinogenesis. Hence, in an experimental animal model, if an effect on the promotion stage can be demonstrated at a high carcinogen dose, it is expected that a more pronounced effect would be demonstrable at a lower "more realistic" dose. It was found that the tumor-inhibiting effect of voluntary activity was most pronounced in the high-dose group when assessed in terms of total tumor number/group or tumor multiplicity; no effect on tumor incidence or latency was observed[49] (Table 7). In the low-dose group (Table 8), activity significantly decreased total tumor number and latency but failed to suppress either tumor multiplicity or incidence when compared to sedentary controls. In the DMBA model, therefore, voluntary activity was equally or perhaps more effective as an anti-promoter under high- as compared to low-dose conditions. That the inhibitory effect of exercise was exerted throughout the experiment can be seen in Figure 6. At all points from the onset of tumor appearance, the active group exhibited lower tumor numbers than the sedentary groups.

Table 7. Effect of Voluntary Exercise on Incidence, Multiplicity and Number of DMBA-Induced Mammary Tumors: High DMBA

Group	DMBA	Tumor-bearing rats/ rats at risk	%	Total number of tumors/group	# Tumors/rat
HF EX[a]	10 mg	28/30	93	90[b]	3.0 ± 2.1^c
HF Sed[d]	10 mg	30/30	100	160	5.3 ± 3.23

[a] HF EX = High-fat diet and exercised.
[b] Exercise group significantly less than sedentary (p<0.001) by chi square test.
[c] Exercise group significantly less than sedentary (p<0.05) by Armitage's test.
[d] HF Sed = High-fat diet and sedentary.

Table 8. Effect of Voluntary Exercise on Incidence, Multiplicity and Number of DMBA-Induced Mammary Tumors: Low Dose

Group	DMBA	Tumor-bearing rats/ rats at risk	%	Total number of tumors/group	# tumors/rat
HF EX[a]	5 mg	24/30	80	75[b]	2.5 ± 2.0^c
HF Sed[d]	5 mg	26/30	87	102	3.4 ± 2.5

[a] HF EX = High-fat diet and exercised.
[b] Exercise group significantly less than sedentary (p<0.05) by chi square test.
[c] Difference between exercise and sedentary groups N.S. by Armitage's test.
[d] HF Sed = High-fat diet and sedentary.

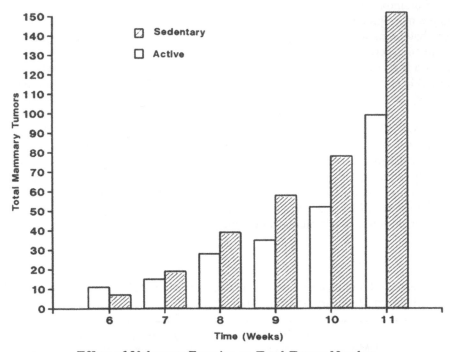

Effect of Voluntary Exercise on Total Tumor Number
DMBA Mammary Tumor Model

Figure 6. Rats were initiated with 10 mg DMBA on day 53 of age and then placed in either activity or conventional cages. Diet was AIN-76A (23% corn oil). Bars represent palpable mammary tumors (after Reference 49).

The activity profiles of Sprague-Dawley females indicate a pattern similar to that found with F344 rats, namely an early rise followed by a gradual decline, though the steepness of the decline was somewhat attenuated (Figures 7 and 8) in the Sprague-Dawley rats. A maximum of 20 miles/day was found in the Sprague-Dawley females, which is considerably greater than observed in the F-344 rats (maximum, 13 miles/day). Body composition data (not shown) indicated a non-significant trend towards decreased body fat content in the active vs. the sedentary group. In contrast to the NMU model, when tumor incidence was assessed after segregation of activity data into tertiles, no differences in tumor incidence were found between the tertiles.

In summary, the results from the DMBA model support the general premise that voluntary activity inhibits the development of mammary tumors in animals fed high-fat diets. However, significant differences were seen between the NMU and DMBA models including: (a) activity exerted different effects on specific parameters of tumorigenesis, (b) lack of an inverse association between the amount of exercise and the anti-promoting effects of activity; and (c) minor effects of activity on overall weight gain and body fat content in the DMBA compared to the NMU model.

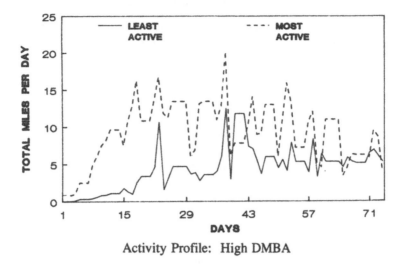

Activity Profile: High DMBA

Figure 7. Plot of activity vs. time for Sprague-Dawley rat, depicting the activity profile, in revolutions/day, for the most and least active animal in the active group. Note, as in the F-344 rat, that early interest in wheel running subsided over time. All animals exhibited a similar chronological pattern of activity. One complete revolution of the wheel is equivalent to 3.53 ft; 1496 revolutions equal 1 mile. Data from Reference 49.

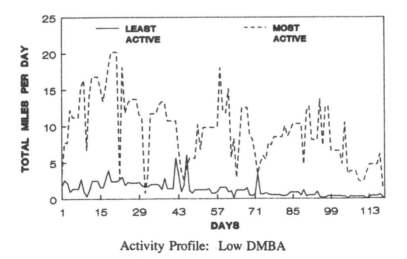

Activity Profile: Low DMBA

Figure 8. Plot of activity vs. time for Sprague-Dawley rat, depicting the activity profile, in revolutions/day, for the most and least active animal in the active group. Note, as in the F-344 rat, that early interest in wheel running subsided over time. All animals exhibited a similar chronological pattern of activity. One complete revolution of the wheel is equivalent to 3.53 ft; 1496 revolutions equal 1 mile. Data from Reference 49.

IV. The C3H/oµJ Mouse Mammary Tumor Model (MMTV)

The MMTV is an RNA-containing retrovirus unique in that it requires glucocorticoids for its integration into the cellular genome.[50,51] After integration via a DNA intermediate the provirus evidently activates a series of oncogenes which result over a period of time in the development of a mammary tumor.[50,51] As seen in Figure 9, when 9-week-old female mice were placed in activity cages, the onset of tumors was similar in both sedentary and active animals. However, tumor incidence was suppressed in the active group throughout the experiment. After 48 weeks, 93% of the sedentary rats had 1 or more tumors, while only 67% of the active rats bore tumors. Interestingly, no difference was seen in the number of tumors/tumor-bearing animal in these two groups. Weight gain data indicate that active animals gained weight at similar rates and at termination were only slightly lighter than sedentary animals (46.4±5.55 vs. 47.6±5.89, mean ± SD g respectively). Activity profiles and body composition data have not yet been assessed. The results of this study suggest that voluntary activity may exert effects on molecular events such as provirus integration or oncogene activation. Although human breast cancers have not been associated with a virus, a number of mutated oncogenes have been isolated from human breast cancers.[51] Hence, our findings with the MMTV model may have implications with regard to the control of oncogene expression by activity in human cancer.

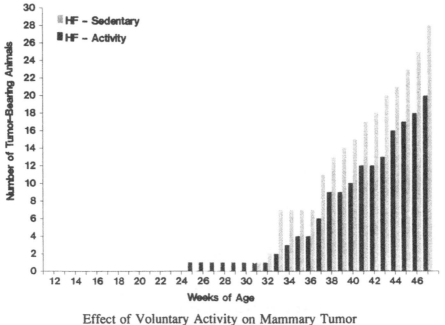

Effect of Voluntary Activity on Mammary Tumor
Development in the C3H Mouse

Figure 9. Histogram depicting cumulative tumor incidence. Mice were placed in conventional and activity cages at 9 weeks of age and experiment terminated at 48 weeks of age. Test for overall trend (p<0.05, Cox's test). (Palpable mammary tumors.)

V. The R13762 Metastasizing Mammary Tumor

The R13762 tumor model[52] has been used in studies designed to assess the effects of dietary fat on the metastatic process. Katz and Boylan [53] discovered that dietary fat stimulated dissemination to the lung in older retired breeders but not in young rats. While the reason for this discrepancy remains to be determined, it suggests that endogenous hormonal differences, associated with age/parity, may be key determinants of the tumor response to exogenous agents. Based on these considerations, we decided to introduce fat content as a secondary variable, along with activity as the primary variable. The experiment, therefore, consisted of two HF (23%) groups (active vs. sedentary) and two MF (11.5%) groups (active vs. sedentary).

After implantation of a 2 mm^3 tumor fragment into the subcutaneous fat pads of 9- to 12- month-old retired breeders, each animal was allocated to one of 4 experimental groups (N=30 per mouse). Growth of the primary tumors was monitored over an 8-week period. At this time, approximately one-half of the rats in all 4 groups exhibited metastatic foci in the lungs. As seen in Figure 10, voluntary exercise had no effect on the growth of the primary tumor implant. Animals fed high-fat diets exhibited an early stimulation of primary tumor growth but the medium-fat group caught up by the end of the experiment.

The volume of lung metastases was determined as described by Katz & Boylan.[53] Foci with diameters under 1 mm were assumed to have a radius of 0.5 mm, those with diameters from 1-3 mm were assigned a radius of 1.5 mm and those over 3 mm in diameter were

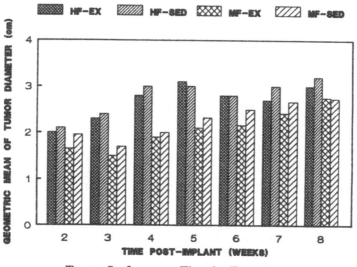

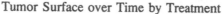

Tumor Surface over Time by Treatment

Figure 10. Histogram depicting growth of R13762 implant in F344 retired breeders under high-fat-Active, high-fat-Sedentary, medium-fat-active, and medium-fat-Sedentary conditions. Diet of high-fat and meduim-fat groups was initiated 5 weeks before tumor implantation. The two largest tumor diameters were measured biweekly and tumor surface expressed as the mean square root of (d_1 x d_2) (geometric mean). Difference between high-fat and medium-fat significant at week 4 (p<0.05). All other comparisons, NS.

from 1-3 mm were assigned a radius of 1.5 mm and those over 3 mm in diameter were measured indiviually and their radii calculated. Individual focus volumes were then calculated using the formula $(4/3 \pi R^3)$ for a sphere and then summed to produce an overall value of total lung foci volume for each animal.

Voluntary activity did not influence the incidence of rats with pulmonary metastases. However, when the number or volume of pulmonary lesions/rat was summed for each of the four groups, a definite trend could be seen with the high-fat active group exhibiting a four-fold greater total number of lesions and a ten-fold greater volume of metastases. The medium-fat groups exhibited the opposite trend, with activity tending to lower both the number and volume of pulmonary metastases (Table 9). Statistical analysis of the data, however, revealed that the differences between mean metastasis volume were not significant. The failure to achieve significance could be due to (a) the possibility that there was no actual difference, (b) the high variance typical of metastasis volumes, and (c) small population samples (N=30) (Tables 10 and 11).

When the high-fat active group was segregated into two subgroups, namely those below and those above the median activity level for the group as a whole, it became apparent that the major part of the total metastatic burden would be attributed to the group above the median activity level (Table 12). In fact, when the more active subgroup was compared to the sedentary group, the former exhibited significantly higher metastatic volumes than the latter, suggesting that under high-fat conditions high levels of activity actually enhance the metastatic process in this model. In the medium-fat groups, there was no obvious association between activity level and metastatic burden (data not shown).

Table 9. Effect of Exercise on Pulmonary Metastases[a]

	HF EX[b]	HF SED[c]	MF EX[d]	MF SED[e]	
Incidence of metastasis	$\frac{16}{30}$	$\frac{14}{30}$	$\frac{16}{30}$	$\frac{12}{30}$	$\frac{(15)}{(30)}$[f]
Total number of nodules by class (diam.)					
(a) <1 mm	235	69	163	321	
(b) 1-3 mm	161	21	31	22	
(c) >3 mm	13	0	3	5	
Total nodules	409	90	197	348	
Total volume of nodules by class (mm³)					
(a) <1 mm	123	36.1	85.3	168.1	
(b) 1-3 mm	674.4	88	129.9	92.2	
(c) >3 mm	351.3	65.4	61.8	90.0	
Total volume (mm³)	1148.7	189.5	277.0	350.3	

[a] The volume of lung metastases was determined as described by Katz and Boylan.[53] Foci with diameters under 1 mm were assigned a radius of 1.5 mm, those with diameters from 1-3 mm were assigned a radius of 1.5 mm and those over 3 mm in diameter were measured individually and their radii calculated. Individual tumor volumes were then calculated using the formula $(4/3 \pi R^3)$ for a sphere and then summed to produce an overall value of lung tumor volume for each animal.
[b] HF EX = High-fat diet and exercised.
[c] HF SED = High-fat diet and sedentary.
[d] MF EX = Medium-fat diet and exercised.
[e] MF SED = Medium-fat diet and sedentary.
[f] Three animals in this group exhibited uncountable mammary lesions which could not be described with certainty as metastatic lesions.

Table 10. Pulmonary Metastases Volume[a]

	HF EX[b]		HF SED[c]	MF EX[d]		MF SED[e]
1. Total volume						
Mean ± SD	95.2 ± 176		21.1 ± 31.8	23.0 ± 34.7		35.7 ± 6.4
Median	38.9		6.6	8.0		36.1
Wilcoxon P		0.11			0.60	
ANOVA P		0.13			0.34	
2. Class a						
Mean ± SD	12.6 ± 13.4		4.8 ± 7.7	7.5 ± 8.7		18.6 ± 21.8
Median	9.0		1.74	5.6		9.4
Wilcoxon P		0.22			0.48	
ANOVA P		0.11			0.85	
3. Class b						
Mean ± SD	81.3 ± 136		13.0 ± 11.5	27.3 ± 14.8		23.9 ± 11.5
Median	22.2		5.6	5.6		11.1
Wilcoxon P		0.09			0.74	
ANOVA P		0.15			0.85	
4. Class c						
Mean ± SD	93.2 ± 107		65.6 ± 30	27.3 ± 14.8		23.9 ± 11.5
Median	44.4		65.6	18.8		28.8
Wilcoxon P		0.69			0.69	
ANOVA P		0.75			0.72	

[a]Animals with no pulmonary metastases excluded from analysis.
[b]HF EX = High-fat diet and exercised.
[c]HF SED = High-fat diet and sedentary.
[d]MF EX = Medium-fat diet and exercised.
[e]MF SED = Medium-fat diet and sedentary.

Table 11. Pulmonary Metastases Volume[a]

	HF EX[b]		HF SED[c]	MF EX[d]		MF SED[e]
1. Total volume						
Mean ± SD	50.8 ± 135		9.9 ± 30	12.2 ± 28		15.5 ± 30
Median	44.8		0	0.69		0
Wilcoxon P		0.28			0.60	
ANOVA P		0.11			0.66	
2. Class a						
Mean ± SD	5.4 ± 10.7		1.6 ± 4.8	3.8 ± 7.2		7.4 ± 16.3
Median	0		0	0		0
Wilcoxon P		0.28			0.62	
ANOVA P		0.08			0.58	
3. Class b						
Mean ± SD	29.8 ± 89.5		3.9 ± 8.5	5.7 ± 13.5		4.1 ± 9.7
Median	0		0	0		0
Wilcoxon P		0.36			0.61	
ANOVA P		0.12			0.58	
4. Class c						
Mean ± SD	15.5 ± 53		4.3 ± 17.6	2.7 ± 9.2		4.0 ± 10.0
Median	0		0	0		0
Wilcoxon P		0.24			0.47	
ANOVA P		0.28			0.62	

[a]All animals with (and without) pulmonary metastases included in analysis.
[b]HF EX = High-fat diet and exercised.
[c]HF SED = High-fat diet and sedentary.
[d]MF EX = Medium-fat diet and exercised.
[e]MF SED = Medium-fat diet and sedentary.

Table 12. Pulmonary Metastases Volume.

Groups	$\bar{x} \pm$ SD	ANOVA		Wilcoxon's nonparametric T statistic	
		F	P	F	P
1. High-fat Low ex[a] High ex	11.4 ± 21 90.1 ± 185	2.69	0.11	2.76	0.10
2. High-fat Low ex Sedentary	11.4 ± 21 9.9 ± 24	0.05	0.83	0.02	0.89
3. High-fat High ex Sedentary	90.1 ± 185 9.9 ± 23	5.61	0.002*	3.5	0.06

[a] The high-fat active group was segregated into two subgroups after ranking by activity status: Group 1, 15 animals below the median activity level (low exercise) and Group 2, 15 animals above the median (high exercise). Pulmonary foci volumes among groups 1 and 2 and the high-fat sedentary controls were then compared pairwise.

VI. Summary and Conclusions

The results of these studies indicate that voluntary activity suppresses the development of chemically and virally induced primary mammary tumors in rats and mice fed high-fat diets. These diets were chosen to mimic the current U.S. fat consumption of approximately 40% of calories as fat.[54] It remains to be seen if activity exerts a similar suppressive effect on animals fed their customary low-fat diet (10% calories as fat). In general, the activity profiles of the female Fischer F-344 and Sprague-Dawley rat and the C3H/ouj mouse exhibited a similar pattern with an early peak followed by a gradual plateau over time. The effects of activity on body fat composition showed a trend toward a decreased percent of body fat when compared to sedentary animals but a statistically significant decrease was found only in the F-344 female rat.

In the DMBA model, carcinogen dose did alter outcome parameters. For example, time to first tumor was extended under low- but not high-DMBA conditions, and, conversely, tumor multiplicity was significantly decreased in the high- but not low-DMBA group.

In the NMU model, an inverse association was found between the amount of activity and tumor incidence. A similar association was not found with the DMBA model. The reason for this is uncertain, but further analysis in terms of other parameters such as total tumor number may shed more light on this discrepancy.

The suppressive effect of activity on the MMTV-induced mouse mammary tumor is of particular interest since it raises the possibility that activity may exert effects on the process of provirus insertion, and/or oncogene activation—an area of great potential promise in cancer prevention.

Activity appeared to enhance the volume and to a lesser degree the number of metastatic foci in the lungs of F-344 retired breeders under high-fat but not medium-fat conditions. In addition, the most active animals in the high-fat group exhibited the greatest volume of metastases. These results, together with those in the NMU model, point to the critical importance of the quantity of voluntary activity an animal engages in and its relation to both primary and secondary cancer prevention. They imply that beyond a certain point of either frequency or intensity, the beneficial effect of exercise may be nullified by competing deleterious effects. The metastases study has also brought to light the importance of dietary fat as a potential intervening variable. Animals fed medium-fat diets exhibited lower activity levels, in general, and lower levels of pulmonary metastases when compared to high-fat animals.

The results described here and by Thompson *et al.* (Chapter 6, this volume) indicate that a key area of future research interest will be determination of the type and amount of exercise that confers protection. There are various forms (anaerobic/aerobic; isometric/isotonic) and measures (VO_2, body heat production, lean body mass) of physical activity, and more systematic analyses using such measures together with mechanistic studies will be necessary before a full understanding of the anti-cancer effects of exercise can be gained.

Acknowledgments

This study was supported by NCI Grant #RO1-CA48741 and NIH Division of Research Resources Grant RR-05775. The author wishes to thank Dr. C. Meschter for pathology support, Dr. E. Katz for generously providing her expertise in the R13672 study, Ms. V. Saa and Mr. T. Baxter for their expert technical assistance, and Ms. A. Banow for assistance in the preparation of this manuscript.

References

1. B. Jowett, translation, "Dialogues of Plato," Random House, New York, (1937).
2. I. Sivertsen and W.H. Hastings, Preliminary report on the influence of food and function on incidence of mammary tumor in "A" stock albino mice, *Minn Med.* 21:873 (1938).
3. S. Milone, Fatigue, effect of prolonged fatigue in rat on development of sarcoma, *Giornale Academia Medicine di Torino.* 91:231 (1928).
4. H.P. Rusch and B.E. Kline, The effect of exercise on the growth of a mouse tumor, *Cancer Res.* 4:116 (1944).
5. S.A. Hoffman, K.E. Paschkis, and D.A. DeBias, The infuence of exercise on the growth of transplanted rat tumours, *Cancer Res.* 22:597 (1962).
6. C. Moore and P.W. Tittle, Muscle activity, body fat, and induced rat mammary tumors, *Surgery (St. Louis)* 73:329 (1973).
7. J.A. Norton, S.F. Lowry, and M.F. Brennan, Effect of work-induced hypertrophy of skeletal muscle on tumour and non-tumour bearing rats, *J Appl Physiol.* 46:654 (1979).
8. P.A. Deuster, S.D. Morrison, and R.A. Ahrens, Endurance exercise modifies cachexia of tumor growth in rats, *Med Sci Sports Exer.* 17:385 (1985).
9. M.R. Bennink, H.J. Palmer, and M.J. Messina, Exercise and caloric restriction modify rat mammary carcinogenesis, *Fed Proc.* 45:1087 (1986).
10. R.A. Yedinak, D.K. Layman, and J.A. Milner, Influences of dietary fat and exercise on DMBA-induced mammary tumors, *Fed Proc.* 46:436 (1987).
11. H.J. Thompson, A.M. Ronan, R.A. Ritacco, A.R. Tagliaferro, and L.D. Meeker, Effects of exercise on the induction of mammary carcinogenesis, *Cancer Res.* 48:2720 (1988).
12. H.L. Thompson, A.M. Ronan, R.A. Ritacco, and A.R. Tagliaferro, Effect of type and amount of dietary fat on the enhancement of rat mammary tumorigenesis by exercise, *Cancer Res.* 49:1904 (1989).

13. V.E. Baracos, Exercise inhibits progressive growth of the Morris hepatoma 7777 in male and female rats, *Can J Physiol Pharmacol.* 67:864 (1989).

14. G. Andrianopoulas, R.C. Nelson, C.T. Bombeck, and G. Souza, The influence of physical activity in 1,2-dimethylhydrazine-induced colon carcinogenesis in the rat, *Anticancer Res.* 7:849, (1987).

15. L.A. Cohen, K.W. Choi, and C.X. Wang, Influence of dietary fat, caloric restriction, and voluntary exercise on N-nitrosomethylurea-induced mammary tumorigenesis in rats, *Cancer Res.* 48:4276 (1988).

16 B.S. Reddy, S. Sugie, and A. Lowenfels, Effect of voluntary exercise on azoxymethane-induced colon carcinogenesis in male F344 rats, *Cancer Res.* 48:7079 (1988).

17. E. Kreiger, C.D. Youngman, and T.C. Campbell, The modulation of aflatoxin B_1 (AFB_1) induced preneoplastic lesions by dietary protein and voluntary exercise in Fischer F344 rats, *Fed Proc.* 2(5):A3304 (1988).

18. H. Benjamin, J. Storkson, and M.W. Pariza, Effect of voluntary exercise on mammary tumor development, *Fed Proc.* 2(5):A5202 (1988).

19. B.D. Roebuck, J. McCaffrey, and K.J. Baumgartner, Protective effects of voluntary exercise during the postinitiation phase of pancreatic carcinogenesis in the rat, *Cancer Res.* 50:6811 (1990).

20. K. Tokuyama, and H. Okuda, Fatty acid synthesis in adipose tissues of physically trained rats *in vivo*, *Am J Physiol.* 245 (*Endocrinol Metab.* 8):E8-E13 (1983).

21. C.L. Goodrick, Effects of long-term voluntary wheel exercise on male and female Wistar rats, 1. Longevity, body weight, and metabolic rate, *Gerontology* 26:22 (1980).

22. B.C. Shyu, S.A. Anderson, and P. Thoren, Spontaneous running in wheels. A microprocessor assisted method for measuring physiological parameters during exercise in rodents, *Acta Physiol Scand.* 121:103 (1984).

23. J.C. Russell, W.F. Epling, D. Perce, R.M. Amy, and D.P. Boer, Induction of voluntary prolonged running by rats, *J Appl Physiol.* 63:2549 (1985).

24. K. Tokuyama, M. Saito, and H. Okuda, Effect of wheel running on food intake and weight gain of male and female rats, *Physiol Behav.* 28:899 (1982).

25. H.G. Anantharaman-Barr, and J. Decombaz, The effect of voluntary activity on growth and energy expenditure of female rats, *Int J Vit Nutr Res.* 57:341 (1987).

26. M.F.W. Festing, Wheel activity in 26 strains of mouse, *Lab Animals.* 11:257 (1977).

27. K.A. Dawson, D.B. Crowne, C.M. Richardson, and E. Anderson, Effects of age on nocturnal activity rhythms in rats, *Prog Clinical Biol Res.* 227B:107 (1987).

28. J. Dearman, and K.T. Francis, Plasma levels of catecholamines, cortisol and beta-endorphins in male athletes after running 26, 6 and 2 miles, *J Sports Med.* 23(1):30 (1983).

29. H. Galbo, The hormonal response to exercise, *Proc Nutr Soc.* 44:257 (1983).

30. K. De Meirleir, M. L'Hermite-Baleriaux, M. L'Hermite, R. Post, and W. Hollman, Evidence for serotoninergic control of exercise, *Horm Met Res.* 17:380 (1985).

31. J. Fishman, R. Boyar, and L. Hellman, Influence of body weight on estradiol metabolism in young women, *J Clin Endocrinol Metab.* 41:989 (1975).

32. L. Bernstein, R.K. Ross, R.A. Lobo, R. Hanisch, M.D. Krailo, and B.E. Henderson, The effects of moderate physical activity on menstrual cycle patterns in adolescents. Implications for breast cancer prevention, *Br J Cancer.* 55:681 (1987).

33. R. Rauramaa, Physical activity and prostanoids, *in:* "Physical activity in health and disease," P.O. Astrand and G. Grimby, eds., *Acta Med Scand Symposium Series No 2.* Almquist & Wiksell Intern, (1986).

34. M. Allen, Activity generated endorphins: A review of their roles in sports science, *Can J App Sports Sci.* 8:115 (1983).

35. L. Fitzgerald, Exercise and the immune system, *Immunol Today.* 9:337 (1988).

36. J.G. Cannon, W.J. Evans, V.A. Hughes, C.N. Meredith, and C.A. Dinarello, Physiological mechanisms contributing to increased interleukin-1 secretion, *J Appl Physiol.* 61(5):1869 (1986).

37. L.T. Mackinnon, Exercise and natural killer cells. What is the relationship?, *Sports Med.* 7:141 (1989).

38. E.R. Eichner, Exercise, lymphokines, calories and cancer, *The Physician and Sports Medicine.* 15:109 (1987).

39. A.J. Trembley, P. Després, and C. Bouchard, The effects of exercise training on energy balance and adipose tissue, morphology and metabolism, *Sports Med.* 2:223 (1986).

40. R.R. Jenkins, Free radical chemistry: relationship to exercise, *Sports Med.* 5:156 (1988).

41. L. Cordain, R.W. Latin, and J.J. Behnke, The effects of an aerobic running program on bowel transit time, *J Sports Med.* 26:101 (1986).

42. C.W. Welsch, and H. Nagasawa, Prolactin and murine mammary tumorigenesis: A review, *Cancer Res.* 37:951 (1977).

43. H. Nagasawa, Prolactin and human breast cancer: A review, *Europ J Cancer.* 15:167 (1979).

44. D.M. Lawson, N. Sensui, D.H. Haisenleder, and R.R. Gala, Rat lymphoma cell bioassay for prolactin: observations on its use and comparison with radioimmunoassay, *Life Sci.* 31:3063 (1982).

45. F.C. Leung, S.M. Russel, and C.S. Nicoll, Relationship between bioassay and radioimmunoassay activities, *Endocrinol.* 103:1619 (1978).

46. J. Klindt, M.C. Robertson, and H.G. Friesan, Episodic secretory patterns of rat prolactin determined by bioassay and radioimmunoassay, *Endocrinol.* 111:350 (1983).

47. L.A. Cohen, K. Choi, J-Y Backlund, R. Harris, and C-X Wang, Modulation of N-nitrosomethylurea-induced mammary tumorigenesis by dietary fat and exercise, *In Vivo.* 5:333 (1991).

48. P.W. Sylvester, S. Forczek, M.M. Ip, and C. Ip, Exercise training and the differential prolactin response in male and female rats, *J Appl Physiol.* 67:804 (1989).

49. L.A. Cohen, C. Meschter, and E. Zang, Inhibition of rat mammary tumorigenesis by voluntary exercise, *Proc Amer Assoc Cancer Res.* 32:125, Abstract 747 (1991).

50. C.A. Kozak, Retroviruses as chromosomal genes in the mouse, *Adv Cancer Res.* 44:295 (1985).

51. M.J. Van de Vijver, and R. Nusse, The molecular biology of breast cancer, *Biochem Biophys Acta.* 1072:33050 (1991).

52. A. Neri, D. Welch, T. Kawaguchi, and G.L. Nicolson, Development of biologic properties of malignant cell sublines and clones of a spontaneously metastasing rat mammary adenocarcinoma, *J Natl Cancer Inst.* 68:507 (1982).

53. E.B. Katz, and E.S. Boylan, Stimulatory effect of a high polyunsaturated fat diet on lung metastasis from the 13762 mammary adenocarcinoma in female retired breeder rats, *J Natl Cancer Inst.* 79:351 (1987).

54. National Research Council, Committee on Diet and Health, "Diet and health: implications for reducing chronic disease risk," National Acad. Press, Washington, DC (1989).

Chapter 6

Effect of Amount and Type of Exercise on Experimentally Induced Breast Cancer

HENRY J. THOMPSON

I. Introduction

Epidemiologic and laboratory data indicate that certain patterns of physical activity may alter the risk for cancer. Exercise is a type of physical activity being promoted for its health benefits. The influence of exercise on the induction of breast cancer in an animal model for the disease was investigated. The data presented indicate that both the intensity and duration of exercise affect the promotion stage of chemically induced mammary carcinogenesis. Whereas certain patterns of exercise inhibited the tumorigenic response and yielded a protective effect that was sustained even after exercise was discontinued, others had either no effect or accelerated the rate of mammary tumor appearance. It is concluded that further characterization of patterns of physical activity that alter the tumorigenic process in the breast and at other cancer sites is warranted. Experiments are also needed to identify the mechanisms that underlie cancer-preventive as well as cancer-enhancing effects of exercise. A goal of research in this area should be to determine if the quantity and quality of exercise needed to attain cancer preventive effects differs from that which is recommended for health-fitness benefits.

Physical activity is defined as bodily movement due to skeletal muscle contraction that results in quantifiable energy expenditure.[1] Both epidemiologic and laboratory data indicate that certain patterns of physical activity may alter the risk for cancer.[2-4] However, the amount of scientific evidence concerning this relationship is still quite limited and there are conflicting reports about the nature of the association.[2-5] The fact that the trend in industrialized societies is for an increasingly sedentary lifestyle with the promotion of a regular regimen of exercise as a means to attain appropriate levels of energy expenditure raises a number of important questions. Does the habit of regular exercise protect an individual against the occurrence of cancer? If the answer is yes, then how much exercise is enough and what type of exercise is best? An ongoing effort in my laboratory during the last several years has attempted to address these questions and is the topic of this paper. Breast cancer

Henry J. Thompson ● Laboratory of Nutrition Research, AMC Cancer Research Center, Denver, Colorado

Exercise, Calories, Fat, and Cancer, Edited by M.M. Jacobs
Plenum Press, New York, 1992

has been the subject of these investigations since both epidemiologic and laboratory data indicate that the course of this disease may be altered by physical activity status as well as diet.[2-6] A long-term goal of this program of research is to identify mechanisms by which exercise modulates the tumorigenic process.

II. General Comments on Methodology

A. Model for Experimentally Induced Breast Cancer

A large number of laboratory investigations that have contributed to the development of existing treatments for breast cancer were initially conducted in the 7,12-dimethylbenz-(a)anthracene (DMBA)-induced rat mammary tumor system. An exhaustive review of this tumor model and the similar N-methyl-N-nitrosourea (MNU)-induced mammary tumor system is provided by Welsch.[7] Although no rodent model of mammary cancer has yet been found in which the morphology of the tumors is identical to human breast cancers, the DMBA and the MNU models appear to be the most suitable experimental systems currently available.[7,8] These model systems were used in the experiments discussed in this paper.

B. Model for Physical Activity

Of the several elements of research methodology that should be considered by those investigating the influence of exercise on tumorigenesis, the selection of the type of activity and the apparatus by which it is induced deserve special attention. Although there may be other options, the majority of published work has been conducted using either free access to an activity wheel (voluntary exercise) or involuntary exercise induced by swimming or by running animals in a motor-driven activity wheel, rotating drum, or on a treadmill.[5] Voluntary exercise has the advantage that it is self-determined and spontaneous. However, the inherent problem is that of variability in the amount and intensity of activity performed within and among the animals during the time course of an experiment and the decline in activity level with increasing duration of an experiment.[9] Several approaches can be used to address this problem, but they require an extensive array of equipment and the use of operant behavioral-conditioning techniques.[10] If a voluntary activity regime is desired, certain strains of rat, e.g., Fisher 344, and mice display higher levels of spontaneous activity, a fact that also must be taken into account. An additional factor in the use of the activity wheel relates to the nature of the exercise and the degree to which it achieves and/or sustains a "training effect." Thus, the actual correlation between revolutions run, energy expended, and improvement in aerobic capacity needs to be assessed.

Various approaches to the involuntary exercise of rodents have been reported and several have inherent problems. A drawback encountered when swimming is used to exercise rodents is the buoyancy of the animal due to its fur. Rats also display diving behavior in order to avoid swimming and they may experience an increased risk of respiratory diseases. An alternate approach is the use of a motorized activity wheel and/or tumbling drum. However, rats sometimes cling to the wheel and revolve with it to avoid running or they may not run continuously in a revolving drum. As mentioned above, it is unclear how revolutions run in a wheel correlate with work load and intensity of exercise. Another method of involuntary exercise frequently chosen by experimentalists working with rats is running them on a motorized, adjustable-incline, variable-speed treadmill. Despite the fact that exercise is involuntary, this method has several important advantages. Duration and intensity of physical activity can be varied and uniformly applied to all animals in a treatment group. A high degree of compliance can be achieved and maintained throughout an experiment and changes in aerobic capacity can be quantified and used as a basis for developing a progressive exercise training protocol. The great utility gained in using the treadmill also is reflected in that the same apparatus can be used to model different types of physical activity. Because of these advantages, the treadmill was used in the work presented in this chapter.

C. Diet Formulation

The composition of the diets used in the work reported is shown in Table 1 and is referred to as AIN-76A. This formulation is discussed elsewhere.[10-11] When diets of differing fat content were used, they were formulated to maintain equality of nutrient density per kcal.

III. Presentation of Experimental Findings

In the initial experiment designed to study the effect of exercise on mammary tumor induction, female Sprague-Dawley rats were intubated with 5 mg DMBA at 50 days of age and randomized into experimental groups 14 days after carcinogen administration.[12] In this experiment, it was hypothesized that mammary tumor development in rats fed a high-fat diet (24.6% wt/wt) formulated with corn oil would be reduced by exercise to a level similar to that observed when rats were fed a low fat (5% wt/wt) corn oil-formulated diet. Animals were exercised on a motorized treadmill at a speed of 20 m/min, 1° incline, for 15 min/day, 5 days a week for an 18-week experimental period. This speed and duration was chosen since the results of a preliminary experiment indicated that this exercise regime could be implemented and sustained without the use of aversive stimuli and had no effect on animal

Table 1. Diet Formulations[a]

| Ingredient[b] | Diet composition (%) | |
	Low fat	High fat
Corn oil	5.0	24.6
Casein	20.0	24.6
D,L-Methionine	0.3	0.5
Cerelose[c]	15.0	9.0
Corn starch[c]	50.0	29.3
Fiber	5.0	6.2
Mineral mix[d]	3.5	4.3
Vitamin mix[d]	1.0	1.2
Choline chloride	0.2	0.3
Total	100.0	100.0
Caloric density (kcal/g)	3.8	4.8
Calories from fat (%)[e]	11.0	46.0

[a] Diets were formulated to have essentially the same nutrient density per kcal.
[b] Ingredients are of the grade specified in References 10 and 11.
[c] Source of carbohydrate was modified to avoid the complications that can result from feeding a high-sucrose diet in long-term experiments.
[d] AIN-76A formulations specified in Reference 10 as modified in Reference 11.
[e] These levels were selected on the basis of the suggested nutrient requirements for the rat and the estimated amounts of fat consumed by humans at the lowest and highest ranges of intake in the United States.

growth rates. As shown in Figure 1 and Table 2, it was observed that rather than being inhibitory, the tumorigenic response in exercised rats was significantly enhanced in comparison to sedentary rats fed a low- or a high- fat diet. The exercised rats had a growth rate indistinguishable from that of the sedentary rats, had no differences in carcass composition, and had normal estrous cycle periodicity.

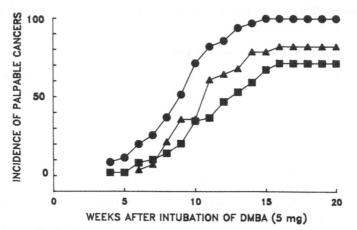

Figure 1. Incidence of palpable mammary cancers expressed as a percentage. These data are plotted vs. time in weeks after administration of 5 mg DMBA/rat. Treatment groups are: low fat and sedentary (■); high fat and sedentary (▲); high fat and exercised (●). Latency curves were significantly different from one another (p < 0.01).

Table 2. Effect of Exercise and Dietary Fat on Mammary Tumor Induction[a]

Diet[b]	Exercise[c]	No. of Rats	Cancer incidence (%)	Average no. of cancers/rats	Median cancer-free time (weeks)
Low fat	Sedentary	49[d,e]	71.4[f]	2.1[f]	12.5[i]
High fat	Sedentary	28[e]	82.1[f]	4.0[g]	10.0
High fat	Exercised	35	100.0[g]	6.1[h]	8.9

[a] Animals were given 5 mg DMBA at 50 days of age. They were randomized into one of three groups 14 days after carcinogen administration.

[b] The low-fat diet is 5% fat (wt/wt) provided as corn oil; the high-fat diet is 24.6% corn oil (wt/wt).

[c] Animals either were placed on a treadmill and not exercised or were exercised 15 min/day, 5 days/week, at a beltspeed of 20 m/min and an incline of 1°.

[d] Twenty-five of these rats were maintained as described in Reference 11. The remaining rats were as an out-of-room control. They were maintained identically with three exceptions: a normal phase light cycle, no human activity in the room during the dark cycle, and no sham handling for exercise on a treadmill. The tumor response in these animals was indistinguishable from that of rats maintained in the room in which exercise was conducted.

[e] One rat in the low-fat sedentary group and 2 rats in the high-fat sedentary group were eliminated from the study within 30 days of carcinogen treatment due to injuries sustained from hooking their teeth in the perforated food followers used in food cups to limit spilling of diet.

[f,g,h] Values within a column with different superscripts are statistically different, p < 0.05.

[i] Life table analysis test for trend indicated a significant promotional effect of both high-fat diet and exercise on time to tumor, p < 0.01.

In a follow-up study, the results of the initial experiment were further evaluated.[13]   The experiment was designed to determine whether the enhancement of mammary tumorigenesis by exercise would be observed in rats fed a low-fat as well as a high-fat diet.   Female Sprague-Dawley rats were intubated with 5 mg DMBA at 50 days of age.   At 64 days of age these rats were assigned to experimental groups fed a low-fat (5% wt/wt) or a high-fat (24.6% wt/wt) corn oil-formulated diet.   One-half the rats in each diet group were exercised on a motorized treadmill at a beltspeed of 20 m/min, 1° incline for 15 min/day, 5 days/week for 20 weeks.   Exercise under these conditions enhanced the rate of mammary tumor appearance irrespective of the level of dietary fat that was fed (Figure 2).   Consistent with the results of the first experiment, exercise had no effect on growth, carcass composition or estrous cycle periodicity, but did result in a training effect measured as the maximal ability of the animals to consume oxygen (Table 3).

The objective of the next experiment[14] was to determine the effect of increasing intensity of exercise on mammary tumor development but under the same conditions of speed and duration of treadmill running shown in the previous two experiments to enhance the rate of mammary tumor development.[12,13]   Female Sprague-Dawley rats were injected with 50 mg MNU/kg body weight at 50 days of age.   At 57 days of age these rats were assigned to one of three exercise treatments.   Rats were run at an incline of 1°, 7.5°, or 15° at a constant belt-speed of 20 m/min.   Exercise duration was 15 min/day, 5 days/week.   Throughout the experiment, rats were fed a low-fat diet (5% wt/wt).   The experiment was terminated 16 weeks after injection of MNU.   The effect of these exercise conditions on the tumorigenic

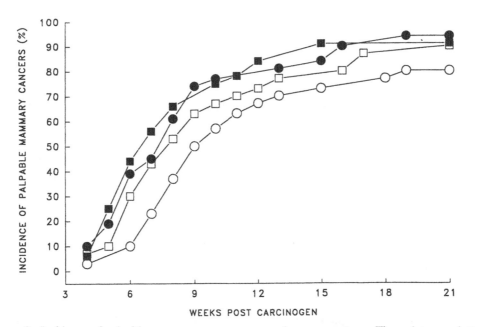

Figure 2. Incidence of palpable mammary cancer expressed as a percentage. These data are plotted vs. time in weeks after administration of 5 mg DMBA/rat. Treatment groups are: low-fat and sedentary (O); high-fat and sedentary (□); low-fat and exercised (●); and high-fat and exercised (■). Exercise accelerated the rate of appearance of mammary tumors (p < 0.05).

Table 3.   Effect of Exercise on the Maximal Capacity of Animals to Consume Oxygen (VO$_2$ max)

Exercise[a]	VO$_2$ max ml/min per kg[b,c]
No	55.1 ± 1.9
Yes	72.8 ± 2.1

[a] Exercised rats ran on a treadmill inclined to 1° at a beltspeed of 20 m/min, 15 min/day, 5 days/week.
[b] Maximal capacity to consume oxygen (VO$_2$ max) is measured as ml oxygen consumed per min per kg body weight. Each is a mean ± SEM.
[c] Difference between groups was statistically significant, $p < 0.05$.

Table 4.   Relative Risk for Mammary Tumor Occurrence among Treadmill-Exercised Rats

Treadmill incline (degree)[a]	Relative risk[b] months		
	1	2	3
1	—	—	—
7.5	5.3	1.0	1.3
15.0	5.0	0.9	1.1

[a] Rats were exercised on a treadmill at a beltspeed of 20 m/m, 15 min/day, 5 day/wk for 17 weeks. The incline at which animals ran was varied.
[b] Risk for the ocurrence of the first palpable mammary cancer in a rat on a monthly basis for rats running at the two highest intensities was compared to the risk for first tumor occurrence in rats running at the lowest intensity.

Table 5.   Effect of Exercise Intensity on VO$_2$ Max and Body Composition of Female Rats

Treadmill incline (degree)[a]	VO$_2$ max[b] ml/min per kg	Body composition[b]			
		Moisture	Protein %	Fat	Ash
1.0	78.8 ± 5	62.6 ± 0.6	20.6 ± 0.7	13.1 ± 1.1	3.8 ± 0.1
7.5	81.3 ± 3	63.4 ± 1.5	21.4 ± 0.5	11.1 ± 1.8	4.1 ± 0.2
15.0	93.7 ± 4	63.1 ± 0.8	22.3 ± 0.5	9.5 ± 0.7	5.1 ± 0.5

[a] Each rat was exercised 15 min/day, 5 days/wk at a beltspeed of 20 m/min.
[b] Each value is a mean ± SEM. VO$_2$ max and ash increased and body fat decreased with increasing treadmill incline, $p. < 0.05$.

response is shown in Figure 3 and Table 4. During the first month of exercise the relative risk for tumor appearance was increased five-fold in the two highest exercise intensity groups (7.5° and 15° treadmill incline) in comparison to animals exercised at the lowest intensity (Table 4). However, relative risk for tumor appearance declined in subsequent months and

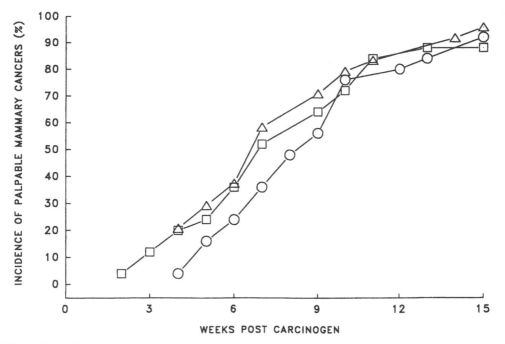

Figure 3. Incidence of palpable mammary cancers expressed as a percentage. These data are plotted vs. time in weeks after injection of 50 mg MNU/kg body weight. All rats were fed a low-fat diet and were exercised at a beltspeed of 20 m/min for 15 min/day, 5 days/week for 15 weeks. Exercise was on a treadmill that was inclined at an angle of 1° (O); 7.5° (△); or 15° (□). Latency curves were significantly different only during the first month of exercise (p < 0.05).

was not different from unity. As indicated by the data presented in Table 5, the levels of exercise to which the animals complied had a profound effect on body composition and aerobic capacity measured as VO_2 max. Within the constraints of interpretation imposed by the rapid tumorigenic response induced by the 50-mg dose of MNU, it was surprising that the increasing exercise intensity, although sufficient to improve aerobic capacity and alter body composition, failed to inhibit tumor development. The results of this experiment also indicated the existence of a time-related dimension to the effect of exercise on the tumorigenic response.

In a recently completed experiment,[14] the effects of duration (15 vs. 30 min), intensity (beltspeed: 2m/min, 20m/min or 40m/min), and type (continuous vs. interval running) of treadmill activity on the promotion phase of mammary tumorigenesis were evaluated. Female Sprague-Dawley rats were injected with 25 mg MNU/kg body weight at 50 days of age. At 57 days of age rats were randomized into one of four exercise treatment groups. They were either run at a speed of 2 m/min or 20 m/min at 1° incline 30 min/day, 5 days/week or at a beltspeed of 40 m/min at 1° incline continuously for 15 min/day or for 1-min intervals alternating with 1-min intervals of rest 15 times per day. Thus all rats other than those that walked at 2 m/min ran the same distance but under different conditions of intensity and duration. Exercise was continued for a 15-week period after carcinogen injection and then stopped. Throughout the experiment, rats were fed a low-fat (5% wt/wt) diet. The experiment was terminated 32 weeks after the administration of MNU. As shown in Figure 4, exercise at a speed of 20 or 40 m/min delayed tumor appearance in comparison to rats walking 2 m/min. Furthermore, the protective effect of exercise was sustained even after the discontinuation of exercise. These results are potentially significant in that they indicate that duration and intensity of exercise may be important factors in altering the tumorigenic response. However, further work is necessary to confirm and extend these observations.

IV. Discussion

In evaluating laboratory studies of the relationship between physical activity and cancer, particularly those published prior to 1988, it is notable that the majority of protocols involved intense, long-duration and/or exhaustive exercise.[5] In none of those studies was the influence of exercise on tumor development shown to be independent of an effect on caloric intake. The importance of this issue is reflected in the work of Moore and Tittle[15] in which complete inhibition of DMBA-induced mammary tumorigenesis was observed with either prolonged daily exercise or a level of caloric restriction equivalent to that occurring in

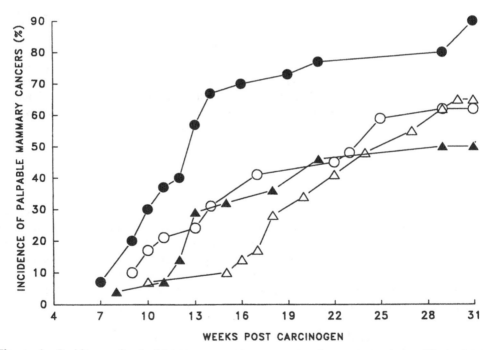

Figure 4. Incidence of palpable mammary cancers expressed as a percentage. These data are plotted vs. time in weeks after injection of 25 mg MNU/kg body weight. All rats were fed a low-fat diet throughout the experiment. Exercise was conducted for only the first 15 weeks of the study. The experiment was terminated 32 weeks after carcinogen injection. Exercise was on a treadmill set at an incline of 1° at one of four beltspeed and duration combinations. The combinations were: 2 m/min for 30 min (●); 20 m/min for 30 min (○); 40 m/min for 15 min (▲) and 40 m/min for 1 min with intervals of 1 min of rest for a total of 15 exercise events each day (△). Exercise at 20 or 40 m/min caused a significant delay in mammary tumor appearance in comparison to rats exercised at 2 m/min ($p < 0.05$).

exercised rats. These observations provide strong evidence that imposition of an energy deficit may be involved when exhaustive exercise has been reported to inhibit tumor occurrence. That caloric restriction inhibits tumorigenesis is clearly supported by the findings of Tannebaum[16] and many others.[7] However, the results presented in this paper indicate that exercise may exert calorie-independent effects on mammary tumorigenesis. This observation is suggested by the data shown in Table 6. The energy expended in performing the exercise routine reported to stimulate mammary tumorigenesis[12,13] or to inhibit its development[17] was calculated. The exercise protocol observed to accelerate mammary tumorigenesis, required a 250-g rat to expend 0.5 kcal. That energy expenditure is 1.5% of the animal's daily maintenance energy requirement. In the work of Cohen in which inhibition of mammary tumorigenesis by exercise was observed,[17] rats were reported to run an average distance of 1.8 miles/day. The energy expenditure for this activity is estimated to be 4.6 kcal, which is 15% of a female rat's maintenance energy requirement. Thus the level of exercise achieved via voluntary running in an activity wheel and that has been reported to inhibit tumorigenesis was on average 10 times greater than the level that was observed to accelerate tumorigenesis. However, the fact that exercise conditions requiring an energy expenditure of 3-5% of the maintenance energy requirement have been found to have either no effect or to inhibit mammary tumorigenesis suggests that qualitative aspects of an exercise regime that are independent of effects on energy balance may also be important in determining the effect of exercise on tumor development.

Several mechanisms could account for a calorie-independent effect of exercise on the tumorigenic process. Sylvester et al.,[18] working with treadmill-exercised female rats, reported that exercise of a magnitude that our laboratory found to stimulate mammary tumor appearance, alters the sensitivity of the hypothalamic-pituitary axis to prolactin-releasing factors and increases prolactin secretion. Elevated secretion of prolactin is consistent with our observation of enhanced mammary tumor induction in exercised rats whose caloric intake was unaltered by exercise. On the other hand, more intensive exercise has been reported to result in a dysfunction of the hypothalamic-pituitary axis that parallels the occurrence of amenorrhea

Table 6. Energy Expenditure Attributed to Exercise

Activity		Estimated energy expenditure (kcal)	Percent of maintenance energy expenditure
Running wheel	1.8 miles/day	4.6[a]	15[b]
Treadmill	20 m/min for 15 min	0.5[c]	1.5[b]
Treadmill or	40 m/min for 15 min 20 m/min for 30 min	1.0[c]	3.0[b]

[a] Estimated for a 200-g female Fisher 344 rat running at 24 m/min at an incline of 1°.
[b] Maintenance energy expenditure was calculated based on a resting rate of oxygen consumption of 21 ml/min per kg body weight.
[c] Estimated for a 250-g female Sprague-Dawley rat.

in some athletes[19]; it has been proposed that this effect would reduce breast cancer risk.[20] However, it is unclear if exercise induces endocrine dysfunction directly or if it is primarily a caloric effect and linked to the state of energy equilibrium of an individual.

Another potentially energy-independent activity of exercise that could influence the tumorigenic process is its effect on immune function. Exercise exerts pleiotropic effects on the immune system that are related to training intensity and to length of time over which an exercise training program has been maintained.[21,22] Initially, the net effects of exercise are considered to enhance immune function. However, there are an increasing number of reports that endurance training for extended periods can impair immune function. The possible implications of such effects of exercise on immune activity and their relationship to cancer risk clearly may merit consideration.

V. Summary

It appears that exercise derived by treadmill running can enhance or inhibit the development of mammary cancer depending on the intensity and duration of the activity. The effects of timing of exercise relative to the phases of carcinogenesis and the frequency of exercise on the tumorigenic response in the mammary gland have yet to be studied. What is needed are further investigations of a spectrum of exercise conditions that exert differential effects on measures of physical fitness, energy intake, body composition, and/or the efficiency of utilization of carbohydrate, fat, and protein as energy substrates. This should facilitate identification of critical relationships between physical activity and the risk for cancer. This goal can best be achieved initially through carefully controlled laboratory studies using appropriate experimental systems. There are several mechanisms by which exercise could alter the course of tumor development. A goal in this field should be to first characterize the influence on tumorigenesis of amount and type of exercise that have differential effects on metabolism and thereafter proceed to investigate the basis for the effects observed. Experiments should be designed to dissociate effects of exercise related to local and/or systemic changes induced by skeletal muscle contraction from those attributable to changes in energy expenditure. Ultimately, investigations of the type proposed should allow for determination of whether the quantity and quality of exercise needed to attain health-related benefits for chronic diseases such as cancer differs from what is recommended for fitness benefits.[23] This should also permit formulation of a specific set of recommendations about the amount and type of physical activity that in concert with appropriate dietary practices can significantly reduce the risk for cancer.

Acknowledgments

The author wishes to thank Anne Ronan, Kazuko Sakamoto, Jack Sneddin, and Anthony Tagliaferro for their technical assistance and Joyce Manley and Connie Ryan for their assistance in preparing this manuscript. This work was supported by Grant #86B09 from the American Institute for Cancer Research and PHS CA52626 from the National Cancer Institute. Address all correspondence to Dr. Thompson, Laboratory of Nutrition Research, AMC Cancer Research Center, 1600 Pierce Street, Denver, CO 80214.

References

1. C.J. Casperson, K.E. Powell, and G.M. Christenson, Physical activity, exercise and physical fitness: definitions and distinctions for health related research, *Public Health Reports.* 100:126 (1985).

2. H.W. Kohl, R.E. LaPorte, and S.N. Blair, Physical activity and cancer: an epidemiological perspective, *Sports Med.* 6:222 (1988).

3. R.J. Shephard, Exercise and malignancy, *Sports Med.* 3:235 (1986).

4. R.J. Shephard, Physical activity and cancer, *Internat J Sports Med.* 11:413 (1990).

5. H.J. Thompson, Modulation of carcinogenesis by physical activity: a critical analysis, (submitted).

6. National Research Council, "Diet and Health," National Academy Press, Washington, D.C. (1989).

7. C.W. Welsch, Host factors affecting the growth of carcinogen-induced rat mammary carcinomas: a review and tribute to Charles Brenton Huggins, *Cancer Res.* 45:3415 (1985).

8. H.J. Thompson and H. Adlakha, Dose-responsive induction of mammary gland carcinomas by the intraperitoneal injection of 1-methyl-1-nitrosourea, *Cancer Res.* 51:3411 (1991).

9. Report of the American Institute of Nutrition Ad Hoc Committee on Standards for Nutritional Studies, *J Nutr.* 107:1340 (1977).

10. F.H. Bronson, Puberty in female rats: relative effect of exercise and food restriction, *Am J Physiology.* 252:R140 (1987).

11. Second Report of the American Institute of Nutrition Ad Hoc Committee on Standards for Nutritional Studies, *J Nutr.* 110:1726 (1980).

12. H.J. Thompson, A.M. Ronan, K.A. Ritacco, A.R. Tagliaferro, and L.D. Meeker, Effect of exercise on the induction of mammary carcinogenesis, *Cancer Res.* 48:2720 (1988).

13. H.J. Thompson, A.M. Ronan, K.A. Ritacco, and A.R. Tagliaferro, Effect of type and amount of dietary fat on the enhancement of rat mammary tumorigenesis by exercise, *Cancer Res.* 49:1904 (1989).

14. H.J. Thompson, Unpublished observations.

15. C. Moore and P.W. Tittle, Muscle activity, body fat and induced rat mammary tumors, *Surgery.* 73:329 (1973).

16. A. Tannenbaum, Genesis and growth of tumors. II effects of caloric restriction, *Cancer Res.* 2:460 (1942).

17. L.A. Cohen, K. Choi, and L. Wang, influence of dietary fat, caloric restriction and voluntary exercise on N-nitrosomethylurea-induced mammary tumorigenesis in rats, *Cancer Res.* 48:4276 (1988).

18. P.W. Sylvester, S. Forczek, M.M. Ip, and C. Ip, Exercise training and the differential prolactin response in male and female rats, *J Appl Physiol.* 7:804 (1989).

19. A.B. Loucks, and S.M. Horvath, Athletic amenorrhea: a review, *Med Sci Sports Exerc.* 17:56 (1985).

20. R.E. Frisch, G. Wyshak, and N.L. Albright, Lower lifetime occurrence of breast cancer and cancers of the reproductive system among former college athletes, *Am J Clin Nutr.* 45:328 (1987).

21. E.R. Eichner, Exercise, lymphokines, calories and cancer, *Physician Sport Med.* 15:109 (1987).

22. M.A. Pahlavani, T.H. Cheung, J.A. Chesky, and A. Richardson, Influence of exercise on the immune function of rats of various ages, *J Appl Physiol.* 64:1997 (1988).

23. American College of Sports Medicine, The recommended quantity and quality of exercise for developing and maintaining cardiovascular and muscular fitness in healthy adults, *Med Sci Sports Exer.* 22:265 (1990).

2. D.W. Reid, R.E. LaPorte, and S.N. Blair. Physical activity and cancer: an epidemiological perspective. Sports Med. 8:222 (1988).

3. R.J. Shephard, Exercise and malignancy. Sports Med. 3:324 (1986).

4. R.J. Shephard, Physical activity and cancer. Exercise? Sports Med. 13:413 (1992).

5. K.E. Thompson, Moderation of the response to physical activity by diet.

Chapter 7

Modulation of Chemical Toxicity by Modification of Caloric Intake

RONALD W. HART, JULIAN E. A. LEAKEY,
MING CHOU, PETER H. DUFFY,
WILLIAM T. ALLABEN and RITCHIE J. FEUERS

I. Introduction

Nutrition is known to play a major role in the etiology of many disease states. Heart disease and cancer are both influenced by dietary factors, and chronic diseases, with their long latencies, appear to be especially susceptible to the influence of diet. Diet affects the pathogenesis of coronary heart disease, gallstones, appendicitis, varicose veins, obesity, hiatus hernia, and cancer.[1] Indeed, in the last case, it has been suggested that at least 36% of all causes can be attributed to dietary factors.[2]

It is now well established that in laboratory animals *caloric restriction* (i.e., the restriction of caloric intake to 60-70% of what the animal would normally consume) is an extremely powerful modulator of a spectrum of degenerative diseases and is the only known intervention that has been conclusively shown to increase maximum achievable lifespan.[3-6] Caloric restriction has been found to delay the occurrence of most age-associated diseases or to slow their progression, often to the extent that clinical expression is eliminated.[5,7] These effects appear to be dependent upon a specific reduction in calories, since reducing dietary components such as protein or fat without reducing the overall caloric intake is much less effective in increasing longevity or suppressing neoplasia.[5-8] Although there is a large amount of evidence suggesting that caloric restriction may be acting on primary aging processes themselves rather than directly modulating the pathogenic processes underlying specific degenerative diseases, the precise molecular and biochemical mechanisms by which caloric restriction influences the aging process remain elusive. It seems likely that caloric restriction may act, in part, by modifying chemical toxicity.

In 1930, McCay showed that caloric restricted mice lived much longer than animals fed *ad libitum* and that the onset of senescence was delayed. Tannenbaum and Silverstone[9] then demonstrated that chemically induced toxic endpoints were reduced or even eliminated in

Ronald W. Hart, Julian E. A. Leakey, Ming Chou, Peter H. Duffy, William T. Allaben and Ritchie J. Feuers • National Center for Toxicological Research, Jefferson, Arkansas

Exercise, Calories, Fat, and Cancer, Edited by M.M. Jacobs
Plenum Press, New York, 1992

caloric restricted animals. Low-protein diets retarded morbidity due to malignant lymphomas, and pancreatic and lung tumors were rarely found, whereas they routinely appeared in the high-protein diet groups. Rats fed 70% of *ad libitum* for their life span, or 60-70% for 7 weeks past weaning exhibited significant reductions in tumor formation. When divided into lighter/heavier subgroups for each treatment regime, the lighter groups had the lowest tumor incidences even within groups. In each case, the lighter subgroups had less tumors. Thus, body weight was suggested to be a factor in tumor susceptibility.

Kritchevsky *et al.*[10] demonstrated that the protective effects of caloric restriction do not begin until you achieve about a 30% reduction level. At 40% restriction, significant protective effects against cancer were seen. Recently, numerous other studies have shown the powerful affects of caloric restriction on chemical toxicity.[11-15] However, the mechanisms through which caloric restriction produced these remarkable effects has not been delineated.

In 1985, the United States *National Institute of Aging* (NIA) and the *National Center for Toxicological Research* (NCTR) initiated an extensive collaborative program (*Project Caloric Restriction*, PCR) to establish a colony of aged, closely controlled and tightly regulated rodents for use in both gerontological and toxicological research.[3,16] We present here a brief overview of the results of studies concerning modulation of chemical toxicity by caloric restriction at the NCTR.

II. Animals and Diets

The PCR study has used four genotypes of mouse and three of rat. They are listed in Table 1. Since different pathologies arise in different strains and species, the use of different genotypes allows the comparison of the effects of Caloric Restriction on degenerative pathologies that are specific to individual genotypes to pathologies that are common to all genotypes. The B6C3F$_1$ mouse and Fischer 344 rat were selected for the additional reason that they predominate in chronic toxicity studies. Thus, a large data base already exists on their response to a wide range of toxic substances as a function of dose and endpoint.

The animals are maintained under specific pathogen-free conditions on a 12-hour light/dark cycle. In most cases the restriction (to 60% of *ad libitum* consumption) is started at 14-16 weeks. The restricted diets are fortified with vitamins and minerals equivalent to what would be received by the animals on the *ad libitum* diet. All animals are singly housed and, except during certain experiments, they are fed during the early light phase. Over the initial 9-year experimental period, the study is expected to produce over 100,000 animals

Table 1. Rodent Genotypes and Diets Used in the NCTR/NIA PCR Program

Rat	Diet[a]	Mouse	Diet[a]
Fischer 344	NIH-31	B6D2F$_1$	NIH-31
Fischer 344	Masoro	DBA/2NNia	NIH-31
Brown-Norway	NIH-31	B6C3F$_1$	NIH-31
Brown-Norway x Fischer-344 F1 hybrid	NIH-31	C57Bl/6NNia C57Bl/6NNia	NIH-31 EM-911A

[a]NIH-31 is the autoclavable form of NIH-06. EM-911A is Emory-Morse 911A developed by the Emory Morse Co., Guildford, CT. Masoro is Masoro Diet C from Ralston Purina.

with up to 22,000 being maintained at any one time. The bulk of these animals are being utilized by NIA-funded projects at the NIH and at universities throughout the United States and Canada. Additional details on the animals, their housing conditions, and diets have been published elsewhere.[3,16,17]

III. Body Weight, Survival, and Pathology

The 60% caloric restriction that is used in the PCR study appears to stabilize body weight for the genotypes used on the study. Data for the Fischer 344 rat on the NIH-31 diet is summarized in Table 2. In both sexes body weight stops increasing once the restriction starts, but it does not significantly decrease until senescence. Thus, the restricted animals do not appear to be suffering from under-nutrition. The *ad libitum*-fed rats continue to gain weight until middle age, but they also lose weight in old age.

As can be seen from Table 2, caloric restriction significantly increases the median length of life in both male and female Fischer 344 rats. Similar increases have been observed in the other genotypes.[3,18] Maximally achievable lifespan is also increased by caloric restriction in all the genotypes used in the PCR study. For example, none of the male, *ad libitum*-fed Fischer 344 that were used for longevity assessment survived past 140 weeks, whereas approximately 10% of the restricted male rats were still living at 150 weeks and several survived to 170 weeks.[18]

Pathological studies have demonstrated that for all the genotypes on the study caloric restriction reduced both the frequency and severity of age-associated lesions. In the Fischer 344 rat for example, chronic nephropathy, which effects all *ad libitum*-fed animals in the NCTR colony by 24 months, developed later and did not attain the same severity in the restricted animals.[18] The frequency and severity for the most common neoplasms in this strain (e.g., pituitary adenoma, testicular interstitial cell hypoplasia, and mononuclear cell leukemia) were also reduced by caloric restriction.[18] Thus, as expected from previous research,[5,7] the caloric restriction as performed on the PCR study is successful at extending lifespan and reducing susceptibility to several degenerative diseases.

IV. Free Radical Detoxification

Active oxygen species, or free radicals which are byproducts of normal metabolic processes, have been speculated to be involved in the aging process. It is thought that

Table 2. Body Weight Changes and Longevity in *Ad Libitum*-Fed and Calorically Restricted Fischer 344 Rats[a]

Age (weeks)	Male *Ad libitum*	Male restricted	Female *Ad libitum*	Female restricted
20 Weeks	320.5 g	251.3 g	142.7 g	106.8 g
52 Weeks	420.5 g	227.4 g	200.0 g	109.4 g
80 Weeks	456.4 g	253.0 g	213.7 g	102.6 g
120 Weeks	367.5 g	272.6 g	192.3 g	120.5 g
152 Weeks	–	228.2 g	154.7 g	75.2 g
175 Weeks	–	–	136.8 g	74.4 g
MLL[b]	103 Weeks	126 Weeks	116 Weeks	133 Weeks

[a] Taken from Witt *et al.*[18] for rats on NIH-31 diet.
[b] MLL refers to median length of life.

accumulation of free-radical induced damage to any number of important macromolecules might also be involved in certain toxic events. Circumstantial evidence suggests that free radical production is reduced by caloric restriction. We have shown that several important enzymes of lipid metabolism (therefore, potential for lipoperoxidation) are reduced by caloric restriction.[19-21] Additionally, we have shown that the activity of the major male-specific cytochrome P4502C11 that produces oxygen radicals during bioactivation of several drugs and carcinogens, including aflatoxin is reduced by caloric restriction (see below and References 22 and 23). Table 3 shows that caloric restriction increases the activity of superoxide dismutase and also increases the "effective" activity of catalase. Catalase is susceptible to oxidation by its substrate; H_2O_2, which results in its inactivation and accumulation as complex I. caloric restriction increases catalase activity by limiting accumulation of inactive complex I. These studies are being extended to examine support systems for free radical detoxification, including NADPH and GSH levels, as well as glucose 6 phosphate dehydrogenase and glutathione reductase activities. This will allow for a more accurate evaluation of the role of caloric restriction in the mechanism for improved free radical detoxification.

V. Caloric Restriction and Drug Metabolism in the Liver

One of the most striking effects of caloric restriction in the rat is its suppression of sex-specific hepatic enzymes. The expression of many liver enzymes is sexually dimorphic in adult rats.[24] The enzymes that are most affected are the microsomal cytochrome P450s and other enzymes that are associated with the metabolism of steroid hormones and xenobiotics. For example cytochrome P4502C11 is expressed predominantly in male rat liver, whereas testosterone-5α-reductase is expressed predominantly in female rat liver.[25]

In several cases sex-specific expression of these enzymes has been shown to be regulated by serum growth hormone.[25] The male rat growth hormone secretory pattern is characterized by a pulsatile serum profile, having relatively high pulse amplitudes and low interpulse concentrations, whereas the female serum growth hormone profile exhibits greater pulse frequency, lower pulse amplitude, and interpulse concentrations that are significantly higher than those of males.[25,26] Sexually dimorphic pituitary growth hormone secretion develops around puberty,[26] and its pulsatility decays in senescence.[27] Many of the changes in liver enzyme expression that occur during senescence can be correlated with changes in growth hormone secretion. For example, expression of cytochrome P4502C11 decreases in aging male rats, but expression of cytochrome testosterone-5α-reductase increases.[28] Thus, the senescent male rat liver appears to be feminized.

Table 3. Effective Catalase and Superoxide Dismutase Activities in 10-Month-Old Fischer 344 Rats

	Activity	
Diet	Catalase[a]	Superoxide dismutase[b]
ad libitum	2324 ± 420	14 ± 4
caloric restriction	3710 ± 318	4 ± 2

[a] Catalase activity = pmol/min per g liver (sec^{-1}).
[b] Superoxide dismutase activity is the percentage of inhibition of maximal free radical formation.

Caloric restriction also feminizes male-specific enzyme activities in young and middle-aged Fischer 344 rats by decreasing male-specific activities and increasing female-specific activities (Reference 29 and Table 5). Furthermore, recent data from our laboratory suggests that caloric restriction masculinizes female-specific activities in young female rats (Table 4). However, in old rats, where the liver has already lost its sex-specific differentiation, caloric restriction appears to remasculinize the male-specific activities.[22,23,29] This latter effect is most probably due to the general retardation of physiologic aging delaying age-dependent hepatic de-differentiation in the restricted rats.

It is probable that restriction-induced hypercortism is responsible for the suppression of sex-specific enzyme expression in the calorically restricted rat. We have found that surgical stress or glucocorticoid treatment causes similar effects on these enzymes. Moreover, glucocorticoids are well known mediators of pituitary growth hormone secretion.[30] If indeed hypercortism does prove to be responsible for these effects on hepatic differentiation, then it is possible that the glucocorticoid-induced suppression of the hypothalamic-pituitary-hepatic axis during early and midlife protects this axis from degeneration in old age.

VI. Chemical Carcinogenesis

Caloric restriction reduces cancer incidence and progression, but the biochemical mechanisms involved remain unclear. Early work by Tannenbaum and Silverstone[9] using a chemically induced mammary carcinoma model suggested that the primary effect of caloric restriction was on tumor promotion. More recent data from our laboratories suggest that for some chemical carcinogenesis models, caloric restriction is also affecting the initiation stage of carcinogenesis.[31] Aflatoxin B_1 is an extremely mutagenic and carcinogenic mycotoxin which has been implicated epidemiologically as a causative agent in human liver cancer.

Table 4. Effect of Caloric Restriction on Sex-Specific Liver Enzymes[a]

Enzyme[b]	Specificity	*Ad libitum*-fed	Caloric Restriction
9-Month-old males:			
Testosterone 16α-Hydroxylase [PC4502C11]	Male	2.78 ± 0.20	1.70 ± 0.30
Testosterone-5α-reductase	Female	2.01 ± 0.21	4.13 ± 0.79
Corticosterone sulfotransferase	Female	4.96 ± 0.32	18.0 ± 1.1
18-Week-old-females:			
Corticosterone sulfotransferase	Female	145.6 ± 6	110 ± 4

[a] Taken in part from Leakey *et al.*[29]
[b] Activities assayed in microsomal and cytosol fractions of liver from Fischer 344 rats.

Table 5. Effect of Caloric Restriction on Concentrations of Hydrolysis Products of Aflatoxin B_1-Modified Hepatic Nuclear DNA[a]

Diet	Adduct concentration [pmol/mg DNA][b]	
	AFB-N^7-G	AFB-N^7-F
Ad Libitum (N = 4)	44.2 ± 2.3	11.7 ± 2.0
Restricted (N = 4)	19.3 ± 1.9	3.4 ± 0.3

[a] Taken from Chou *et al.*[31]
[b] Male Fischer 344 rats were dosed with 0.1 mg/kg aflatoxin B_1 3 hours before killing.

AFB1 is metabolically activated by microsomal drug-metabolizing enzymes. The result is formation of a reactive epoxide that binds to cellular macromolecules such as DNA. Caloric restriction has been shown to decrease the binding of aflatoxin B_1 to hepatic nuclear DNA following exposure either *in vivo* or *in vitro*. These effects may be partly explained by the suppressive effects of caloric restriction on hepatic cytochrome P4502C11, since this cytochrome P450 isoform plays a major role in converting aflatoxin B_1 to its toxic epoxide.[32] Caloric restriction has also been shown to increase the rate of DNA repair in rodent liver[33] and this may also contribute to the observed decreases in DNA binding. The major adducts formed by exposure to aflatoxin B_1 are 8,9-dihydro-8-(N^7-guanyl)-9-hydroxyaflatoxin B_1 (AFB-N^7-G) and 8,9-dihydro-8-(2,6-diamino-4-oxo-3,4-dihydropyrimid-5-yl formamido)-9-hydroxyaflatoxin B_1 (AFB-N^7-F). As shown in Table 5, the production of both these adducts is reduced by caloric restriction.

    Oxygen radicals such as superoxide and the hydroxyl radical have been implicated to play a role in both the initiation and promotion stages of cancer.[34] As discussed above, data from our laboratories suggest that oxygen radical concentrations may be reduced in calorically restricted animals for a number of reasons. First, both catalase and superoxide dismutase, which detoxify free radicals, appear to be increased in liver and other tissues by caloric restriction. Furthermore, recent data has shown that hepatic glutathione concentrations are increased during the early stages of caloric restriction, but only at circadian timepoints where body temperature and metabolic activity are also low. It is also possible that free radical production is also decreased by caloric restriction since several cytochrome P450 isoforms, which produce free radicals as a byproduct of their actions, are also decreased.[29] Moreover, the observed decreases in body temperature and oxygen consumption that occur in caloric restriction rodents at certain circadian timepoints may also lower oxygen radical production due to lowered rates of mitochondrial respiration.

VII. Consequences for Human Nutrition

    It has been established that caloric restriction extends the lifespan of many invertebrate and lower vertebrate species as well as rodents,[6] but as yet there is no definitive evidence whether or not caloric restriction will increase longevity, decrease neoplastic and degenerative diseases, or have a positive impact on toxicologic events in higher mammals or in man. There is some evidence that reduced caloric intake in man reduces urinary output of thymidine glycol and 8-hydroxyguanidine, which implies reduced free radical-mediated DNA damage.[35] Additionally, the evidence presented herein suggests that caloric restriction has potential for reducing toxic affects. However, until the molecular and biochemical mechanisms by which caloric restriction evokes its effects on disease and longevity is fully understood, the only way that it can be conclusively proved that caloric restriction does work in prolonging life in higher animals is to perform longevity studies in these species. Such experiments, using non-human primates, have been sponsored in the United States by the NIA and are already underway,[36] but it will be some time before any definitive data will be available.

However, if we assume that caloric restriction does evoke similar effects in man as it does in rodents—and as yet there is no evidence that it does not, then the consequences of caloric restriction will be highly relevant to health care issues worldwide. The rodent data would suggest that the degenerative diseases of the elderly that afflict the developed countries may have much less impact on the elderly of the developing countries, due to existing conditions of dietary restriction in the latter through economic necessity or cultural preferences. The data would also suggest that when setting nutritional guidelines throughout the world that nutritional quality should take precedence over quantity.

VIII. Summary

Caloric restriction increases maximum achievable lifespan and offsets the time to development of degenerative disease. Part of these desirable effects may result from positive modulation of toxic events. We have shown that when rodents are placed on a diet that is reduced in total calories by 40%, several beneficial changes on biochemical systems which impact on toxicologic processes are positively enhanced. Lipid metabolism is reduced and, therefore, the potential for lipoperoxidation is reduced. Additionally, activity of enzymes that produce free radicals as byproducts (cytochrome P4502C11) are also reduced. Concurrently, we have shown that the "effective" activity of catalase and the activity of superoxide dismutase (which are required for the detoxification of toxic oxygen radicals) are significantly increased by caloric restriction. The activities of enzymes of drug and xenobiotic metabolism are also altered by caloric restriction. The effect upon activity may be to either decrease or increase activity, dependent upon whether the enzyme activates compounds to intermediates which may be more toxic or whether the enzyme acts to reduce toxicity. We have also shown that caloric restriction may affect the initiation stage of carcinogenesis. Aflatoxin B_1 binding to hepatic nuclear DNA was reduced by caloric restriction (caloric restriction reduced both major adducts that are formed upon exposure to aflatoxin B_1). caloric restriction also reduced cytochrome P4502C11 which converts aflatoxin B_1 to its toxic epoxide, and may partly explain the reduction in binding. These results suggest that caloric restriction may, in part, extend the time to development of degenerative disease by altering basic biochemical mechanisms of toxicity.

Acknowledgment

Address correspondence to Ritchie J. Feuers, National Center for Toxicological Research, Jefferson, Arkansas 72079

References

1. D.P. Burkitt, Diseases of affluence, *in*: "Nutrition and Killer Diseases: The effects of dietary factors on chronic diseases," J. Rose, ed. Noyes, Park Ridge, N.J. (1982).
2. R. Doll and R. Peto, The causes of Cancer: Quantitative estimates of avoidable risks of cancer in the United States today, *J Natl Cancer Inst.* 66:1191 (1981).

3. W.T. Allaben, M.W. Chou, R.A. Pegram, J. Leakey, R.J. Feuers, P.H. Duffy, A. Turturro, and R.W. Hart, Modulation of toxicity and carcinogenesis by caloric restriction, *Korean J Toxicol*. 6:167 (1990).

4. L. Fishbein, "Biological Effects of Dietary Restriction," Springer-Verlag, New York (1991).

5. E.J. Masoro, Nutrition and aging — A current assessment, *J Nutri*. 115:842 (1985).

6. R. Weindruch and R.L. Walford, "Retardation of aging and disease by dietary restriction," Thomas Press, Springfield, Ill. (1988).

7. E.J. Masoro, Food restriction in rodents: an evaluation of its role in the study of aging, *J Gerontol*. 43:B59 (1988).

8. I. Shimokawa, B.P. Yu, and E.J. Masoro, Influence of diet on fetal neoplastic disease in male Fischer 344 rats, *J Gerontol*. 46:B228 (1991).

9. A. Tannenbaum and H. Silverstone, Effect of limited food intake on survival of mice bearing spontaneous mammary carcinomas and on the incidence of lung metastases, *Cancer Res*. 13:532 (1953).

10. D. Kritchevsky, M.M. Webber, and D.M. Klurfeld, Dietary fat versus caloric content in initiation and promotion of 7,12-dimethylbenz[a]anthracene-induced mammary tumorigenesis in rats, *Cancer Res*. 44:3174 (1984).

11. D. Kritchevsky, M.M. Webber, C.L. Buck, and D.M. Klurfeld, Calories, fat and cancer, *Lipids*. 21:272 (1986).

12. S.P. Kumar, S.J. Roy, K. Tokumo, and B.S. Reddy, Effect of different levels of caloric restriction on azoxymethane-induced colon carcinogenesis in male F344 rats, *Cancer Res*. 50:5761 (1990).

13. L. Lagopoulos and R. Stadler, The influence of food intake on the development of diethylnitrosamine-induced liver tumors in mice, *Carcinogenesis*. 8:33 (1987).

14. G.A. Boissonnealt, C.E. Elson, and M.W. Pariza, Net energy effects of dietary fat on chemically-induced mammary carcinogenesis in F344 rats, *J Natl Cancer Inst*. 76:335 (1986).

15. S. Rehm, K.G. Rapp, and F. Deerberg, Influence of food restriction and body fat on life span and tumor incidence in female outbred Han:NMRI mice and two sublines, *Z Versuchtierk*. 27:249 (1987).

16. W.M. Witt, C.D. Brand, V.G. Atwood, and O.A. Soave, A nationally supported study on caloric restriction in rodents, *Lab Anim*. 18:37 (1989).

17. P.H. Duffy, R.J. Feuers, J.E.A. Leakey, K.D. Nakamura, A. Turturro, and R.W. Hart, Effect of chronic caloric restriction on the physiological variables related to energy metabolism in the male Fischer 344 rat, *Mech Aging Dev*. 48:117 (1989).

18. W.M. Witt, W.G. Sheldon, and J.D. Thurman, Pathological endpoints in dietary restricted rodents—Fischer 344 rats and B6C3F$_1$ mice, *in*: "Biological Effects of Dietary Restriction," L. Fishbein, ed., Springer-Verlag, New York (1991).

19. R.J. Feuers, P.J. Duffy, J.E.A. Leakey, A. Turturro, R.A. Mittelstaedt, and R.W. Hart, Effect of chronic caloric restriction on hepatic enzymes of intermediary metabolism in the male Fischer 344 rat, *Mech Aging Dev*. 48:179 (1989).

20. R.J. Feuers, J.D. Hunter, P.J. Dutty, J.E.A. Leakey, R.W. Hart, and L.E. Sceving, ^{125}I-Insulin binding in liver and influence of insulin on blood glucose in calorically restricted B6C3F$_1$ male mice, *Ann Rev Chronopharmacol*. 7:193 (1989).

21. R.J. Feuers, J.D. Hunter, D.A. Casciano, J.G. Shaddock, J.E.A. Leakey, P.J. Duffy, L.E. Sceving, and R.W. Hart, Modifications in regulation of intermediary metabolism by caloric restriction in rodents, *in*: "Biological Effects of Dietary Restriction," L. Fishbein, ed., Springer-Verlag, New York (1989).

22. J.E.A. Leakey, H.C. Cunny, J. Bazare, Jr., P.J. Webb, R.J. Feuers, P.J. Duffy, and R.W. Hart, Effects of aging and caloric restriction on hepatic drug metabolizing enzymes in the Fischer 344 rat. I. The Cytochrome P-450 dependent monooxygenase system, *Mech Aging Dev*. 48:145 (1989).

23. J.E.A. Leakey, H.C. Cunny, J. Bazare, Jr., P.J. Webb, J.C. Lipscomb, W. Slikker, Jr., R.J. Feuers, P.H. Duffy, and R.W. Hart, Effects of aging and caloric restriction on hepatic drug metabolizing enzymes in the Fishcer 344 rat. II. Effects on conjugating enzymes, *Mech Aging Dev*. 48:157 (1989).

24. P. Skett, Biochemical basis of sex differences in drug metabolism, *Pharmacol Rev.* 38:269 (1988).

25. P.G. Zaphiropouos, A. Mode, G. Norstedt, and J-A. Gustafsson, Regulation of sexual differentiation in drug and steroid metabolism, *Trends Pharmacol Sci.* 10:149 (1989).

26. S. Eden, Age- and sex-related differences in episodic growth hormone secretion in the rat, *Endocrinology* 105:555 (1979).

27. W.E. Sonntag, R.W. Steger, L.J. Forman, and J. Meites, Decreased pulsatile release of growth hormone in old male rats, *Endocrinology.* 107:15 (1980).

28. T. Kamataki, K. Maeda, M. Shimada, K. Kitani, T. Nagai, and R. Kato, Age-related alteration in the activities of drug-metabolizing enzymes and contents of sex-specific P-450 in liver microsomes from male and female rats, *J Pharmacol Exp Ther.* 233:222 (1985).

29. J.E.A. Leakey, J.J. Bazare, J.R. Harmon, R.J. Feuers, P.H. Duffy, and R.W. Hart, Effects of caloric restriction on hepatic drug metabolizing enzyme activities in the Fischer-344 rat, *in*: "Biological Effects of Dietary Restriction," L. Fishbein, ed., Springer-Verlag, New York (1991).

30. G.P. Ceda, R.G. Davis, and A.R. Hoffman, Glucocorticoid modulation of growth hormone secretion *in vitro.* Evidence for a biphasic effect of GH-releasing hormone mediated release, *Acta Endocrinol.* 114:465 (1987).

31. M.W. Chou, R.A. Pegram, P. Gao, and W.T. Allaben, Effects of caloric restriction on aflatoxin B_1 metabolism and DNA modification in Fischer 344 rats, *in*: "Biological Effects of Dietary Restriction," L. Fishbein, ed., Springer-Verlag, New York (1991).

32. T. Shimada, S. Nakamura, S. Imaoka, and Y. Funae, Genotoxic and mutagenic activation of aflatoxin B_1 by constitutive forms of cytochrome P-450 in rat liver microsomes, *Tox Appl Pharmacol.* 91:13 (1987).

33. J. Lipman, A. Turturro, and R.W. Hart, The influence of dietary restriction on DNA repair in rodents: a preliminary study, *Mech Aging Dev.* 48:135 (1989).

34. T.F. Slater, K.H. Cheeseman, and K. Proudfoot, Free radicals, lipid peroxidation and cancer, *in*: "Free Radicals in Molecular Biology, Aging and Disease," D. Armstrong, ed., Academic Press, New York (1984).

35. M.G. Simic, and D.S. Bergtold, Urinary biomarkers of oxidative DNA-base damage and human caloric intake, *in*: "Biological Effects of Dietary Restriction," L. Fishbein, ed., Springer-Verlag, New York (1991).

36. G.S. Roth, D.K. Ingram, and R.G. Cutler, Primate models for dietary restriction research, *in*: "Biological Effects of Dietary Restriction," L. Fishbein, ed., Springer-Verlag, New York (1991).

Chapter 8

Calories, Fat, Fibers, and Cellular Proliferation in Swiss Webster Mice

DAVID B. CLAYSON, ERIC LOK, FRASER W. SCOTT,
ROGER MONGEAU, WALISUNDERA M. N. RATNAYAKE,
EDUARDO A. NERA and PENNY JEE

I. Introduction

Doll and Peto[1] suggested that 35% (range 10-70%) of all human cancers among the U.S. population were associated in some way with diet or nutrition. Despite this alarming statistic, there is very little firm understanding of the factors present in the diet that lead to cancer development. This arises for several reasons. First, the literature on diet and cancer is both vast and self-contradictory. Two committees sponsored by the U.S. National Academy of Sciences (U.S. National Research Council[2]; U.S. National Academy of Sciences[3]) reached different conclusions about the relative importance of the amount of diet consumed and the level and type of fat in the diet. Second, there has been, until recently, a prudent reluctance to base anti-cancer recommendations for the modification of human diets on well founded and repeated observations in experimental animals. Epidemiologic evidence on the nature of the human diet and the incidence of cancer is often unreliable because of difficulties patients and controls have in recalling what they ate years or decades ago. The value of animal experiments is now being recognized by the massive research program on the beneficial effects of dietary restriction being undertaken by Dr. Hart and his colleagues at the National Center for Toxicological Research.[4-9] Third, there has been a reluctance to examine food components for their carcinogenic potential. This has arisen because the only remedial action following discovery of a naturally occurring carcinogen as a component of an important food crop has, until the past few years, been to cease using the food crop, an action that might substantially reduce the human food supply. Biogenetic engineering now provides the opportunity to reduce the levels of undesirable substances naturally occurring

David B. Clayson, Eric Lok, Eduardo A. Nera and Penny Jee • Toxicology Research Division, Bureau of Chemical Safety, Food Directorate, Health Protection Branch, National Health and Welfare, Ottawa, Ontario, Canada; Fraser W. Scott, Roger Mongeau and Walisundera M. N. Ratnayake • Nutrition Research Division, Bureau of Nutritional Sciences, Food Directorate, Health Protection Branch, National Health and Welfare, Ottawa, Ontario, Canada;

Exercise, Calories, Fat, and Cancer, Edited by M.M. Jacobs
Plenum Press, New York, 1992

in food crops or, if it is used unwisely, to increase this level and thus increase human cancer risk. This problem is far from theoretical. It has recently been shown that background sister chromatid exchanges, a genotoxic event sometimes linked to carcinogenesis, are dependent in primary rat hepatocytes on the diet to which the rats were previously exposed.[10] The background rate of sister chromatid exchanges in hepatocytes was lower when a purified diet was fed to the rats than when a commercial chow was used.

Increased knowledge of the effects of dietary modification at the biologic and biochemical level in experimental animals has the potential for application in a meaningful way to humans. As a contribution to this perceived problem, a study was initiated, in Ottawa, on the effects of dietary modification on cellular proliferation. This was believed to be a useful approach since there is considerable information in experimental animals that enhancement of cellular proliferation increases the expression of several of the stages in the process of chemical carcinogenesis.

II. The Experimental Approach

Groups of 10 (range 8-15) female Swiss Webster mice (Charles River, St. Constant, Quebec) were used in the restriction and fat studies, while similar groups of males of the same colony were employed in the fiber studies. Mice were fed for 30 days with a modified AIN-76A diet[11,12] (Table 1) designed to illustrate the effects of the desired dietary modification. Occasionally, a powdered laboratory diet (Number 5001, Ralston Purina, Woodstock, Ontario) was used. Vaginal smears were obtained from female mice from 15 days on diet to the end of the experiment. Males were killed after 30 days, females 2 days following the first estrus to follow 30 days feeding. This was done to minimize effects of cyclic variations in hormone levels that might introduce variability in the observed labeling indices, especially when hormone responsive tissues such as the mammary gland were investigated. One hour before death, mice were injected ip with 0.25 uCi/g body weight 3[H]-thymidine (specific activity 20 Ci/mmol). Slides were prepared from appropriate tissues for radioautography and histopathology. Finally, all results were analyzed for statistical significance by appropriate techniques.

Cell proliferation studies are labor intensive and, in some views, tedious. More rapid methodology, such as flow cytometry, loses certain important items of information and cannot be usefully employed with specific tissues. In studies on BHA using this method, for example, it is difficult to prepare separate cell suspensions from the lesser and greater curvatures of the rodent forestomach, with the result that the higher sensitivity to BHA of

Table 1. Composition of the Basic AIN 76A Semi-Purified Diet

Component	Percentage in diet	
Fat	15	
Carbohydrate	55	
(Corn starch)		(37)
(Sucrose)		(18)
Casein, vitamin-free	20	
Cellulose-type fiber	5	
AIN 76 mineral mix	3.5	
AIN 76A vitamin mix	1.0	
DL-methionine	0.3	
Choline bitartrate	0.2	

cells in the lesser curvature is lost.[13,14] Similarly, preparations of cell suspensions from the intestinal epithelial crypt cells are not adequate, since it is not possible to examine separately cells from the proliferative and non-proliferative compartments of this tissue.[15]

III. Dietary and Caloric Restriction

Dietary restriction consists of reducing the amount of food provided to the test animal whereas caloric restriction involves reducing the level of energy in the diet, usually by reducing the amount of carbohydrate, while maintaining the levels of other nutrients at a constant level.[15-19] The effects of 25% dietary restriction, using both a cereal-based laboratory diet and the AIN-76A semi-purified diet, were examined in seven tissues: ductal cells of the mammary gland, lining cells of the urinary bladder, skin, esophagus, and crypt cells of the duodenum, jejunum, and colo-rectum (0.5 to 1 cm above the anal orifice). In each case there was a statistically significant reduction in the degree of labeling. Restricting calorie intake by 25% also resulted in lower labeling indices. A third study in which graded levels of calorie restriction were investigated in the mammary gland, urinary bladder, skin, esophagus, and colo-rectum demonstrated that levels of calorie restriction of 0, 10, 20, 30, and 40% led to an approximately log-linear inhibition in cell labeling with the duct cells of the mammary gland being the most markedly affected (Figure 1). It was observed that there was only one estrus in the 10 mice restricted at the 40% level compared to the approximately 40 that occurred in the other groups. This suggests that 40% caloric restriction has a profound effect on hormonal rhythms in the highly restricted animals.

These results closely parallel long-term studies on the effect of dietary and caloric restriction on the incidences of naturally and chemically induced tumors. Tannenbaum and Silverstone[20] first stressed the correlation between dietary or calorie restriction and, particularly, mammary tumors in mice. Others have confirmed and extended their seminal results.[21-23]

IV. Fibers and Bulking Agents

Specific fibers and bulking agents are widely believed to protect humans from colo-rectal cancer. A series of studies has been conducted that were designed to demonstrate the effects of modifying the fiber content of the AIN-76A diet on cellular proliferation in the male Swiss Webster mouse duodenum, upper colon, proximate to the cecum, and colo-rectal areas of the intestinal tract. The only consistent results obtained have been in the duodenal crypts. Fibers or bulking agents in specific cases reduced the number of labeled cells in each crypt but changes in the proliferative compartment labeling index were less apparent because these fibers also reduced the size of the proliferative compartment. (The proliferative compartment is the group of cells lining the crypt from the highest labeled cell on one side to the highest labeled cell on the other side.) This is in contrast to observations with restricted diets in which the number of labeled cells was reduced but the height of the proliferative compartment was less affected by treatment.

Two fiber-free diets were used in which the levels of starch and sucrose were 2:1 (high-starch fiber-free) and 1:2 (high-sucrose fiber-free) in a total 67.5% dietary carbohydrate. The high-starch fiber-free diet consistently led to a lower number of tritium-labeled duodenal cells/crypt than the high-sucrose fiber-free diet (Figure 2). There was little if any consistent difference in effects in the colon or colo-rectum.

Fibers form a variable amount of the various fiber sources and, in consequence, it was not possible to maintain a constant dietary level of 10% without altering the nutritional balance of the diet. The amounts of dietary fiber (bran) or bulking agents actually administered varied (Table 2). Fibers and bulking agents in some cases induced reductions in

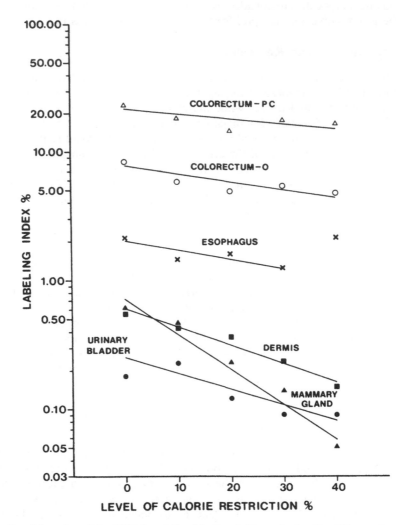

Figure 1. Semi-log plot of the 3[H]-thymidine labeling indices obtained in different tissues of female Swiss Webster mice under various levels of caloric restriction. Lines were drawn by eye to enable the reader to connect points obtained from each tissue. O = overall labeling indices of the crypt cells of the colo-rectum. PC = proliferative compartment labeling indices of the colo-rectum. (Reproduced from Lok *et al.*, 1990).[15]

labeling in the duodenal crypts but few changes of a consistent nature were discovered in the lower levels of the gastro-intestinal tract. It is noteworthy that, in the duodenum, oat bran and oat gum led to the largest inhibiting effect, while wood cellulose (alphacel) had no effect (Figure 3).

Jacobs and his colleagues in California, and many others, have made extensive studies on the effect of fibers and related materials in the rat intestinal tract.[24-27] In specific experiments in rats, Lupton and Jacobs[27] noted an increase in cell proliferation when certain fibers were added to the diet. The present results in combination with the extensive literature suggest that if fibers do indeed have a beneficial effect as anti-cancer agents in the sigmoid-rectum of humans, either humans behave differently to rodents insofar as the

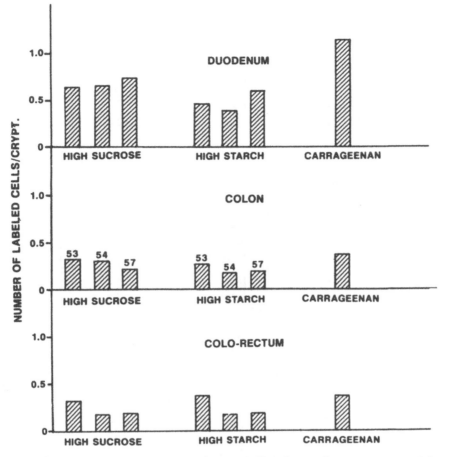

Figure 2. Effect of high-sucrose fiber-free, high-starch fiber-free, and carrageenen-containing AIN 76A semi-purified diets on the number of 3[H]-thymidine labeled cells/crypt in the male Swiss Webster mouse duodenum, colon and colo-rectum. The number of labeled cells/crypt is shown since these lead to variations in crypt anatomy including the proliferative compartment height.

Table 2. Levels of Fibers and Bulking Agents Used in Experiments Reported in Figures 2 and 3.[a]

10% Added fiber or bulking agent	6% Added fiber or bulking agent
Wood cellulose	Oat bran
Polydextrose	Rice bran
Wheat bran	Guar gum
(hard or soft wheat)	
Corn bran	
Oat gum	

[a]These amounts refer to the amount of fiber, not the amount of fiber source.

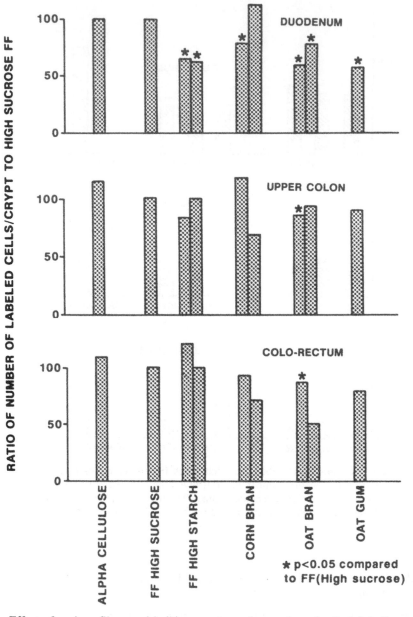

Figure 3. Effect of various fibers and bulking agents on the number of cells labeled/crypt in the duodenum, colon, and colo-rectum of male Swiss Webster mice following feeding an AIN-76A semi-purified diet (reproduced from Clayson *et al.*, 1991).[19]

intestinal tract is concerned or fibers and bulking agents exert their effects by a completely different mechanism in these species. Reddy *et al.*[28] demonstrated that dietary wheat bran, oat bran, or corn bran ingestion led to a reduction in fecal mutagenicity, in *S. typhimurium* tests, in healthy human subjects. Nevertheless, it is possible that the approach described here may, in the future, be valuable as a means of identifying fibers and bulking agents that have an irritant effect on the intestinal tract and may thus "promote" the development of human colo-rectal cancers.

V. Fat

The modified AIN-76A semi-purified diet used in these studies contained 15% fat. The effects of varying the nature of this fat on cellular proliferation in the ductal cells of the mammary gland and the colo-rectal crypts is being investigated. No anti-oxidants were added to the fats used in these studies.[29] The effects of using 100% lard, 68% lard + 32% safflower seed oil, 50% lard + 50% soybean oil, 100% soybean oil, 87% menhaden oil + 13% safflower seed oil, 80.6% cod liver oil + 19.4% safflower seed oil, or 59% cod liver oil + 41% safflower seed oil were investigated in the first two experiments. It was clearly demonstrated that the animals fed diets rich in lard, menhaden oil, or cod liver oil demonstrated a significantly higher level of labeling in both the ductal cells of the mammary gland (Figure 4) and the colo-rectal crypts than did those treated with the vegetable oils. Moreover an analysis of possible factors in the fats that might lead to these changes in labeling index demonstrated that in both tissues (Figure 5) the higher the level of linoleic acid in the fat, the lower the number of labeled cells. This was confirmed by designing diets with progressively lower levels of linoleic acid and showing that, with the exception of one apparently aberrant point, there was a relation between the linoleic content of the fat and the degree of cell labeling in both tissues (Figure 5). Experiments are now in progress to determine whether these results are due to autooxidation of the fats before they are eaten or are due to the direct action of the fats on the organism. Either conclusion is of importance to the safety of the human food supply. The importance of dietary anti-oxidants will be emphasized if environmental rancidization is the driving force behind the results so far obtained.

It must be emphasized that these "fat" experiments are based on "normal" female Swiss Webster mice rather than on those that have received massive doses of carcinogens to initiate tumors. The possibility that carcinogen-swamped tissues in rodents may react differently to dietary stimuli needs to be investigated if the relevance of rodent studies to humans, who are generally exposed to much lower levels of carcinogens in their environment, is to be better understood. In the meantime the most that can be safely pointed out is that the effect of high levels of animal fats such as lard and fish fats as menhaden oil or cod liver oil, increases cell proliferation in certain mouse tissues and this may ultimately offer an explanation of why animal fats, in excess, appear to be deleterious in the genesis of human sigmoid-rectal and mammary cancer. This, again, needs more thorough investigation.

VI. Overview

Cell proliferation studies are not new to research on the effects of diet. They have, for example, been previously employed in attempts to explain the action of dietary factors such as fibers on the crypt cells of the intestinal tract[25] as well as many other dietary modifications. Our earlier results concerning the carcinogenicity of butylated hydroxyanisole (BHA)[13,14] and the failure to obtain useful results with the putative rodent hepatocarcinogen butylated hydroxytoluene (BHT)[30] suggested to us that cell proliferation studies might be valuable in the solution of problems arising from dietary modification of physiological or toxicological processes. The results presented in this report confirm its potential usefulness in certain, but not all, situations.

The critical importance of cell proliferation in the carcinogenic process has recently been emphasized by Ames and Gold[31] who stressed the fact that excessive proliferation is associated with mutation, another critical process in the genesis of cancer. While this is true, it must not be overlooked that carcinogenesis, in specified circumstances is associated with other mechanistic factors and that the inability of a particular mechanistic route to account for such factors does not necessarily mean that this particular route is not vital to carcinogenesis in other cases.[17,18] The present results, which stress the important consequences of

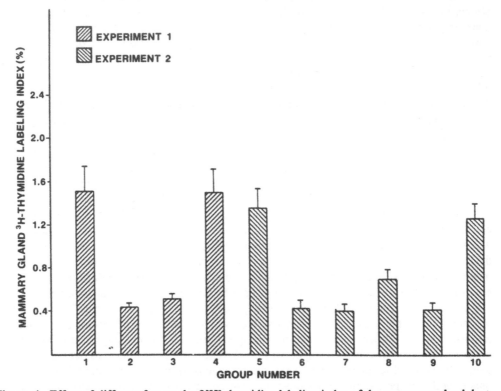

Figure 4. Effect of different fats on the 3[H]-thymidine labeling index of the mammary gland duct cells of female Swiss Webster mice. The 15% fat in the semi-purified AIN-76A diet consisted of: Groups 1, 5: 100% lard; Groups 2, 6: 50% lard + 50% soybean oil; Groups 3, 7: 100% soybean oil; Group 4: 87% menhaden oil + 13% safflower seed oil; Group 8: 68% lard + 32% safflower seed oil; Group 9: 59% cod liver oil + 41% safflower seed oil, and Group 10: 80.6% cod liver oil + 19.4% safflower seed oil.

dietary or energy restriction on cellular proliferation, promise to help in understanding the action of fats in the genesis of mammary and colo-rectal cancers, but, at present, do nothing to explain the perceived beneficial effects of specific fibers and bulking agents in the colon.

VII. Summary

Increased cellular proliferation has been associated with the enhanced expression of several key stages in carcinogenesis. A standard protocol was used to investigate the effect of specific dietary regimens on cellular proliferation. Young adult Swiss Webster mice were fed for 30 days with modified AIN-76A semi-purified diets designed to illustrate the effects of the levels of dietary or calorie restriction, different fibers and bulking agents, and different fats on cellular proliferation. Female mice were used for the restriction and fat studies, males for the fiber and bulking agent studies. Vaginal smears were taken from females from treatment day 15, and the mice killed 2 days following the first estrus following 30 days feeding; males were killed on the 30th day. One hour before death, mice were injected ip with 0.25 uCi/g 3[H]-thymidine. Slides were prepared for radioautography and histopathology. Both dietary and calorie restriction led to reduced 3[H]-thymidine labeling indices in

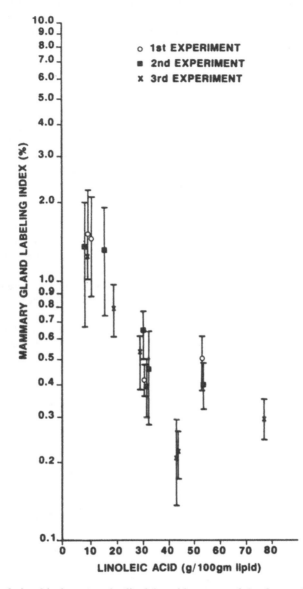

Figure 5. The relationship between the linoleic acid content of the fat used in the AIN-76A diet (g/100 g fat) and the 3[H]-thymidine labeling index of the ductal cells of the mammary gland of female Swiss Webster mice. This figure shows the combined results of the experiments illustrated in Figure 4 (O and ■) and a separate linoleic acid level-response study (x).

each of the seven tissues studied, the mammary gland being the most severely affected. Different fibers and bulking agents, in specific cases, reduced labeling in the duodenum but not to a consistent statistically significant extent in the colon or colo-rectal region. In the duodenum, oat bran and oat gum were the most effective while wood cellulose (alphacel) had no effect. Investigations on the effects of different fats is continuing. High levels of lard, menhaden oil, or cod liver oil as the fat component of the AIN-76A diet, led to much higher levels of labeled cells in the mammary gland or colo-rectal region than did fat components rich in vegetable oils. The labeling indices appeared to be inversely correlated with the level of linoleic acid in the diet, a presumption that has been confirmed by investigating a series of diets containing different levels of this acid. Anti-oxidants were not used in any of these fat-modified diets. The overall results obtained in these studies clearly indicate the utility of cellular proliferation studies in investigating the effects of dietary modifications.

Acknowledgments

The authors warmly thank Drs. K. Khera, P. Fischer, and F. Iverson for reviewing the manuscript and making valuable suggestions. Address correspondence to David B. Clayson, Toxicology Research Division, Bureau of Chemical Safety, Health Protection Branch, National Health and Welfare, Ottawa, Ontario KIA OL2, Canada.

References

1. R. Doll and R. Peto, "The Causes of Cancer. Quantitative Estimates of Avoidable Risks of Cancer in the United States today," Oxford University Press, Oxford (1981).
2. U.S. National Research Council, Food and Nutrition Board, "Toward Healthful Diets," National Academy of Sciences, Washington, D.C. (1980).
3. U.S. National Academy of Sciences, "Diet, Nutrition and Cancer," Committee on Diet, Nutrition and Cancer, National Research Council, National Academy Press, Washington, D.C. (1982).
4. M.G. Kolta, R. Holson, P.H. Duffy, and R.W. Hart, Effect of long-term caloric restriction on brain monoamines in aging male and female Fischer 344 rats, *Mech Aging Devolop.* 48:191 (1989).
5. J.E.A. Leakey, H.C. Cunny, J. Bazare, F.J. Webb, R.J. Feuers, P.H. Duffy, and R.W. Hart, Effects of aging and caloric restriction on hepatic drug metabolizing enzymes in the Fischer 344 rat, I. The cytochrome P450 dependent monooxygenase system, *Mech Aging Develop.* 48:145 (1990).
6. K.D. Nakamura, P.H. Duffy, M-H. Lu, A. Turturro, and R.W. Hart, The effect of dietary restriction on myc protooncogene expression in mice: a preliminary study, *Mech Aging Develop.* 48:199 (1989).
7. W.M. Witt, D. Brand, V.G. Attwood, and O.A. Soave, A nationally supported study on caloric restriction of rodents, *Lab Animal.* 18:37 (1989).
8. P.H. Duffy, R.J. Feuers, and R.W. Hart, Effect of chronic caloric restriction on the circadian regulation of physiological and behavioral variables in old male B6C3F1 mice, *Chronobiol Internat.* 7:291 (1990).
9. P.H. Duffy, R.J. Feuers, K.D. Nakamura, J. Leakey, and R.W. Hart, Effect of chronic calorie restriction on the synchronization of various physiological measures in old female Fischer 344 rats, *Chronobiol Internat.* 7:113 (1990).
10. P.M. Eckl, T. Alati, and R.L. Jirtle, The effects of a purified diet on sister chromatid exchange frequencies and mitotic activity in adult rat hepatocytes, *Carcinogenesis* 12:643 (1991).
11. American Institute of Nutrition, Report of the American Institute for Nutrition *ad hoc* Committee on Standards for Nutritional Studies, *J Nutr.* 107:1340 (1977).
12. American Institute of Nutrition, Second report of the *ad hoc* Committee on Standards for Nutritional Studies, *J Nutr.* 110:1726 (1980).
13. D.B. Clayson, F. Iverson, E. Nera, E. Lok, C. Rogers, C. Rodrigues, D. Page, and K. Karpinski, Histopathological and radioautographical studies on the forestomach of Fischer 344 rats treated with butylated hydroxyanisole and related chemicals, *Food Chem Toxicol.* 24:1171 (1986).
14. E.A. Nera, F. Iverson, E. Lok, C.L. Armstrong, K. Karpinski, and D.B. Clayson, A carcinogenesis reversibility study of the effects of butylated hydroxyanisole on the forestomach and urinary bladder in male Fischer 344 rats, *Toxicology* 53:251 (1988).

15. E. Lok, F.W. Scott, R. Mongeau, E.A. Nera, S. Malcolm, and D.B. Clayson, Calorie restriction and cellular proliferation in various tissues of the female Swiss Webster mouse, *Cancer Letts.* 51:67 (1990).

16. E. Lok, E.A. Nera, F. Iverson, F. Scott, Y. So, and D.B. Clayson, Dietary restriction, cell proliferation and carcinogenesis: a preliminary study, *Cancer Letts.* 38:249 (1988).

17. D.B. Clayson and D.L. Arnold, The classification of carcinogens identified in the rodent bioassay as potential risks to humans: what type of substance should be tested next? *Mutat Res.* 257:91 (1991).

18. D.B. Clayson and D.J. Clegg, Classification of carcinogens: polemics, pedantics or progress, *Regulat Toxicol Pharmacol.* 14:147 (1991).

19. D.B. Clayson, F.W. Scott, R. Mongeau, E.A. Nera, and E. Lok, Dietary and caloric restriction: its effect on cellular proliferation in selected mouse tissues, *in:* "Biological Effects of Dietary Restriction," L. Fishbein, ed. *ILSI Monograph*, Springer Verlag, Berlin, (1991).

20. A. Tannenbaum and H. Silverstone, Nutrition and the genesis of tumours, *in:* "Cancer," R.W. Raven, ed., Butterworth, London, (1957).

21. F.R. White, The relationship between underfeeding and tumor formation, transplantation and growth in rats and mice, *Cancer Res.* 21:281 (1961).

22. M.H. Ross and G. Bras, Influences of protein under- and overnutrition on spontaneous tumor prevalence in the rat, *J Nutr.* 103:944 (1973).

23. K.K. Andreou and P.R. Morgan, Effect of dietary restriction on induced hamster cheek pouch carcinogenesis, *Arch Oral Biol.* 26:525 (1981).

24. L.R. Jacobs, Effects of dietary fiber on mucosal growth and cell proliferation in the small intestine of the rat: a comparison of oat bran, pectin and guar gum with total fiber derivatives, *Amer J Clin Nutr.* 37:954 (1983).

25. L.R. Jacobs, Fiber and colon cancer, *Gastroenterol Clin N Amer.* 17:747 (1988).

26. L.R. Jacobs and J.R. Lupton, Dietary wheat bran lowers colonic pH in rats, *J Nutr.* 112:592 (1982).

27. J.R. Lupton and L.R. Jacobs, Fiber supplementation results in expanded proliferative zones in rat gastric mucosa *Amer J Clin Nutr.* 46:980 (1987).

28. B. Reddy, A. Engle, S. Katsifis, B. Simi, H-P. Bartram, P. Perrino, and C. Mayan, Biochemical epidemiology of colon cancer: effects of types of dietary fiber on fecal mutagens, acid, and neutral sterols in healthy subjects, *Cancer Res.* 49:4629 (1989).

29. K.L. Fritsche and P.V. Johnston, Rapid autoxidation of fish oil in diets without added antioxidants, *J Nutr.* 118:425 (1988).

30. D. Briggs, E. Lok, E.A. Nera, K. Karpinski, and D.B. Clayson, Short-term effects of butylated hydroxytoluene on the Wistar rat liver, urinary bladder and thyroid gland, *Cancer Letts.* 46:31 (1989).

31. B.N. Ames and L.S. Gold, Too many rodent carcinogens: mitogenesis increases mutagenesis, *Science* 249:970 (1990).

Chapter 9

Caloric Intake, Dietary Fat Level, and Experimental Carcinogenesis

ROSWELL K. BOUTWELL

I. Introduction

The percentage of calories provided by the fat content of the diet is a major public health issue. In order to lessen the probability of developing certain types of cancers, one of the most frequently recommended dietary changes is to lessen the percentage of calories provided by fat. The question that will be addressed herein is: What is the evidence for a *specific* role for dietary fat as a factor determining the incidence of cancer in laboratory animals? Because of the limitations inherent in epidemiology attributable to very large differences in life-style, human data on the role of nutrition on cancer incidence/mortality are often inconclusive.

A critical appraisal of animal studies reveals that four experiments have been published that were specifically designed to provide evidence on the relative importance on the amounts of dietary fat *vis à vis* calories in carcinogenesis. Specifically, in the case of carcinogenesis of the mammary glands in rats and skin in mice, the incidence of neoplasms is not determined by the percentage of fat in the diet nor by the amount of fat consumed but rather by the caloric balance of the animal.

In the context of current concerns on the role of nutrition in human health, interestingly, the first investigation on the impact of dietary fat level on carcinogenesis was a component of a series of experiments to determine whether tissue cholesterol levels played a role in tumor development in mouse skin caused by ultraviolet light. Although no effects attributable to cholesterol levels were observed, Baumann and Rusch[1] reported in 1939 that higher levels of fat incorporated into the stock diets that were fed to the mice enhanced skin carcinoma incidence caused by ultraviolet light. A follow-up study by Lavik and Baumann[2] confirmed that higher levels of dietary fat enhanced skin tumor incidence induced by methylcholanthrene. In 1942, Tannenbaum[3] extended the investigation of the effect of diets high in fat content to spontaneous mouse mammary tumors, a model system that was found to be responsive to diets high in fat. Subsequent to these first three reports, a huge number

---

Roswell K. Boutwell ● McArdle Laboratory for Cancer Research, University of Wisconsin Medical School, Madison, Wisconsin

Exercise, Calories, Fat, and Cancer, Edited by M.M. Jacobs
Plenum Press, New York, 1992

of papers and books have been published on the role of the level and nature of dietary fat in the susceptibility of animals and humans to cancer.

Meanwhile, evidence that caloric restriction reduced the incidence of spontaneous and induced neoplasms of mice appeared. Sivertsen and Hastings reported in 1938[4] a reduction of spontaneous mammary tumor incidence in mice from 88% to 16% attributable to caloric restriction, an observation that was confirmed by Tannenbaum in 1940.[5] This phenomenon, too, is well documented in the cancer literature. It is important to recognize that the degree of caloric restriction required to reduce the probability of the appearance of neoplasms is no more than that required to maintain the experimental animal at the weight of a young adult. The obesity that is common in pathogen-free animals fed *ad libitum* is the most important exogenous factor favoring susceptibility to carcinogenesis if the exposure level is not overwhelming.

II. Fat Level, Energy Balance, and Cancer Incidence

Data from four experiments from four independent laboratories will be presented. These experiments were selected because in each case a comparison was made of the effect on carcinogenesis of feeding a low-fat diet *ad libitum* with a high fat diet restricted in the level of calories. In each case, the quantity of fat consumed per animal per day was either stated or calculable from the data in the publication.

The results of an insightful and pivotal yet largely overlooked experiment were published by Lavik and Baumann in 1943.[6] They established that mice fed diets high in fat at a lowered level of caloric intake developed fewer hydrocarbon-induced skin tumors than those mice that were fed the low-fat diet *ad libitum*. At the *ad libitum* feeding level for the 5% fat diet, the mice consumed 0.06 g of fat per mouse per day on average over the duration of the experiment and 54% developed skin carcinomas in response to methylcholanthrene applications. In contrast, mice fed a 15% fat diet restricted to 66% of the caloric intake of the *ad libitum*-fed mice, consumed 0.24 g of fat per mouse per day (a four-fold increase) yet the carcinoma incidence was reduced by one-half to 28% (Table 1). Clearly, the incidence of skin carcinomas was not dependent on the percentage of fat in the diet nor on the amount of fat consumed per day. Rather, the incidence of skin carcinomas was dependent on the caloric intake of the mice.

Data confirming the results that were reported by Lavik and Baumann[6] were published in 1949.[7] In this experiment, skin cancer was induced in mice by twice weekly applications of benzo[a]pyrene. Mice, restricted in calories (carbohydrate only) to 83% of the *ad libitum* controls were fed a diet containing 27% corn oil, a very high level. The control diet contained 2% corn oil, a very low level that was adequate to provide the minimal requirement for the essential fatty acids. The *ad libitum*-fed control group consumed an average of 0.07 g of fat per mouse per day and the skin cancer incidence was at 82% at 24 weeks. The mice on the high-fat diet consumed 0.54 g of fat per day, yet the tumor incidence was lower: 72% (Table 2).

Table 1. Restriction of Caloric Intake Modulates the Enhancing Effect of Fat on Mouse Skin Carcinogenesis[6]

Caloric intake (% of *ad libitum*)	Fat level (% of diet)	Fat intake (g/mouse per day)	Skin carcinomas (%)
100	5	0.06	54
66	15	0.24	28

Table 2. Moderate Restriction of Caloric Intake Modulates the Enhancing Effect of Fat on Mouse Skin Carcinogenesis[7]

Caloric intake (% of *ad libitum*)	Fat level (% of diet)	Fat intake (g/animal per day)	Neoplasms (%)
100	2	0.07	82
83	27	0.54	72

The degree of restriction was moderate; the mice fed the high-fat diet at a calorie level reduced to 83% of *ad libitum* gained an average of 8.4 g per mouse beginning at the young adult weight of 24.5 g. The *ad libitum*-fed mice gained 10.2 g per mouse. In retrospect, based on experience gained subsequently from hundreds of carcinogenesis experiments, the dose of benzo[a]pyrene was too high. A lower dose of carcinogen requiring a period of observation longer than 24 weeks would have resulted in decreased toxicity and allowed the *ad libitum*-fed mice to gain more weight and increased the difference in carcinoma incidence between the two groups. The effect of factors modulating carcinogenesis is, in general, decreased as the carcinogenic stimulus is increased, a point that is not widely recognized.

The third experiment to be considered was published by Boissonneault, Elson, and Pariza in 1986.[8] They examined the relationship between the level of dietary fat and the caloric intake of rats on the incidence of mammary cancer caused by a single dose of 7,12-dimethylbenz[a]anthracene at 7 weeks of age. The high-fat diet (30%) was fed to rats at a level of caloric intake reduced to 81% of the amount that was consumed by the animals fed the low-fat (5%) diet *ad libitum*. The *ad libitum*-fed rats consumed an average 0.6 g of fat per day and the incidence of mammary tumors was 43%. In contrast, the animals fed the diet high in fat but calorically restricted to 81%, consumed 2.2 g of fat per day and only 7% developed mammary neoplasms at 24 weeks after administration of the carcinogen (Table 3). It is important to emphasize that while the rats fed *ad libitum* gained an average of approximately 105 g, the calorically restricted rats gained 75 g in the 24 weeks of the experiment (4 g per rat per day vs. 3 g per rat per day). The explanation for these data is that mammary tumor incidence does not depend on the percentage of fat in the diet but rather depends on an energy balance that allows an optimal growth but not obesity.

The final example to be cited was published by Welsch *et al.* in 1990.[9] Tumors were induced in rats by a single iv dose of 7,12-dimethylbenz[a]anthracene at 55 days of age. As in all of the previously cited experiments, the fat component of the diet was corn oil. In all of the experiments except the first one that was cited,[6] restriction was in carbohydrate only. The diet fed *ad libitum* contained 5% of fat whereas the high-fat diet contained 20% fat and consumption was restricted to 88% of the *ad libitum* level. The level of fat consumption by the two groups was 0.62 g vs. 1.9 g per rat per day for the low- and high-fat diets, respec-

Table 3. Moderate Restriction of Caloric Intake Modulates the Enhancing Effect of Fat on Mammary Carcinogenesis of Rats[8]

Caloric intake (% of *ad libitum*)	Fat level (% of diet)	Fat Intake (g/animal per day)	Mammary Neoplasms (%)
100	5	0.6	43
81	30	2.2	7

tively. In spite of a three-fold greater fat consumption, the number of mammary neoplasms per rat did not differ significantly (Table 4).

These data are of particular interest because the enhancing effect of the 20% fat diet was obliterated by a very small degree of restriction (12%). This effect of that degree of restriction on the rats was minimal as manifest by the fact that the average gain in weight per rat over the 16-week experiment was 65 g and 60 g for the *ad libitum* and calorically restricted rats, respectively; the initial weights averaged 168 g and 173 g, respectively.

The incidence of rats bearing one or more mammary carcinomas at 16 weeks was high, 93% to 97%, and thus the dose of carcinogen was obviously high. It is likely that the high dose masked the protective effect of the modest degree of caloric restriction. Therefore, the fact that there was no significant increase in the number of neoplasms in the group fed the 20% fat diet at a level only 12% less than the *ad libitum* group is indicative of the dominance of the protective effect of a minimal degree of caloric restriction over the enhancing effect of fat.

Finally, a series of papers from the group headed by Kritchevsky and Klurfeld[10-13] support the evidence of the afore-described experiments, namely that the quantity of fat consumed per day does not determine the incidence of neoplasms; the level of caloric intake is the determinant. The data from this series of papers are not presented because the experimental design differs from the four experiments that have been described. The design was such that calorie-restricted groups consumed the same amount of fat per day as the *ad libitum* controls; the groups were pair-fed with respect to the amount of fat consumed per animal per day. Under these conditions, it was clear that moderate inhibition of weight gain that was accomplished by control of caloric intake significantly reduced mammary and colon tumorigenesis even when the rats were fed a major portion of their calories as fat.

III. Discussion

Ample evidence was presented to prove that the major determinant of carcinogenesis in specific model systems is attributable to caloric intake and that the quantity of fat consumed per day is not important if caloric intake is controlled. This fact was established in animals fed diets that were nutritionally adequate in protein, minerals, and micronutrients.

The experiments were designed specifically to address the role of the relative importance of dietary fat level vs. caloric intake as determinants of carcinogenesis. However, even sophisticated statistical analysis applied to data from as many as 82 published experiments that were designed to reveal only the effect of caloric restriction in mice revealed that tumor incidence increased with increasing caloric intake and body weight regardless of the level of dietary fat.[14] Although meta-analysis is a valuable tool to evaluate certain issues in human epidemiology, human diet-related issues are complicated by diverse life-styles. Data obtained from animals that are specifically designed with a single variable are incontestable.

Table 4. Moderate Restriction of Caloric Intake Modulates the Enhancing Effect of Fat on Mammary Carcinogenesis of Rats[9]

Caloric intake (% of *ad libitum*)	Fat level (% of diet)	Fat intake (g/animal per day)	Neoplasms (number/rat)
100	5	0.62	4.1
88	20	1.9	4.1

The question of a *calorie-independent*, tumor-enhancing effect of fat itself, as opposed to an intentional alteration in total caloric intake, is not resolved by the experiments that are cited; more work is required to answer the question. This question will not be discussed except to state that evidence that the Atwater values of 4, 4, and 9 kcal per gram of carbohydrate, protein, and fat oversimplify the biologic values of these macronutrients under the multitude of biologic variables that exist. The issue of the caloric values of these macronutrients independently and in combination was explored by Forbes and colleagues[15-18] in the 1940s and more recently by others including Donato and Hegsted.[19] The principles established by Forbes *et al.*, namely that fat is utilized more efficiently by the growing and adult rat, was applied to the enhancing effect on carcinogenesis of increased levels of dietary fat when substituted for carbohydrate *isocalorically* according to the Atwater values for the nutrients.[7] It was concluded that it is likely that the efficiency of utilization conferred by higher fat levels was sufficient to account for the enhancing effect of a high-fat diet on carcinogenesis. However, the point that is established by the four experiments presented in this review is much more important and is not subject to debate: The quantity of fat consumed per day did not determine the incidence of neoplasms of the skin or mammary gland; the level of caloric intake was the determinant. There is no independent effect of fat *per se* that enhances carcinogenesis if the total caloric intake is not in excess of that required to maintain the animal at the body weight of a young non-obese adult.

The question of the molecular mechanisms by which caloric balance predominates remains for future research. A number of possibilities were discussed by Welsch[20] and it is likely that several or all of them as well as others not yet considered play a role. However, there is evidence for physiologic changes that characterize the calorically restricted animal that are often overlooked.[21] Animals that are subject to caloric restriction are meal-eaters and therefore fast intermittently. As a result, a part of the energy consumed when the animal is fed is deposited as glycogen after the animals are "trained" to meal eating.[21] Rather than fluctuating within narrow limits as in animals that are free to eat frequently to fulfill body energy needs, liver glycogen rises to above normal levels as a storage mechanism and this reserve is called upon later in the between-meal period and glycogen levels fall to near zero, far below levels seen in fully fed animals.[21] There is also the phenomenon called the labile liver protein reserve that serves a similar function. As a means of establishing and controlling these functions, the adrenal cortex hypertrophies[21] and circulating adrenal steroids increase. It has been shown that a topically applied or ingested adrenal cortical steroid inhibits skin carcinogenesis.[22] Furthermore, there is a decrease in available polypeptide growth hormones in the calorically restricted animal. This is manifest by a decrease in gonadotropes[21] and in the fasting serum insulin levels reported by Klurfeld *et al.*[13]

Thus in animals that become obese, the hormone balance that protects against cancer is upset: The adrenal cortical steroid levels are decreased and the levels of the growth stimulating polypeptide hormones that enhance or promote cancer are available in excess. This is also true for the eicosanoids. Elevated levels of prostaglandin E_2, which may be more readily available from essential fatty acids in the over-fed animal, is an essential component of the mechanism of promotion.[23] There is no competition for the essential fatty acids, amino acids, and other metabolites for energy; they are available in excess in the over-fed animal. These facts provide a basis for studying the mechanism of caloric restriction in carcinogenesis.

A consideration of the extrapolation to humans of the animal data that have led to the conclusion that caloric balance is critical to carcinogenesis follows. The interrelationship between the metabolism of carbohydrate, fat, and protein and the fate of these macronutrients as sources of energy and as carbon and nitrogen sources for the synthesis of specific essential molecules as well as for storage as fat are basically similar for all animals including human beings. Therefore, there is no doubt that the data presented herein are applicable to the problem of decreasing the risk of human cancer, even in those individuals that are genetically predisposed to cancer. Early childhood cancer is a different issue; the level of endogenously produced promoting agents such as polypeptide hormones is necessarily high during early stages of growth and development.

IV. Epilogue

What should the advice for the human population be, based upon data from animal experiments? It is not so simple as a recommendation to maintain a non-obese, young adult weight. Rather, emphasis should be broader, including the importance of consuming fruits, vegetables, and whole-grain cereals. Over 30 compounds that are components of these foods have been shown to protect against carcinogenesis in experimental animals. Rapid assays for their detection are being used (e.g., Reference 23) and the details are beyond the scope of this discussion. The importance of the dietary sources of protective agents must be emphasized. Furthermore, consumption of appropriate levels of fruits, vegetables, and whole-grain cereals tends to displace some of the more calorie-dense foods. Effort must be exercised to lower the consumption of "empty calories," specifically sugar and the pure fats such as the vegetable oils, especially those high in polyunsaturated fatty acids, and animal fats (e.g., lard) and the consumer products high in these fats such as most snack foods, candies, and rich desserts. However, meat, milk, and eggs are essential for optimal health and should be consumed in moderate amounts. The life of people in the real world is not as simple as is the case for laboratory animals in well-designed experiments. However, it is clear that despite wide variation in life-style and genetic background, weight control through a combination of exercise, control of caloric intake, and proper diet as advised by the USDA, NRC, and NCI/NIH should be encouraged in the strongest terms for all people without compromise. Implementation of that advice would have a major impact on the quality of life and on the cost of health care.

References

1. C.A. Baumann and H.P. Rusch, Effect of Diet on Tumors Induced by Ultraviolet Light, *Am J Cancer.* 35:213 (1939).
2. P.S. Lavik and C.A. Baumann, Dietary Fat and Tumor Formation, *Cancer Res.* 1:181 (1941).
3. A. Tannenbaum, The Genesis and Growth of Tumors III. Effects of a High Fat Diet, *Cancer Res.* 2:468 (1942).
4. I. Sivertsen and W.H. Hastings, A Preliminary Report on the Influence of Food and Function on the Incidence of Mammary Gland Tumor in A Stock Albino Mice, *Minn Med.* 21:873 (1938).
5. A. Tannenbaum, The Initiation and Growth of Tumors, *Am J Cancer.* 38:335 (1940).
6. P.S. Lavik and C.A. Baumann, Further Studies on the Tumor Promoting Action of Fat, *Cancer Res.* 3:749 (1943).
7. R.K. Boutwell, M.K. Brush, and H.P. Rusch, The Stimulating Effect of Dietary Fat on Carcinogenesis, *Cancer Res.* 9:741 (1949).
8. G.A. Boissonneault, C. Elson, and M.W. Pariza, Net Energy Effects of Dietary Fat on Chemically Induced Mammary Carcinogenesis in F344 Rats, *J Nat Cancer Inst.* 76:335 (1986).
9. C.W. Welsch, J.L. Hoase, B.L. Herr, S.S. Eliasberg, and M.A. Welsch, Enhancement of Mammary Carcinogenesis by High Levels of Dietary Fat: A Phenomenon Dependent on *Ad Libitum* Feeding, *J Nat Cancer Inst.* 82:1615 (1990).
10. D. Kritchevsky, M.M. Weber, C.L. Buck, and D.M. Klurfeld, Calories, Fat, and Cancer, *Lipids.* 21:272 (1986).

11. D. Kritchevsky, M.M. Weber, and D.M. Klurfeld, Dietary Fat *versus* Caloric Content in Initiation and Promotion of 7,12-dimethylbenzanthracene-Induced Tumorigenesis in Rats, *Cancer Res.* 44:3174 (1984).

12. D.M. Klurfeld, M.M. Weber, and D. Kritchevsky, Inhibition of Chemically Induced Mammary and Colon Tumor Promotion by Caloric Restriction in Rats Fed Increased Dietary Fat, *Cancer Res.* 47:2759 (1987).

13. D.M. Klurfeld, C.B. Welch, L.M. Lloyd, and D. Kritchevsky, Inhibition of DMBA-Induced Mammary Tumorigenesis by Caloric Restriction in Rats Fed High Fat Diets, *Int J Cancer.* 43:922 (1989).

14. D. Albanes, Total Calories, Body Weight, and Tumor Incidence in Mice, *Cancer Res.* 47:1987 (1987).

15. E.B. Forbes, R.W. Swift, R.E. Elliot, and W.H. James, Relation of Fat to the Economy of Food Utilization. I. By the Growing Albino Rat, *J Nutr.* 31:203 (1946).

16. E.B. Forbes, R.W. Swift, R.F. Elliot, and W.H. James, The Relation of Fat to the Economy of Food Utilization. II. By the Mature Albino Rat, *J Nutr.* 31:213 (1946).

17. E.B. Forbes, R.W. Swift, W.H. James, and J.W. Bratzler, Further Experiments on the Relation of Fat to the Economy of Food Utilization. I. By the Growing Albino Rat, *J Nutr.* 32:387 (1946).

18. E.B. Forbes, R.W. Swift, E.J. Thacker, V.F. Smith, and C.F. French, Further Experiments on the Relation of Fat to the Economy of Food Utilization. II. By the Mature Albino Rat, *J Nutr.* 32:397 (1946).

19. K. Donato and D.M. Hegsted, Efficiency of Utilization of Various Sources of Energy for Growth, *Proc Nat Acad Sci USA.* 382:4866 (1985).

20. C.W. Welsch, Enhancement of Mammary Tumorigenesis by Dietary Fat: Review of Potential Mechanisms, *Am J Clin Nutr.* 45s:192 (1987).

21. R.K. Boutwell, M.K. Brush, and H.P. Rusch, Some Physiological Effects Associated with Chronic Caloric Restriction, *Am J Physiol.* 154:517 (1948).

22. R.K. Boutwell, Some Biological Aspects of Skin Carcinogenesis, *Prog Exptl Tumor Res.* 4:207 (1964).

23. A.K. Verma, C.L. Ashendel, and R.K. Boutwell, Inhibition by Prostaglandin Synthesis Inhibitors of the Induction of Epidermal Ornithine Decarboxylase Activity, the Accumulation of Prostaglandins, and Tumor Promotion Caused by Tetradecanoylphorbolacetate, *Cancer Res.* 40:308 (1980).

Chapter 10

A Model System for Studying Nutritional Interventions on Colon Tumor Growth: Effects of Marine Oil

SELWYN A. BROITMAN and FRANCIS CANNIZZO, JR.

I. Introduction

In the U.S. colonic cancer is the second and third leading cause of death in men and women, respectively. While colonic cancer is multifactorial, a growing body of evidence implies that this disease may be preventable to a significant degree. Epidemiologic evidence[1,2] indicates that populations consuming diets high in fat are at greater risk for colon cancer than are populations consuming diets low in fat. Concordance for these findings has been obtained in a number of animal models[3-6] using a variety of carcinogens for bowel tumor induction, these workers noted that rats fed diets high in fat had a greater incidence and/or greater number of bowel tumors than rats fed diets low in fat. Sakaguchi *et al.*[7] indicated that the type of dietary fat was important in AOM (azoxymethane)-induced colon tumorigenesis with 5% polyunsaturated-fat (PUFA) diets resulting in a higher tumor incidence, tumor number, and greater degree of histologic malignant differentiation, than in rats fed saturated-fat diets. Studies from this lab a few years ago[4] and work of Reddy and Maeura[8] indicated that dietary PUFA were also more effective in increasing carcinogen-induced bowel tumor yields than saturated fat.

A variety of mechanisms have been proposed to explain the effects of dietary lipids on colon tumor promotion[3,9-11] and include: 1) immune suppression by PUFA, 2) lipid oxygen/peroxy radicals as tissue proliferation stimulants, 3) increased fecal bile acids augmenting tissue proliferation, 4) enhanced membrane fluidity by essential fatty acids in tissue proliferation/immune mechanisms, 5) net energy (kcal) retention for tumor growth and 6) enhanced prostaglandin synthesis. It is appreciated that certain effects ascribed to tumor promotion may be distinguished from the events during tumor initiation. However, the line demarcating promotional events from mere enhancement of tumor growth is considerably less clear.

Selwyn A. Broitman and Francis Cannizzo, Jr. ● Departments of Microbiology and Pathology, Boston University School of Medicine, Boston, Massachusetts

Exercise, Calories, Fat, and Cancer, Edited by M.M. Jacobs
Plenum Press, New York, 1992

For the most part these studies have been derived from carcinogen-induced tumors of the large bowel and involve 1,2-dimethylhydrazine (DMH), azoxymethane (AOM), nitrosomethylurea (NMU), or N-methyl-N'-nitro-N-nitrosoguanidine (MNNG). Conventionally, these bowel carcinogens are given on a multiple-dose schedule over a period of time. Consequently, each dose of carcinogen may serve to promote each previous dose. As a result, nutritional events that have been ascribed to the promotional phase of carcinogenesis must be at least additive to the promotional effects of carcinogen in order to be detected. In addition, nutrients that may inhibit tumorigenesis to some extent must counteract the promotional effects of carcinogens so that these effects may be detected by the termination of the studies.

In delineating a role of lipid in colon carcinogenesis, the incorporation of nutritional lipids into various cellular components of bowel tumors has been accomplished by a number of investigators to provide insights on their mechanism of action. Control tissues to evaluate tumor lipids have included non-involved bowel, liver, serum, etc. Unfortunately, cell types from these sites are clearly different and may not be appropriate controls for the effects of lipid nutriture on tumor development. This current report utilizes a transplantable colon tumor model system in which these problems may be circumvented. By implanting CT-26[12] at various sites it was noted that certain sites were lipid nutrition responsive and others were non-responsive. To evaluate this system, two dietary lipids known to have promotional effects on bowel tumors and a third shown to be inhibitory for bowel tumors were utilized.

II. Materials and Methods

A. Animal Care and Feeding

Weanling BALB/c BYJ mice (The Jackson Laboratory, Bar Harbor, ME) were placed at random into each diet group upon arrival. The numbers of animals in each dietary group varied according to each experiment and is detailed separately. Temperature, humidity, and light-dark cycle were carefully controlled. Guidelines promulgated in the Guiding Principles in the Care and Use of Animals, approved by the American Physiological Society, are strictly adhered to.

Mice were fed commercial mouse chow and water *ad libitum* for 4 to 7 days and then fed experimental diets. All diets conform to the AIN-76 standard[13] and were modified[14] to provide identical amounts of kcal, protein, vitamins, and minerals at all levels of fat. All diets provided adequate essential fatty acids to prevent EFA (essential fatty acid)-deficiency.[15-17] "Low-fat" diets contained 5 g of fat, or 5% fat by weight, providing 11.6% kcal as fat; "high-fat" diets contained 20 g of fat, or 24.7% fat by weight, providing 46.5% of calories as fat (Table 1). Lipids used were 1) hydrogenated coconut oil, a saturated fat; 2) safflower oil, an n-6 polyunsaturated fat high in EFA; and 3) marine oil, an n-3 polyunsaturated fat high in eicosapentaenoic acid (EPA) and docosahexaenoic acid (DHA).

B. Tissue Culture

Tissue culture techniques have been adapted from Brattain[17] and modified[18] as follows: Frozen CT-26 cells were thawed, seeded at 1×10^6 cells per 75 cm^2 flask, and grown in RPMI-1640 medium supplemented with 10% fetal bovine serum and a 1% glutamine, 1% penicillin/streptomycin combination. Confluent (7-day) cultures of approximately 2×10^7 cells were harvested and used to seed an appropriate number of flasks to perform the scheduled inoculations. Cells of passage 8 were used to perform all studies.

Confluent cultures were harvested by trypsinization, washed, and pelleted at 250 xg. Tumor implantation into the flank or mid-scapular area utilized serial dilutions of cells from 1×10^3 to 1×10^6 in a volume of 0.1 ml given subcutaneously. Intracolonic (subserosal in the mid-descending colon) inoculations of mice for tumor growth assay and time to death groups were performed using 1 x 10^6 cells suspended in 0.05 ml serum-free medium. Intravenous inoculations of mice for the colonization assay were performed using 1 x 10^5 cells suspended in 0.1 ml serum-free medium. Cell suspensions were maintained at 4°C during the surgical procedure; survival of cells after 9 hours at this temperature was >95%, as determined by trypan blue exclusion.

Table 1. Composition of Experimental Diets

	Low fat (g)	High fat (g)
Ingredients[a]		
Lipid[b] – marine oil, safflower oil,	5.00	20.00
or hydrogenated coconut oil	4.03	18.80
Casein[c]	20.00	20.00
Corn starch	15.00	7.17
Sucrose	50.00	23.90
Fiber	5.00	5.00
D,L-methionine	0.30	0.30
Choline bitartrate	0.20	0.20
AIN mineral mix	3.50	3.50
AIN vitamin mix	1.00	1.00
Total weight	100.00	81.07
Energy value (kcal/g)[a]	3.965	4.877
% kcal as fat	11.6%	46.5%
Anticipated daily intake for adult BALB/c mice/100 g body weight		
Energy (kcal/day)	88.00	88.00
Food	22.20	18.00
Protein	4.00	4.00
Fat	1.11	4.44
Carbohydrate	14.43	6.89
Fibre	1.11	1.11
Choline bitartrate	0.04	0.04
AIN mineral mix	0.78	0.78
AIN vitamin mix	0.22	0.22

[a] Diets were formulated according to guidelines set forth by Newberne.[14]

[b] Marine oil contains 5.51% essential fatty acids by weight, safflower oil contains 77.0% essential fatty acids by weight, hydrogenated coconut oil contains less than 0.1% essential fatty acids by weight (GLC analysis). 0.97g and 1.20g of safflower oil were added to the low- and high-fat hydrogenated coconut oil diets to provide a total of 5 g and 20 g of fat with 1.7% and 1.7% essential fatty acids, respectively.

[c] Casein is assumed to be 90% protein.

[d] Calculated as 4.1 kcal/g for starch, sucrose, and casein, and 9.2 kcal/g for marine, safflower, and coconut oils.

C. Tumor Implantation into the Bowel

Animals were anesthetized with sodium pentobarbital, ip approximately 78 mg/kg body weight, and the abdomen was swabbed with 70% ethanol. A standard 1.5-cm, mid-clavicular, laparotomy incision was used to visualize the descending colon. A 1-ml syringe outfitted with a 27-gauge needle was used to inject the cell bolus subserosally, on the anti-mesenteric side, being careful not to puncture the lumen. Following implantation of tumor cells, the gut was replaced in the abdominal cavity and swabbed with 70% ethanol. Wound clips (9 mm; Clay Adams, Harvard Bioscience, So. Natick, MA) were used to close muscle and skin layers together. To prevent post-operative hypothermia, mice recovered under a heat lamp until active. Incision scars were observed for pus or necrosis, exudate or excessive tenderness, or other healing abnormalities. At necropsy, gross external and internal appearance of the scar was noted.

Animals were thoroughly necropsied on post-op days 21 and 28, to ascertain primary tumor size, the number and size of both metastases and direct extensions, and the condition of the non-involved tissue. Measurements of primary tumors were taken and used to calculate total volumes using the formula[19]: length x width^2 x 0.4. Consideration of the number of animals required at each timepoint for statistically valid comparisons predetermined the sizes of the groups to be killed.

D. Colonization Assay[20]

A 30-gauge needle on a 1-ml syringe was used to inoculate tail veins of animals for the pulmonary colonization group by iv injection. After 21 days animals were killed, chests opened, and the trachea visualized. A blunt 18-gauge needle, introduced into the trachea of each animal, was used to infuse 2 to 3 ml of a dye solution (comprising 15% India ink and 2% NH_4 in phosphate-buffered saline), until the lungs fully insufflated. Lungs were immediately excised *en bloc* and immersed in Fakete's solution. Foci were independently counted under magnification by three technicians, and averaged.

The tumor foci from the lungs of random specimens selected from each group were measured with verneer calipers (Manostat, Switzerland; Harvard Bioscience, So. Natick, MA) and the colony diameter was recorded. Foci size distribution was determined in the various diet groups to investigate the possible coalescence of small foci into fewer large ones (yielding lower colony counts) or the presence of a few, fast-growing lesions that could engulf the lung (yielding an equal tumor volume as that obtained for more numerous, small, individual tumors).

E. Time to Death

Tumor cell implantation was conducted exactly as described for the tumor growth assay group. Surgery was performed in a continuous process, alternating the implantations among the various dietary groups at random. Following surgery and recovery, animals were caged and observed twice daily for signs of sepsis or morbidity and time of demise.

F. Statistical Methods

The non-parametric Kruskal-Wallis ANOVA was used to analyze pulmonary colonization assay data to accomodate the data's skew; the Mann-Whitney U Test was applied to identify specific significant differences. Transformed tumor growth assay data at 21, and 28 day timepoint (untransformed data were found to be lognormal) were analyzed using Gaussian ANOVA followed by the Scheffe multiple-comparisons test. These statistical procedures were performed on the university's mainframe computer using the SPSS Statistical Package.

G. Histology

At necroscopy, tumors and other selected tissues were fixed in buffered formalin and stained with hemotoxylin and eosin.

III. Results

Mice fed the various diets, high- or low-fat of different types, consume essentially the same number of calories daily. These data have been reported previously.[18]

It was important to establish a standardized dose of cells of CT-26 with which tumor size and effects of nutritional interventions could be evaluated. Figure 1 illustrates the results of these studies in which 10^3 to 10^6 CT-26 cells were inoculated into the mid-scapular region or flank region in BALB/c mice who were fed a 20-g saturated-fat diet. Some of this data is included in a recent report.[21] The latency time, defined as the period of time from injection of tumor cells to the first palpable tumor (approximately 1.0 mm in diameter) range from approximately 25 days with the smallest number of cells to about 10 days with 10^5 or 10^6 cells at both sites of implantation. The time to death following the appearance of the tumor was also inversely related to the number of cells implanted at either location. For the remaining studies, except where noted, it was elected to use 10^4 cells, which would allow approximately 2 weeks before the tumors appeared and at least 30 days for the animals to succumb. Thus the length of time for the nutritional intervention would be 30 days prior to implantation and an additional 6 weeks or more following implantation of the tumor at either site. The effects of nutritional interventions on tumor latency and time to death following tumors implanted into the flank is also shown (Table 2). Regardless of the level of fat (5 g or 20 g) or the type (saturated or polyunsaturated) of fat, the time for the appearance of the tumor was between approximately 17 to 20 days and was not significantly different among each of the nutritional groups.

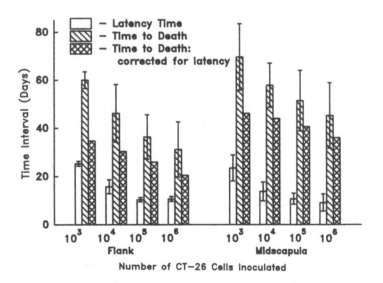

Figure 1. Effect of innoculum size on tumor latency time and time to death. Mice were implanted with CT-26 into the flank (6 mice/group) or in the mid-scapular area (8 mice/group) and fed a 20-g coconut oil diet.

Table 2.   Tumor Latency Time and Time to Death in Mice Fed Varying Levels of PUFA
and Saturated Fat Diets — CT-26 Cells Implanted into Flank

Diet	# of mice	Tumor latency[a] (days)	Time to death[a] (days after implant)
20 g saturated fat	14	16.6 ± 2.6	49.2 ± 14.1
5 g saturated fat	8	19.8 ± 1.0	50.8 ± 12.7
20 g unsaturated fat	8	17.3 ± 0.2	57.4 ± 8.4
5 g unsaturated fat	7	17.3 ± 2.3	58.1 ± 12.7

[a] Figures are expressed as the mean number of days before tumor appearance and time to death respectively, ± SEM, in mice innoculated with 10^4 CT-26 cells.

Growth rates of tumors implanted on the flank in animals fed either a 5- or 20-g saturated or polyunsaturated diet are shown in Figure 2 using data from Reference 21. The time for the first appearance of the measurable tumor was considered as day one for each of the nutritional groups. Since tumors were measured every second day, it is possible that a tumor could have become palpable the day prior to its first detection. Thus, this implies an error in measurement in which any given group could be shifted to the right for a one-day time interval. No significant differences in tumor volume were noted among any of the dietary groupings. Further, the slopes of all of these lines of each dietary group were similar and the doubling time for tumor growth in any group is around 3 days. A survival curve is shown in Figure 3 and illustrates that the number of surviving mice inoculated with 10^4 CT-26 cells on the flank was no different regardless of the level of saturated fat in the diet. Similar findings were obtained when PUFA was utilized at the high and low levels and when the tumor cells were implanted in the mid-scapular area.

Marine oil diets have been used previously in studies in which inhibition of bowel tumor growth relative to other lipids has been demonstrated.[18] In the current studies, CT-26 was implanted in the mid-scapular area and tumor volume measured over a 23-day period. It is apparent in Figure 4 that mice fed high-fat diets containing either coconut oil, safflower oil, or marine oil exhibited tumors that were not significantly different in size.

Table 3 illustrates a comparison of the pulmonary colonization assay in animals fed marine oils or the safflower oil diet. Animals fed the marine oil diet at 5- or 20-g levels exhibited no significant differences in pulmonary colonization. Mice fed the safflower oil diet at the 5-g level exhibited the same number of pulmonary colonies as mice fed marine oil at the low- or high-fat diet. However, mice fed the high-fat safflower oil diet showed greater than a three-fold increase in the number of pulmonary colonies ($p < 0.01$) indicating that the pulmonary bed was responsive to dietary lipids and that increasing levels of polyunsaturated fat increased the number of pulmonary colonies while marine oil fed at an equivalent high-fat level exhibited a reduction in colonies relative to the high-fat safflower oil diet.

When tumors were implanted into the bowel of mice fed the low- and high-fat coconut oil and safflower oil diets (Figure 5) a dose-response effect to the level of dietary lipid was apparent but no significant differences between the type of lipid was noted. After 28 days following implantation into the colon, mice fed the high-fat diets exhibited tumors that were three- to four-fold larger than those fed the low-fat diets ($p < 0.01$). The effects on tumors in animals fed the high-fat diets are somewhat understated, since some mice succumb to their tumors in these groups after 21 days. In time, the tumors are generally larger and have occluded the bowel. The graph depicts only the surviving mice at the 28th day.

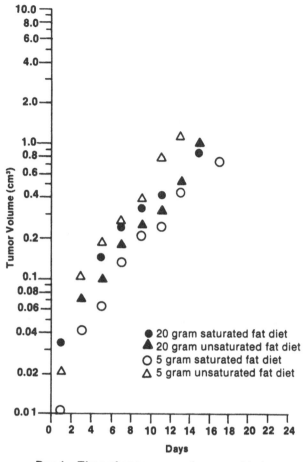

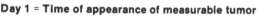

Figure 2. Growth of tumors implanted on the flank of mice fed either a 5- or 20-g coconut or safflower oil diet. Innoculum of 10^4 CT-26 cells was implanted into 14 mice in the 20-g coconut oil group and 8 mice in each other dietary group.

Previously, this lab demonstrated an inhibitory effect of dietary marine oil on post-promotional growth of CT-26 implanted into the bowel.[18] Additional studies are depicted in Figure 6, which also illustrates a marked inhibitory effect of dietary marine oil on tumor growth in the bowel at 28 days. Once again, the size of tumors in mice fed either the 20-g saturated- and unsaturated-fat diets tend to be understated because of mortality. No mortality occured in this marine oil group.

Histologic sections of tumors taken from the three groups revealed that mice fed the marine oil diets had significantly more areas of focal necrosis scattered throughout the colonic tumor than those in the other dietary group. Representative histology is shown in Figures 7a, 7b, 8a, and 8b.

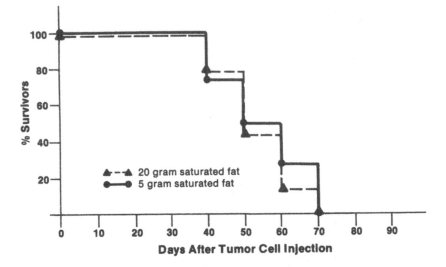

Figure 3. Survival of mice implanted with 10^4 CT-26 cells on the flank and fed a 5- (8 mice) or 20-(14 mice) g coconut oil diet.

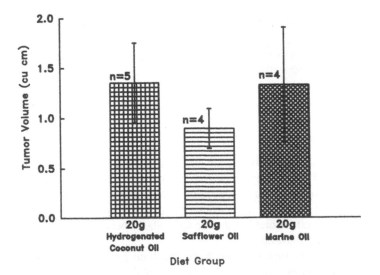

Figure 4. Tumor volumes after 23 days in mice implanted with 10^4 CT-26 cells in the mid-scapular area and fed various high-fat diets.

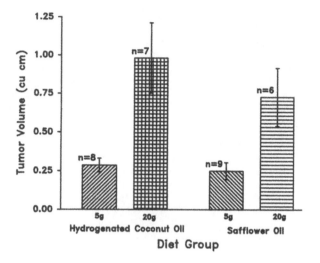

Figure 5. Bowel tumor volumes after 28 days in mice fed various lipid diets.

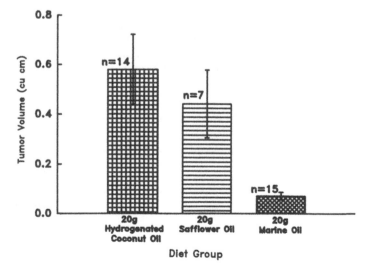

Figure 6. Tumor implantation of 10^6 CT-26 cells in the mid-portion of the decending colon. Mice were killed at 4-day intervals and tumors measured. Findings at 28 days following implantation are depicted.

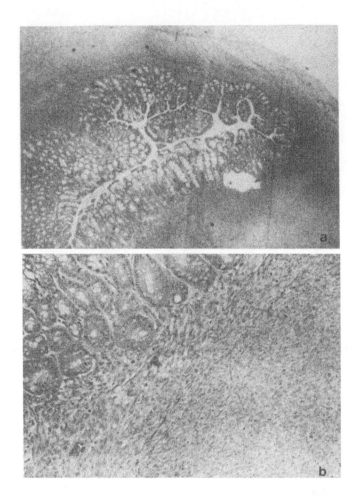

Figures 7a and 7b. Hematoxylin and eosin stain of low and high magnification of CT-26 implanted in mid-descending colon of mice fed a high safflower oil diet after 28 days. Tumor has encircled the lumen with relatively few areas of focal necrosis. On high power, poorly to undifferentiated tumor with areas of acute inflammation. Tumor cells have invaded mucosal glands which exhibit pseudo-polylayerizing.

Table 3.   Pulmonary Colonization in Mice Fed Low- or High-fat Marine or Safflower Oil Diets Implanted with CT-26

Diet group	n	Number of colonies/mouse
5 g marine oil	22	10.2 ± 2.0[a]
20 g marine oil	23	14.3 ± 3.6
5 g safflower oil	22	13.5 ± 4.5
20 g safflower oil	22	55.2 ± 8.0

[a] Mean $\pm$ SEM.

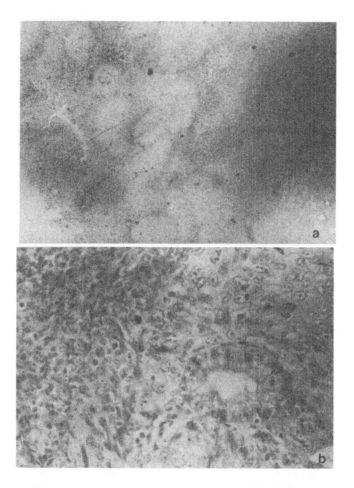

Figures 8a and 8b. Hematoxylin and eosin stain of low and high magnification of CT-26 implanted into the mid-descending colon of mice fed after 28 days. The tumor has encircled the colon; multiple focal areas of necrosis scattered throughout entire cross section of the tumor. At high magnification, necrotic tumor cells and inflammation are surrounded by a margin of viable tumor. Poor to moderate differentiated mucosal glandular elements are visible.

IV. Discussion

In the model system described, it was observed that colon tumor CT-26, implanted in the flank or mid-scapular area grew at the same rate regardless of the level of dietary fat, the type, saturated (with adequate EFA) or polyunsaturated n-6 or n-3. Conversely, the tumor administered iv in a pulmonary colony assay exhibited a higher yield of pulmonary colonies, with an increased level of dietary saturated or n-6 PUFA. Additionally, the inhibitory effects of the n-3 polyunsaturated fat, marine oil, were readily apparent since high levels of dietary marine oils yielded the same number of colonies as low levels. When CT-26 was implanted into the mid-portion of the colon of mice fed various lipid diets, high levels of saturated fat and n-6 PUFA were associated with larger tumor than lower levels of these lipids. Marine oil diets were associated with tumor growth inhibition. Tumors from this latter group yielded histologic findings of focal areas of tumor necrosis that were clearly different from bowel tumors in mice fed the other lipids.

With this model system, it is apparent that the site of implantation determines whether or not the tumor is responsive to lipid nutrients. It is currently not clear why this difference in responsiveness occurs. A number of possibilities currently under exploration include the following potential differences in: blood flow, availability of nutritional substrates, lipid transport, lipid-vitamin interactions, and lipid metabolism between tumors at different sites.

Among the tumor promotional effects ascribed to certain lipids and/or energy in general in mammary and colon sites it has been the repeated observation that tumors in animals fed diets high in lipid (a) occur more rapidly, (b) are often larger, and (c) exhibit a higher incidence than in animals fed diets lower in lipid. Whether these effects are due directly to the effects of lipid or energy on tumors directly or indirectly on carcinogen absorption, activation, detoxification, etc., is not clear. Furthermore, whether the effects of lipid on post-initiation events are exclusively the effects of lipids on tumor growth also has not been discerned.

A possibility bearing on this point had been suggested by King and McCay[22] using 7,12-dimethylbenz(a)-anthracene (DMBA)-induced breast tumorigenesis. High levels of dietary PUFA-enhanced breast tumor incidence compared to saturated fat. They suggested that a given dose of carcinogen would initiate a given number of cells independent of diet. The number of tumors that are palpable within a fixed time would depend on the growth rate of the initiated clone. Consequently, if a higher level of dietary PUFA accelerated clonal growth, the number of tumors reaching palpable size in a fixed time would be greater. Thus the effects of lipid nutrition in accelerating the growth rate of tumors would be interpreted as a tumor-promoting event.

Carroll and Hopkins[23] and Hopkins et al.[24] using DMBA-induced mammary carcinogenesis concluded that EFA is required for maximal mammary carcinogenesis. Ip[10] quantified the EFA for maximal number and incidence of DMBA mammary carcinogenesis at 4-5% linoleic acid (LA) in 20% (by weight) fat diet. Addition of fat, polyunsaturated or saturated, above this dietary level of linoleate failed to augment tumors significantly. Support for the concept that at least one of major promotional effects of dietary fat exclusive of calories[25,26] resides in EFA content (principally linoleic acid) has been provided by a number of others.[21,27,28] In studies conducted over a decade ago with a DMBA-induced mammary tumor cell line Kidwell and Monaco[29] noted that LA was initially required for its survival in culture. Further enhanced growth was obtained by the addition of oleic to LA and inhibition was obtained by saturated fatty acids alone[30]; no attempt was made to keep conditions in tissue culture isocaloric.

Two additional lines of evidence have served to focus attention on LA in tumor growth and promotion. Both relate to alterations in LA metabolism and subsequent tumor inhibition. Linoleic acid, an 18:2, n-6 fatty acid (FA), undergoes a series of elongation and desaturation steps via dihomogamalinoleate to arachidonate (AA) C20:4 n-6. In turn, AA is metabolized by the lipooxygenase pathway via hydroxyeicosatetranoids to a series of leukotrienes.[31,32] Arachidonate is simultaneously metabolized by the cyclooxygenase pathway to prostaglandins principally of the 1 series (PGE_1) and 2 series (PGE_2) and thromboxanes of the 1 and 2 series (TXA_1 and TXA_2). Inhibition of cylooxygenase by modified substrates,[33] or indomethacin[34-37] inhibits PG synthesis coincident with inhibition of spontaneous, carcinogen-induced, or transplantable breast tumor growth.

The other line of evidence is derived from studies concerned with the relationship of dietary fish oils to inhibition of tumorigenesis. Fish oil diets rich in n-3 fatty acids [eicosopentaenoic (EPA) and docosahexaenoic (DHA)] fed to rats inhibits carcinogen-induced tumor incidence and number,[38] transplantable mammary adenocarcinoma,[39-45] a variety of carcinogen-induced colon tumors,[46-49] and, recently, a transplantable colon carcinoma.[18] It is appreciated that EPA in fish oils inhibits formation of PGs (1 and 2 series)[42] and generate PGs of the 3 series. Eicosopentaenoic is a less effective substrate than AA for cylooxgenase, but effectively competes with AA for this enzyme and this effects PG synthesis from AA[50-52] with the resultant reduction in tumor size in rodents fed n-3 lipid compared to those fed n-6 lipid.

These events are associated with tissues exhibiting a diminished proliferative response, and may certainly be a factor in inhibition of CT-26 implanted into the colon of marine oil-fed mice. Additional related effects have been suggested by another conference speaker, Dr. Clifford W. Welsch, who pointed out that tumor peroxidation products in athymic nude mice implanted with human breast carcinomas were more abundant in mice fed marine oil diets than in those fed other lipids.[44] Further, these effects were reversed by the addition of anti-oxidants to the diet. Thus, the findings of focal areas of necrosis in CT-26 colon tumors in mice fed marine oil is consistent with the concept of increased lipid peroxidation products generated via cyclooxygenase and lipoxygenase activity.

Thus it is apparent that certain events described as promotional events utilizing carcinogen-induced tumors cannot be sorted from those lipid nutritional events that modulate the growth of tumors. The current report describes a model system using a transplantable colon tumor, CT-26, in which lipid nutrition as it affects tumor growth can be studied in both cell culture and post-implantation, free of the confounding-variable introduced by carcinogenesis. It also affords certain unique advantages in that, depending on the site of implantation, the colon tumor may be lipid-nutritionally responsive or non-responsive as we have recently described.[18,21] This model system is currently used to evaluate the relationship of EFAs and marine oils to the modulation of tumor growth *in vivo*.

V. Summary

Lipid nutrition effects were evaluated on the growth of a transplantable colon tumor (CT-26) at various sites in the BALB/c mouse. CT-26 implanted into the back or flank of these mice grew well independent of the quality or quantity of fat in the diet. However, when implanted in the mid-portion of the descending colon, tumor growth was related to the level of dietary saturated (coconut oil) or n-6 unsaturated (safflower oil) fat in the diet. Similar findings were obtained when the tumor was utilized in a pulmonary colonization assay. Dietary marine oil (mainly EPA, and DHA n-3 polyunsaturated oils) was found to markedly impair the growth of CT-26 implanted in the bowel and lung, but not in the back.

Thus, CT-26 exhibits nutrition responsiveness at certain sites, but not at others. This may help to explain contradictory findings concerning dietary lipids in certain studies. Inhibition of tumor growth by marine oils may afford preventive or chemotherapeutic implications as its mode of action unfolds. Histologic findings in bowel tumors from mice fed marine oil but not other oils revealed focal areas of necrosis. It is appreciated that arachidonate metabolism is competitively interfered with by EPA in both cyclooxygenase and lipoxygenase pathways. The possibility is raised that the metabolism of marine oils in this model system may generate lipid peroxidation products to a greater extent than n-6 lipids and in turn is associated with focal areas of necrosis.

A model system of nutritionally non-responsive and nutritionally responsive sites for the post-promotional growth of a bowel tumor affords the opportunity to explore lipid effects with control and test tumors in hosts fed identical lipid nutriture.

Acknowledgments

The authors acknowledge the technical assistance of the following members of the laboratory staff who participated in a number of studies from which this report was derived: Mr. John Wilkinson IV, Mr. Paul Colon, Ms. Claudia Kosakolsky-Singer, Ms. Christine O'Conner, Mr. Wayne Saltsman, and Mr. J.Z. Broitman.

The authors thank Dr. Anthony Bimbo of Zapata Haynie Company, Reedville, VA who supplied the marine oil.

The authors also gratefully acknowledge the American Institute for Cancer Research, Grant 85A05, and the National Institutes of Health; National Cancer Institute, Grant CA-38177; and the Oncobiology Training Grant, T32-CA9423, which supported the studies described in this report.

References

1. K.K. Carroll and H.T. Khor, Dietary fat in relation to tumorigenesis, *Prog Biochem Pharmacol.* 10:308 (1975).
2. "Diet, Nutrition and Cancer," National Academy Press, Washington, DC (1983).
3. B.S. Reddy, K. Wanatabe, and J.H. Weisburger, Effect of a high-fat diet on colon carcinogenesis in F344 rats treated with 1,2 dimethylhydrazine, methylazoxymethanol acetate, or methylnitrosourea, *Cancer Res.* 37:4156 (1977).
4. S.A. Broitman, J.J. Vitale, Vavrousek-Jakuba and L.S. Gottleib, Polyunsaturated fat, cholesterol, and large bowel tumorigenesis, *Cancer.* 40:2455 (1977).
5. N.D. Nigro, D.V. Singh, R.L. Campbell and M. Sook, Effects of diet on intestinal tumor formation by azoxymethane in rats. *J Natl Cancer Inst.* 54:439 (1975).
6. B.R. Bansal, E. Rhoads Jr., and S.C. Bansal, Effects of diet on colon carcinogenesis and the immune system in rats treated with 1,2 dimethylhydrazine, *Cancer Res.* 38:3293 (1978).
7. M. Sakaguchi, Y. Hiramatsu, H. Takada, M. Yamamura, K. Hioki, K. Saito, and M. Yamamoto, Effect of dietary unsaturated and saturated fats on azoxymethane-induced colon carcinogenesis in rats, *Cancer Res.* 44:1472 (1984).
8. B.S. Reddy and Y. Maeura, Tumor promotion by dietary fat in azoxymethane-induced colon carcinogenesis in female F344 rats: Influence of amount and source of dietary fat, *J Natl Cancer Inst.* 72:745 (1984).
9. L.M. Braden and K.K. Carroll, Dietary polyunsaturated fat in relation to mammary carcinogenesis in rats, *Lipids* 21:285 (1986).
10. C. Ip, Fat and essential fatty acid in mammary carcinogenesis, *Am J Clin Nutr.* 45:218 (1987).
11. C.W. Welsch, Enhancement of mammary turmorigenesis by dietary fat Review of potential mechanisms, *Am J Clin Nutr.* 45:192 (1987).
12. T.H. Corbett, D.P. Griswold Jr., B.J. Roberts, J.C. Peckham, and F.M. Schabel Jr., Tumor induction relationships in development of transplantable cancers of the colon in mice for chemotherapy assays, with a note on carcinogen structure, *Cancer Res.* 35:2434 (1975).
13. Report of the American Institute of Nutrition Ad Hoc Committee on Standards for Nutritional Studies, *J Nutr* 107:1340 (1977).
14. P.M. Newberne, Control of Diets in Laboratory Animal Experimentation, *in:* "ILAR News" Natl Acad of Sciences, Washington, DC, 21:A1 (1978).
15. R.J. Holman, The ratio of trienoic: tetraenoic acids in tissue lipids as a measure of essential fatty acid requirement, *J Nutr.* 70:405 (1960).
16. R.J. Holman, *in:* "Dietary Fat and Cancer," C. Ip, D.F. Birt, A.E. Rogers and C. Mettlin, eds., Alan R. Liss, Inc., New York, (1986).
17. M.G. Brattain, J. Strobel-Stevens, D. Fine, M. Webb and A.M. Sarrif, Establishment of mouse colonic carcinoma cell lines with different metastatic properties, *Cancer Res.* 40:2142 (1980).
18. F. Cannizzo, Jr. and S.A. Broitman, Post promotional effects of dietary marine or safflower oils on large bowel or pulmonary implants of CT-26 in mice, *Cancer Res.* 49:4289 (1989).
19. A.P. Kyriazis, A.A. Kyriazia, D.G. Scarpelli, M.S. Rao, and R. Lepera, Human pancreatic adenocarcinoma cell line CAPAN-1 in tissue culture and the nude mouse, *Am J Pathol.* 106:250 (1982).

20. H. Wexler, Accurate identification of experimental pulmonary metastasis, *J Natl Cancer Inst.* 36:641 (1966).

21. F. Cannizzo Jr., C.C. O'Connor and S.A. Broitman, Subcutaneously implanted CT-26 in Balb/c mice: Effect of size of inoculum and type and level of dietary lipid, Submitted for publication.

22. M.M. King and P.B. McCay, Modulation of tumor incidence and possible mechanisms of inhibition of mammary carcinogenesis by dietary antioxidants, *Cancer Res.* (Suppl) 43:2485 (1983).

23. K.K. Carroll and G.J. Hopkins, Dietary polyunsaturated fat *versus* saturated fat in relation to mammary carcinogenesis, *Lipids.* 14:155 (1979).

24. G.J. Hopkins, T.G. Kennedy, and K.K. Carroll, Polyunsaturated fatty acids as promoters of mammary carcinogenesis induced in Sprague-Dawley rats by 7,12-dimethylbenz(a)anthracene, *J Natl Cancer Inst.* 66:517 (1981).

25. A. Tannebaum, The genesis and growth of tumors. III. Effects of a high-fat diet, *Cancer Res.* 2:460 (1942).

26. D. Kritchevsky, M.M. Weber and D.M. Klurfield, Dietary fat *versus* calorie content in initiation and promotion of 7,12-dimethylbenz(a)anthracene-induced mammary tumorigenesis in rats, *Cancer Res.* 44:3174 (1984).

27. L.A. Cohen, D.O. Thompson, Y. Maeura, and J.H. Weisburger, Influence of dietary medium chain triglycerides on the development of N-methylnitrosourea-induced rat mammary tumors, *Cancer Res.* 44:5023 (1984).

28. N.E. Hubbard and K.L. Erickson, Enhancement of metastasis from a transplantable mouse mammary tumor by dietary linoleic acid, *Cancer Res.* 47:6174 (1987).

29. W.R. Kidwell and M.E. Monaco, Unsaturated fatty acid requirements for growth and survival of a rat mammary tumor cell line, *Cancer Res.* 38:4091 (1978).

30. M.S. Wicha, L.A. Liotta, and W.R. Kidwell, Effects of free fatty acids on the growth of normal and neoplastic rat mammary epithelial cells, *Cancer Res.* 39:426 (1979).

31. B. Samuelsson, Leukotrienes: Mediators of immediate hypersensitivity reactions and inflammation, *Science.* 220:568 (1983).

32. R.A. Lewis and K.F. Austen, The biologically active leukotrienes. Biosynthesis, metabolism, receptors, functions and pharmacology, *J Clin Invest.* 73:889 (1984).

33. G.A. Rao and S. Abraham, Reduced growth rate of transplantable mammary adenocarcinoma in C3H mice fed eicosa-9,8,11,14-tetraynoic acid, *J Natl Cancer Inst.* 58:445 (1977).

34. V. Hial, Z. Horakova, F.E. Shaff, and M.A. Beavar, Alteration of tumor growth by aspirin and indomethacin: Studies with two transplantable tumors in the mouse, *Eur J Pharm.* 37:367 (1976).

35. G.M. Kollmorgen, M.M. King, S.D. Kosanke, and C. Do, Influence of dietary fat and indomethacin on the growth of transplantable mammary gland tumors in rats, *Cancer Res.* 43:4714 (1983).

36. A.M. Fulton, *In vivo* effects of indomethacin on the growth of murine mammary tumors, *Cancer Res.* 44:2416 (1984).

37. E.A. Carter, R.J. Milholland, W. Shea, and M.M. Ip, Effect of prostaglandin inhibitor indomethacin of 7,12-dimethylbenz(a)anthracene-induced mammary tumorigenesis in rats fed different levels of fat, *Cancer Res.* 43:3559 (1983).

38. J.J. Jurkowski and W.T. Cave Jr., Dietary effects of menhaden oil on the growth and membrane lipid composition of rat mammary tumors, *J Natl Cancer Inst.* 74:1145 (1985).

39. H. Gabor and S. Abraham, Effect of dietary menhaden oil on tumor cell loss and the accumulation of mass of a transplantable mammary adenocarcinoma in Balb/c mice, *J Natl Cancer Inst.* 76:1223 (1986).

40. R.A. Karmali, J. Marsh, and C. Fuchs, Effect of omega-3 fatty acids on growth of a rat mammary tumor, *J Natl Cancer Inst.* 73:457 (1984).

41. G. Poste, J. Doll, T.R. Hart and I.J. Fidler, *In vitro* selection of murine B16 melanoma variants with enhanced tissue-invasive properities, *Cancer Res.* 40:1636, 1980.

42. R.A. Karmali, *in:* "Dietary Fat and Cancer," C. Ip, D.F. Birt, A.E. Rogers and C. Mettlin, eds., Alan R. Liss, Inc., New York (1986).

43. I.J. Fidler, Tumor heterogeneity and the biology of cancer invasion and metastasis, *Cancer Res.* 38:2651 (1978).

44. M.J. Gonzales, R.A. Schemmel, J.I. Gray, L. Dugan Jr., L.G. Scheffield and C.W. Welsch, Effect of dietary fat growth of MCF-7 and MDA-MB 231 human breast carcinomas in athymic nude mice: Relationship between carcinoma growth and lipid peroxidation levels, *Carcinogenesis.* 12:1231 (1991).

45. C.Y. Yang, W.A. Gonnerman, L. Taylor, R.B. Nimberg and P.R. Polgar, Synthetic human parathyroid hormone fragment stimulated prostagladin E_2 synthesis by chick calvariae, *Endocrin.* 120:63 (1987).

46. B.S. Reddy and S. Sugie, Effect of different levels of omega-3 and omega-6 fatty acids on azoxymethane-induced colon carcinogenesis on F344 rats, *Cancer Res.* 48:6642 (1988).

47. P.A. Craven, R. Saito and F.R. DeRubertis, Role of local prostaglandin synthesis in the modulation of proliferative activity of rat colonic epithelium, *J Clin Invest.* 72:1365 (1983).

48. R. Nelson, J.C. Tanure, G. Andrianopoulos, G. Souza and W.E.M. Lands, A comparison of dietary fish oil and corn oil in experimental colorectal carcinogenesis, *Nutr Cancer.* 11:215 (1988).

49. E.E. Deschner, J.S. Lytle, G. Wong, J.F. Ruperto and H.L. Newmark, The effect of dietary omega-3 fatty acids (fish oil) on azoxymethane-induced focal areas of dysplasia and colon tumor incidence, *Cancer* 66:2350 (1990).

50. A.H. Tashjian, E.F. Voelkel, P. Goldhaber and L. Levine, Successful treatment of hypercalcemia by indomethacin in mice bearing a prostaglandin-producing fibrosarcoma, *Prostaglandins* 3:515 (1973).

51. W.T. Cave, Dietary n-3 (omega-3) polyunsaturated fatty acid effects on animal tumorigenesis, *FASEB Jour.* 5:2160 (1991).

52. J.E. Kinsella, K. Shane Broughton and J.W. Whelan, Dietary unsaturated fatty acids: Interactions and possible needs in relation to eicosanoid synthesis, *J Nutr Biochem.* 1:123 (1990).

Chapter 11

Enhancement of Pancreatic Carcinogenesis by Dehydroepiandrosterone

ANTHONY R. TAGLIAFERRO, B. D. ROEBUCK,
ANNE M. RONAN and LOREN D. MEEKER

I. Introduction

Caloric intake and body weight have been established as positive risk factors in the development of several human cancers.[1] Conversely, caloric restriction has been found to significantly inhibit spontaneous[2,3] as well as chemically induced mammary carcinogenesis[4,5] and pancreatic pre-neoplastic foci[6] in laboratory rodents.

The androgenic steroid, dehydroepiandrosterone (DHEA), is synthesized and released primarily from the adrenal cortex. Dehydroepiandrosterone is the most predominant circulating steroid. It is a tissue precursor of androgen and estrogen synthesis, and has been reported to be involved in the modulation of several diverse processes.[7] In man, plasma concentration of DHEA peaks at the end of the second and beginning of the third decades, and declines, reaching its nadir during the eighth decade of the lifespan.[8] Plasma and urinary levels of DHEA have been found to vary inversely with human obesity and cancer.[9] Similarly, plasma levels of DHEAS (the predominant circulating form of the steroid) have been found to be inversely related to the mortality rate associated with heart disease in middle-aged and elderly men studied over a 12-year period.[10] In animal studies, the oral administration of DHEA in pharmacologic doses produces a profound reduction in total mass adiposity in both normal and genetically obese rodents[11]; the inhibition of spontaneous[12] and chemically induced cancers in rodents[13,14]; and a significant protective effect against atherogenic plaque formation in rabbits subjected to mechanical endothelial damage and a high cholesterol dietary challenge.[15]

Typically, DHEA treatment in animals is associated with a food intake to body weight ratio of efficiency[16] or metabolic rate[17] that indicates the state of negative energy balance induced by DHEA is the result of mechanism(s) affecting primarily energy expenditure and

Anthony R. Tagliaferro and Anne M. Ronan ● Department of Animal and Nutritional Sciences, University of New Hampshire, Durham, New Hampshire; B. D. Roebuck ● Department of Pharmacology and Toxicology, Dartmouth Medical School, Hanover, New Hampshire; Loren D. Meeker ● Department of Mathematics, University of New Hampshire, Durham, New Hampshire

Exercise, Calories, Fat, and Cancer, Edited by M.M. Jacobs
Plenum Press, New York, 1992

119

not food intake. In view of its apparent beneficial effects, DHEA has attracted considerable attention as a potential therapeutic agent.[18-22] However, the biochemical and physiologic effects of DHEA administration are not well understood. Perhaps the best known biochemical effect of DHEA that has been used to explain its anti-obesity and anti-carcinogenic effects is its non-competitive inhibition of the enzyme glucose-6-phosphate dehydrogenase (G6PDH),[23] the rate-limiting enzyme in the hexose monophosphate pathway (HMP). Hexose monophosphate pathway is a major source of the reducing equivalent (i.e., NADPH) required for triglyceride synthesis and adipocyte growth and ribose sugar for nucleic acid formation and cell differentiation. However, there is considerable evidence[23-28] that devalues the role of this biochemical mechanism to explain the protective effects of DHEA, and underscores further the complicated function of that steroid in metabolism.

In fact, the biochemical effects of DHEA may not always be beneficial. For example Beamer *et al.*[29] found that DHEA stimulated rather than inhibited the development of spontaneous tumors in ovarian granulosa cells of SWXJ-9 genetic strain of mice. Recently, Thornton *et al.*[30] found that there were no differences in pancreatic pre-neoplastic foci development between control rats and animals that were given an oral administration of DHEA during initiation phase with the chemical carcinogen azaserine (AZA). However, during post-initiation, DHEA treatment produced almost one-and-one-half times more foci per cubic centimeter of pancreas and two times greater occupation of pancreas by focal lesions than control animals treated with AZA alone. At the time of their report, this lab was completing the present study. The findings of our investigation corroborate those of Thornton *et al.*[30] and also provide new evidence that DHEA treatment can produce paradoxical effects on health. In the present investigation, we present evidence that shows DHEA unequivocally promotes pre-neoplastic pancreatic lesions in AZA-treated animals that also were in a nutritional state of negative energy balance produced by an elevation in energy metabolism. These results are particularly dramatic and noteworthy since in previous experiments with this model, Roebuck *et al.*[6] found that when food intake is restricted, the number and size of pancreatic acidophilic foci and neoplasms are significantly less than those in AZA-treated animals fed *ad libitum*. In this paper we will also discuss mechanisms that may explain the apparent promotional and paradoxical effects of DHEA administration on body fatness and carcinogenesis.

II. Materials and Methods

A. Chemicals

Azaserine [AZA CAS:115-02-6; diazoacetate serine ester; Calbiochem-Behring, La Jolla, CA] is an established carcinogen for the pancreas of the rat.[9,18] Dehydroepiandrosterone acetate (Sigma, St. Louis, MO) was added to the diet (6 g DHEA/kg diet or 0.6%).

B. Animals and Treatment Conditions

Lactating Lewis females (Charles River Breeding Laboratories, Inc., Wilmington, MA) with litters comprised of all male pups of 9 days of age were fed a purified diet AIN-76A.[31] At 14 days of age, the pups were initiated ip with a single dose of AZA (30 mg/kg body weight) and weaned at 21 days of age and randomly assigned to one of three post-initiation test groups. For the entire 4-month post-initiation phase, an AIN-76A diet modified to contain 20% unsaturated fat as corn oil,[32] was fed either 1) *ad libitum* (*ad lib* control), 2) *ad libitum* with 0.6% (by weight) DHEA acetate added (DHEA group), or 3) pair-fed to the consumption of the DHEA-supplemented group (PF control). The *ad lib* control group was part of a companion experiment but it was added to this study to permit assessment of the effect of the moderate reduction in food intake expected from the inclusion of DHEA in the diet of the experimental animals. However, we believe the more appropriate control to the DHEA-supplemented group is the PF control group because the pancreas is responsive to food intake.

The rats were housed individually in wire-bottom cages equipped with tunnel feeders and collectors for measuring food spillage. The animals were maintained under reverse 12-h light-dark schedule (0600-1800 hours) at 25°C and 50% relative humidity and were fed fresh food every other day. Food intake was determined every other day and body weights were recorded two times weekly.

At the end of 16 weeks, animals were euthanized by gas inhalation and length from nose to base of tail was measured. Pancreas, kidney, spleen, and epididymal and perirenal fat depots were excised and weighed. Pancreas was fixed in Bouin's solution for analysis by light microscopy. Carcasses (minus pancreas) were weighed, ground, homogenized, and lyophilized for chemical analysis of protein, fat, and moisture using the methods reported previously.[33] Carcass energy was calculated by multiplying total fat and crude protein by their caloric equivalent of 9.45 and 5.4 kcal/g, respectively.

C. Energy Expenditure

Animals were tested individually by indirect calorimetry using methods reported previously.[17] Resting energy expenditure (REE) of fasted animals was measured for 6 hours. (1000-1600 hours) (FREE) and for 14 hours following consumption of a 5-g meal (FDREE). Resting energy expenditure of the DHEA and PF animals was measured individually during week 12 of the post-initiation phase. The thermic effect of food (TEF) is an index of efficiency of energy utilization and represents the increased rate in REE from the fasted to the fed state and was defined as follows:

$$TEF = \frac{FDREE - FREE \ (kcal/kg \ body \ wgt)}{meal \ size \ (kcal)} \times 100$$

D. Quantitative Analysis of Foci

Quantification of lesion number and size was done by light microscopy according to methods described in previous work by Roebuck et al.[34] Briefly, excised pancreas tissue was weighed and fixed in toto. Paraffin sections were cut and stained with hematoxylin and eosin. Atypical acinar cell lesions (i.e., transections of foci) in the tissue sections were measured with an X,Y-digitizing tablet. Two-dimensional measurements were subjected to the stereological calculations of Pugh et al.[35] as adapted for three-dimensional analysis of the pancreas.[33]

E. Statistical Analysis

This experiment resulted in grouped response variables [e.g., pancreatic foci (number and volume), carcass composition (fat, protein, ash), body size (length, mass)] normally exhibiting significant intercorrelations. For this reason, multivariate (MANOVA) statistical techniques were used to test for overall treatment effects, followed by univariate tests to suggest the source of the significant multivariate effects.[36]

III. Results

The DHEA group gained less body mass than the ad lib control or PF control groups (Table 1) and this is reflected in differences in both body length and final body mass between DHEA and PF control animals. The DHEA rats also ate less food than the ad lib-fed control group (12.0 g/day versus 15.2 g/day, respectively). Relative to the PF group, the

DHEA rats had 45% smaller perirenal and 60% smaller (p<0.001) epididymal fat depots (MANOVA p<0.001). On the other hand, organ weights of the DHEA animals, when expressed relative to body mass, were heavier than for the PF controls (data not shown). In particular, liver (65%, p<0.03), kidney (14%, p<0.03), and spleen (22%, p<0.003) were heavier than the PF. On an absolute basis, the pancreas weight (Table 1) of the DHEA group was 29% lighter than that of the PF, but relative to total body mass, the pancreas weights were similar between groups.

Histologically, the acidophilic and basophilic foci observed did not differ from previous observations of these lesions.[32,34] The observed two-dimensional data are shown to demonstrate that large numbers of foci were induced, observed, and measured (Table 2). Statistical analysis of the two-dimensional data is inappropriate.[34,35] The number of basophilic foci was too small to allow accurate calculations of their three-dimensional values. The three-dimensional analysis of the focal volume revealed no difference between the DHEA and PF control groups for the basophilic foci. With respect to the acidophilic foci, the DHEA rats compared to the PF group had significantly more foci per cubic centimeter of pancreas (p=0.01) and more foci per pancreas though not achieving statistical significance. The size of the foci did not differ between groups. The volume of pancreas occupied by foci was significantly greater (p=0.02) in the DHEA group vs. the PF control group. MANOVA of these two variables showed a significant difference (p<0.02). There were no significant differences in either number of lesions or volume occupied by lesions per cubic centimeter between the PF and *ad lib* control groups.

Energy and fat tissue metabolism were evaluated in the DHEA and PF groups. Fasted, fed REE and TEF are shown in Table 3. Rats of the DHEA group had a significantly higher REE in both fasted and fed states as compared to their respective PF control group. However, TEF was not different between DHEA and control rats.

Body composition of the three groups is shown in Figure 1. There was a significant difference in the percentage of body mass as fat, protein, and ash associated with DHEA treatment (MANOVA p<0.001). There were no significant differences in body composition due to food intake (Table 1). On a percentage basis, fatness of the DHEA animals was lower (ANOVA p<0.001) and fat-free components, protein (ANOVA p<0.001), and ash (ANOVA p<0.002), were higher than for the PF and *ad lib* groups. All differences between the DHEA and PF animals were significant. Similarly, the energy content of DHEA carcasses was significantly less (p<0.001) than that of the PF and *ad lib* animals. The carcass contents of the three groups were 549 ± 32 mean + SEM, 742 ± 65, and 1169 ± 42 kcal, respectively. There was no difference in carcass energy content between PF and *ad libitum* groups.

Table 1. Food Intake, Growth Changes, and Pancreas Weight

Experimental group[a]	Rats per group	Food intake (g/day)	Length (mm) crown-rump	Final BW (g)	BW gain (g)	Pancreas total (g)
Ad libitum control	10	15.2	–	451±8	421.0±8	1.16±.03
DHEA	8	12.0	20.81±0.7[b]	271±7	202.3±17	0.69±.06
Pair-fed control	6	12.6	23.33±0.7	406±6	322.5±11	0.97±.09
p values[c]		–	<0.001	<0.001	<0.001	<0.02

[a] All rats were fed a purified diet of 20% unsaturated fat as a modified AIN-76A diet.
[b] All values are mean ± SEM.
[c] Two-tail t-test of DHEA vs. pair-fed groups.

Table 2. Effects of DHEA on the Development of Pancreatic Foci Induced by AZA

Experimental group	Observed transectional data of foci			Calculated volumetric data			
	No. observed per animal	No. per cm^2	Mean area (mm^2 x 100)	No. per cm^3	No. per pancreas	Mean focal diameter (μm)	Volume as percent of pancreas
Acidophilic phenotype							
1. *Ad libitum*	21.5 ± 2.3[a]	16.8 ± 1.6	13.0 ± 0.0	372 ± 57	433 ± 57	462 ± 23	2.2 ± 0.2
2. DHEA	25.4 ± 3.1	21.6 ± 2.1	12.0 ± 1.1	602 ± 105	423 ± 85	386 ± 25	2.6 ± 0.4
3. Pair-fed	15.5 ± 2.7	11.6 ± 2.7	11.8 ± 2.4	338 ± 59	278 ± 60	405 ± 41	1.6 ± 0.6
p value[b]				0.013	ns	ns	0.04
0.05 Basophilic phenotype							
1. *Ad libitum*	4.9 ± 0.8	3.6 ± 0.7	2.2 ± 0.3	—[c]	—	—	0.08 ± 0.02
2. DHEA	1.4 ± 0.5	1.1 ± 0.3	2.5 ± 0.5	—	—	—	0.03 ± 0.02
3. Pair-fed	3.2 ± 1.4	2.1 ± 0.9	1.6 ± 0.3	—	—	—	0.04 ± 0.02
p values							ns

[a] All values are mean ± SEM.
[b] Two tail, t-test of group 2 vs. group 3.
[c] Too few foci were present to accurately calculate these values.

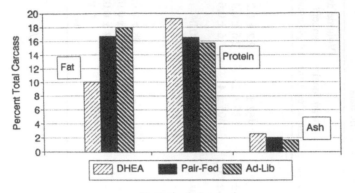

Statistical Analysis
Significant effect due to DHEA (p<0.01) on each component
No significant effect due to diet regime
DHEA vs. PF groups: Significant difference on each component

Figure 1. Carcass percentage of fat, crude protein, and ash of DHEA, PF, and *ad libitum* animals.

Table 3. Resting Energy Expenditure and Thermic Effect of Food of DHEA and Pair-Fed Groups[a]

Group	REE[b]		TEF(%)[c]
	Fasted	Fed	
DHEA n = 8	26.3 ± 1.6	32.4 ± 1.8	36.86 ± 10.7
Pair-fed n = 6	17.9 ± 1.4	25.0 ± 1.9	24.25 ± 8.6
p values[d]	<0.002	<0.018	ns

[a] All values are mean ± SEM.
[b] kcal/kg BW.
[c] TEF = $\dfrac{\text{FDREE–FREE}}{\text{meal size (kcal)}}$ (kcal/kg BW) x 100.

[d] Two tail t-test.

IV. Discussion

The findings of the present investigation corroborate closely with those of Thornton *et al.*[30] who reported almost a 1.5-fold increase in the density of pre-neoplastic focal lesions and a two-fold increase in the percentage of the pancreas occupied by lesions among animals treated with 0.6% DHEA in the diet. In the present study, we found that DHEA treatment increased the number of lesions by 78% and the percentage of pancreas occupied by lesions by 75%. The experimental protocols used in the present study and that of Thornton *et al.*[30] were quite similar. The difference in magnitude of effects of DHEA on foci development between the present study and that of Thornton *et al.*[30] is due largely to the choice of a control group. Thornton *et al.*[30] compared the DHEA group to an *ad libitum*-fed control group. Because DHEA suppresses growth of the rat, the appropriate control group is one initiated with azaserine and restricted in its rate of growth. Although the PF controls ate the same amount of food as the DHEA group, their efficiency of growth was greater. In future experiments, another control would be a group paired in body weight and not food intake. Additionally, Thornton et al.[30] based their measurement of focal lesions on observed two-dimensional procedure focal data. For theoretical reasons outlined by Pugh et al.,[35] the likelihood of bias in measurements of carcinogen-induced foci as observed in tissue sections is high. The stereologic techniques used in the present study to quantitate carcinogen-induced foci minimized the likelihood of that error.

The present findings also confirm the fact that the promotional effects of DHEA on pre-neoplastic lesions were produced in a nutritional state of negative energy balance. That is, young, growing animals were given an oral administration of DHEA mixed in their diets or pair-fed the same amount of food for 4 months. The DHEA animals were 12% shorter, weighed 50% less, and were 6.5% less fat (i.e., 10.2 vs. 16.7% body fat) than the PF animals. Energy expenditure of the DHEA group in the fasted state was 48% higher than that of the PF, which would indicate that DHEA treatment had increased the energy requirements of the animals. The heavier weights observed in liver, spleen and kidney of the DHEA vs. PF animals are consistent with this interpretation. Although FDREE of the DHEA animals was greater than PF, the differences in TEF between groups was not significant due to the high variance within treatment groups. These findings indicate that DHEA treatment did not affect the efficiency of energy production as might be predicted based on other findings that show DHEA stimulates peroxisomal metabolism,[37] substrate cycling,[38] and other bioenergetically wasteful mechanisms.[39] The study of this component of energy metabolism warrants further investigation.

It is known that a mild restriction of food intake will inhibit the development of azaserine-induced pre-neoplastic pancreatic foci. Therefore, it would be expected that a state of negative energy balance created by an increase in energy expenditure would have produced a similar inhibitory effect on foci development. However, the paradoxical effects

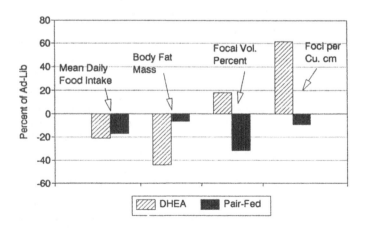

Figure 2. Summary of differences in food intake, body fat gain, and foci development between DHEA (hatched bars) and PF (solid bars) in reference to *ad libitum* animals. A value of 0.0 would indicate no difference from *ad libitum* group.

of DHEA on energy balance and pancreatic cancer summarized in Figure 2 clearly suggest that being in negative energy balance may not be as important as the mechanism(s) through which that nutritional state is achieved for reducing the risk of pancreatic cancer development.

We suggest that the mechanism that may explain DHEA's promotion of pre-neoplastic pancreatic lesions induced by AZA treatment is linked either to the androgenic properties of the steroid, or its effect on lipid metabolism, or both, since the functional properties of androgens and lipid metabolism are not independent of each other.

Dehydroepiandrosterone is a weak androgen, possessing approximately 25% of the potency of testosterone. The chemical model of carcinogenesis used in the present study has been shown to be dependent upon testosterone for pancreatic acidophilic foci development.[40] However, the specific role of this hormone in pancreatic carcinogenesis is not known. Sauer and Dauchy have shown *in vivo* that growth of transplanted hepatic tumors in rats were stimulated dramatically in response to the release of fatty acids induced either by an acute fast[41] or chemically induced diabetes.[42] In two unpublished studies completed recently in our laboratory, we found that DHEA treatment in rats and swine significantly elevated serum fatty acids and their oxidation. We also found that the rate of fatty acid turnover (as measured by glycerol release) measured at basal levels and in response to stimulation by the beta agonist, isoproterenol (10^{-5}M) from isolated adipocytes was significantly greater following DHEA treatment than placebo-treated controls. Xu *et al.*[43] have shown in an *in vitro* study that preadipocytes, exposed to testosterone in primary culture, had an increased capacity for lipolysis in response to isoproterenol or norepinephrine stimulation, and also an increased number of beta-adrenergic receptors on cell membranes. Since exogenous DHEA is converted readily to testosterone,[44] it is possible that in the present study a sufficient amount of DHEA may have been converted to testosterone itself, or mimicked closely the action of that hormone to affect fat cell lipolysis in a similar way.

Another possible mechanism worthy of consideration is the biochemical effects of DHEA on peroxisomal and microsomal metabolism. Dehydroepiandrosterone treatment stimulates the proliferation of peroxisomes in liver.[37,38] We believe that the proliferative response of peroxisomes is related to the influx of fatty acids also induced by DHEA treatment. However, unlike mitochondria, beta oxidation in peroxisomes is not coupled to energy production. Hence, energy is wasted as heat, which would explain in part the elevation in REE. Another mechanism that could explain the apparent promotional effects of DHEA is related to the production of hydrogen peroxide (H_2O_2), a toxic metabolite of peroxisomal beta oxidation. The concentration of H_2O_2 is minimized by the action of several protective enzymes, including catalase in peroxisomes and glutathione peroxidase in the cytosol and mitochondria of cells of several animal tissues.[45] In the case of the latter enzyme, H_2O_2 is reduced readily by the reduced form of glutathione to form water. The chemical reduction of glutathione is dependent upon available NADPH. Concomitantly, DHEA treatment also induces an increase in enzymatic activity of microsomal cytochrome P-450 mono-oxygenase system in liver.[46] This hepatic multiple-enzyme system is normally involved in the detoxification of drugs, carcinogens, the desaturation of fatty acids, as well as the introconversion of steroid hormones. Activity of this microsomal enzyme system is dependent upon available NADPH. Therefore DHEA treatment stimulates simultaneously both glutathione and cytochrome P-450 enzyme activity, to compete for the same limited pool of reducing equivalents that are generated by the HMP. Under these metabolic conditions, the antioxidative capacity of glutathione peroxidase to reduce cellular levels of H_2O_2 would be limited. In the present study, hydroperoxidation by hydroxyl radicals may have exacerbated further the damage or the dysfunction in nuclear and cytosolic processes, that already would have been initiated by AZA.

Common effects of DHEA treatment include hepatomegaly, increased peroxisomal density, and enzyme activity.[47] Those characteristic features resemble quite closely those of other known peroxisome proliferators, particularly the hypolipidic agent, clofibric acid[38] and several of its analogues.[48] Long-term treatment with these agents has been shown to produce hepatocarcinogenesis in rodents.[48] In the present investigation, and that of Thornton *et al.*,[30] there was no evidence of hepatocarcinogenesis in AZA-treated animals. Dehydroepiandrosterone promoted pre-neoplastic lesions only in pancreas. We suspect that the apparent involvement of the pancreas and not liver with foci development does not represent an exclusive effect of DHEA on pancreas. Rather, the promotion of lesions by DHEA may have appeared first in the pancreas since it is a primary target organ for AZA. Also, the experiment was relatively short in duration (4 months), and therefore lesions in the liver may not have been detected. An experiment designed to answer this question is in progress.

In summary, DHEA is a steroid with multiple effects. In view of the fact that there is serious interest in adopting DHEA and its analogues[49] as agents to treat several human conditions including obesity, hypercholesteremia, diabetes mellitus, and chemoprevention of cancer, it is paramount that its mechanism(s) of action and metabolic effects be elucidated first.

Acknowledgments

Authors wish to thank Ms. Kathy Kelley and Janice Warren for their assistance in the preparation of this manuscript. These studies were supported in part from scientific contribution number 1699 New Hampshire Agricultural Experiment Station Project H285 and grant 88A29 from the American Institute for Cancer Research to B.D. Roebuck. Address correspondence to Anthony R. Tagliaferro, Department of Animal and Nutritional Sciences, University of New Hampshire, Durham, NH 03824.

References

1. Cancer In: U.S. Dept of Health and Human Services, Public Health Service, DHHS (PHS) Publication No. 88-50210, *The Surgeon General's Report on Nutrition and Health.* U.S. Government Printing Office, Washington, DC (1988).
2. A. Tannenbaum, Initiation and growth of tumors. I. effects of underfeeding, *Amer. J Cancer.* 38:335 (1940).
3. M.J. Tucker, The effects of long-term food restriction on tumors in rodents, *Int J Cancer.* 23:803 (1979).
4. D. Kritchevsky and D.M. Klurfeld, Calorific effects on experimental mammary tumorigenesis, *Am J Clin Nutr.* 45:236 (1987).
5. M.W. Pariza, Fat, calories and mammary carcinogenesis: net energy effects, *Am J Clin Nutr.* 45:261 (1987).
6. B.D. Roebuck, J.D. Yager, D.S. Longnecker, and S.A. Wilpone, Promotion by unsaturated fat on azaserine-induced pancreatic carcinogenesis in the rat, *Cancer Res.* 41:3961 (1981).
7. G.B. Gordon, L.M. Shantz, and P. Talalay, Modulation of growth, differentiation and carcinogenesis by dehydroepiandrosterone. *Advances in Enzyme Regulation.* 26:355 (1987).
8. N. Orentreich, J.L. Brind, L. Rizer, and J.H. Vogelman, Age changes and sex differences in serum dehydroepiandrosterone sulfate concentrations throughout adulthood, *J Clin Endocrinal Metab* 59:551 (1984).
9. J. Sonka, Dehydroepiandrosterone metabolic effects. *Acta Universitatis Carolinae Medica.* 71:1 (1976).
10. E. Barrett-Connor, K. Khaw, and S.S.C. Yen, A prospective study of dehydroepiandrosterone sulfate, mortality and cardiovascular disease, *N Engl J Med.* 315:1519 (1986).
11. M.P. Cleary, Antiobesity effect of dehydroepiandrosterone in the Zucker rat, *in:* "Hormones and Thermogenesis and Obesity," H. Lardy and F. Strathan, eds., Elsevier, New York (1989).

12. A.G. Schwartz, Inhibition of spontaneous breast cancer formation in female C3H (A^vy/a) mice by long-term treatment with dehydroepiandrosterone, *Cancer Res.* 39:1129 (1979).

13. A.G. Schwartz and R.H. Tanner, Inhibition of 7,12-dimethylbenz(a)anthracene- and urethan-induced lung tumor formation in A/J mice by long-term treatment with dehydroepiandrosterone, *Carcinogenesis.* 2:1335 (1981).

14. J.W. Nyce, P.N. Magee, G.C. Hard, and A.G. Schwartz, Inhibition of 1,2-dimethylhydrazine-induced colon tumorigenesis in Balb/c mice by dehydroepiandrosterone, *Carcinogenesis.* 5:57 (1984).

15. Y. Arad, J. Badimon, and L. Badimon, Dehydroepiandrosterone feeding prevents aortic fatty streak formation and cholesterol accumulation in cholesterol-fed rabbits, *Arteriosclerosis,* 9:159 (1989).

16. M.P. Cleary, A. Shepherd, and B. Jenks, Effect of dehydroepiandrosterone on growth in lean and obese Zucker rats, *J Nutr.* 114:1242 (1984).

17. A.R. Tagliaferro, J.R. Davis, S.T. Truchon, and N. Van Hamont, Effects of dehydroepiandrosterone acetate on metabolism, body weight and composition of male and female rats, *J Nutr.* 116:1977 (1986).

18. J.E. Nestler, C.O. Bartascini, J.N. Clore, and W.G. Blackard, Dehydroepiandrosterone effects on insulin sensitivity, serum lipids levels, and body composition in normal men, *in*: "Hormones and Thermogenesis and Obesity," H. Lardy and R. Stratman, eds., Elsevier, New York (1989).

19. K.S. Usiskin, S. Butterworth, J.N. Clore, Y. Arad, H.N. Ginsberg, W.G. Blackard, and S.E. Nestler, Lack of effect of dehydroepiandrosterone in obese men, *International J of Obesity,* 14:457 (1990).

20. C.W. Boone, G.J. Kelloff, and W.E. Malone, Identification of candidate chemopreventative agents and their evaluation in animal models and human clinical trials: a review, *Cancer Res.* 50:2 (1990).

21. S. Welle, R. Jozefowicz, and M. Statt, Failure of dehydroepiandrosterone to influence energy and protein metabolism in humans, *J. Clin. Endocrinol Metab.* 71:1259 (1990).

22. D.L. Coleman, Therapeutic effects of dehydroepiandrosterone and its metabolites in diabetes-obesity mutants, *in*: "Hormones and Thermogenesis and Obesity," H. Lardy and R. Stratman, eds., Elsevier, New York (1989).

23. P.A. Marks and J. Banks, Inhibition of mammalian glucose-6-phosphate dehydrogenase by steroids, *Proc. Natl. Acad. Sci. USA* 46:447 (1960).

24. A.C. Finan and M.D. Cleary, Lack of an effect of short-term dehydropeiandrosterone treatment on the pentose pathway, *Nutrition Res.* 8:755 (1988).

25. J.P. Casazza, W.T. Schaeffer, and R.L. Veech, The effect of dehydroepiandrosterone on liver metabolites, *J Nutr.* 116:304 (1986).

26. H.M. Tepperman, S.A. De La Garza, and J. Tepperman, Effects of dehydroepiandrosterone and diet protein on liver enzymes and lipogenesis, *Am J Physiol.* 214:1126 (1968).

27. D.A. Diersen-Schadue and M.P. Cleary, No effect of long-term DHEA treatment on either hepatocyte and adipocyte pentose pathway activity or adipocyte glycerol release, *Horm Metabol Res.* 21:356 (1988).

28. M.P. Cleary, The antiobesity effect of dehydroepiandrosterone in rats, *Proc Soc Exp Biol Med.* 196:8 (1991).

29. W.G. Beamer, K.L. Shultz, and B.J. Tennent, Induction of ovarian granulosa cell tumors in SWXJ-9 mice with dehydroepiandrosterone, *Cancer Res.* 48:2788 (1988).

30. M. Thornton, M.A. Moore, and N. Ito, Modifying influence of dehydroepiandrosterone or butylated hydroxytoluene treatment on initiation and development states of azaserine-induced acinar pancreatic preneoplastic lesions in the rat, *Carcinogenesis.* 10:407 (1989).

31. Report of the American Institute of Nutrition *Ad Hoc* Committee on Standards for Nutritional Studies, *J Nutr.* 107:1340 (1977).

32. B.D. Roebuck, D.S. Longnecker, K.J. Baumgartner, and C.D. Thron, Carcinogen-induced lesions in the rat pancreas: effects on varying levels of essential fatty acid, *Cancer Res.* 45:5252 (1985)

33. H.J. Thompson, A.M. Ronan, K.A. Ritacco, A.R. Tagliaferro, and L.D. Meeker, Effect of exercise on the induction of mammary carcinogenesis, *Cancer Res.* 48:2720 (1988).

34. B.D. Roebuck, K.J. Baumgartner, and C.D. Thron, Characterization of two populations of pancreatic atypical acinar cell foci induced by azaserine in the rat, *Lab Invest.* 50:141 (1984).

35. T.D. Pugh, J.H. King, H. Koen, D. Nuchka, J. Chover, G. Wahba, Y. He, and S. Goldfarb, Reliable stereological method for estimating the number of microscopic hepatocellular foci from their transections, *Cancer Res.* 43:1261 (1983).

36. G.W. Snedecor and W.G. Cochran, "Statistical Methods," Ed 6. University of Iowa Press, Ames, IA. (1967).

37. B. Leighton, A.R. Tagliaferro, and E.A. Newsholme, The effect of dehydroepiandrosterone acetate on liver peroxisomal enzyme activities of male and female rats, *J Nutr.* 117:1287 (1987).

38. P.F. Mohan and M.P. Cleary, Comparison of dehydroepiandrosterone and clofibric acid treatment in obese Zucker rats, *J Nutr.* 119:496 (1989).

39. H. Lardy, S. Ching-yuan, N. Kneer, and S. Wielgus, Dehydroepiandrosterone induces enzymes that permit thermogenesis and decrease metabolic efficiency, *in*: "Hormones and Thermogenesis and Obesity," H. Lardy and R. Stratman, eds., Elsevier, New York (1989).

40. C. Sumi, D.S. Longnecker, B.D. Roebuck, and T. Brinck-Johnsen, Inhibitory effects of estrogen and castration on the early stage of pancreatic carcinogenesis in Fischer rats treated with azaserine, *Cancer Res.* 49:2332 (1989).

41. L.A. Sauer, W.O. Nagel, R.T. Dauchy, L.A. Miceli, and J.E. Austin, Stimulation of tumor growth in adult rats *in vivo* during an acute fast, *Cancer Res.* 46:3469 (1986).

42. L.A. Sauer and R.T. Dauchy, Stimulation of tumor growth in adult rats *in vivo* during acute streptozotocin-induced diabetes, *Cancer Res.* 47:1756 (1987).

43. X. Xu, G. DePergola, and P. Bjorntorp, The effects of androgens on the regulation of lipolysis in adipose precursor cells, *Endocrinology.* 126:1229 (1990).

44. E.H. Leiter, W.G. Beamer, D.L. Coleman, and C. Longscope, Androgenic and estrogenic metabolites in serum of mice fed dehydroepiandrosterone: relationship to antihyperglycemic effects, *Metabolism.* 36(9):863 (1987).

45. A. Meisler, Glutathione metabolism and its selective modification, *J Biol Chem.* 263 (33):17205 (1988).

46. H. Wu, J. Masset-Brown, D.J. Tweedie, L. Milewich, and R.A. Frenkel, Induction of microsomal NADPH-cytochrome P-450 reductose and cytochrome P-450IVA1 (p-450 LACO) by dehydroepiandrosterone in rats: a possible peroxisomal proliferator, *Can Res* 49:2337 (1989).

47. R.A. Frenkel, C.A. Slaughter, K. Orth, C.R. Moomaw, and S.H. Hicks, Peroxisome proliferation and induction of peroxisomal enzymes in mouse and rat liver by dehydroepiandrosterone feeding, *J. Steroid Biochem.* 35(2):333 (1990).

48. M.S. Rao and J.K. Reddy, Peroxisome proliferation and hepatocarcinogenesis. *Carcinogenesis.* 8(5):631 (1987).

49. A.G. Schwartz, D.K. Fairman, M. Polansky, M.L. Lewbart, and L.L. Pashko, Inhibition of 7,12-dimethylbenz(a)anthracene-initiated and 12-0-tetradecanoylphorbol-13-acetate promoted skin papilloma formation in mice by dehydroepiandrosterone and two synthetic analogs, *Carcinogenesis.* 10(10):1809 (1989).

Chapter 12

Caloric Restriction and Experimental Carcinogenesis

DAVID KRITCHEVSKY

I. Introduction

Concern over effects of over-nutrition on carcinogenesis is not new. Almost 70 years ago Hoffman[1,2] attributed the rise in cancer incidence of the time to an excess of caloric intake.

Experimentally, Moreschi[3] in 1909 reported that under-feeding of mice bearing a transplanted sarcoma inhibited growth of the tumor. A few years later Rous[4] showed that under-feeding inhibited the development of both spontaneous and transplanted tumors in mice. Sugiura and Benedict[5] showed, in 1926, that under-feeding affected tumor growth in rats as well as mice. Bischoff et al.[6] found that 50% dietary restriction retarded tumor growth in mice. In response to the justifiable criticism that severe dietary restriction could cause deficiencies in some growth factors that could, in turn, be the true cause (rather than reduced calories) of tumor growth they carried out a second study to show that growth inhibition was indeed due to caloric restriction per se.[7]

II. Caloric Restriction and Carcinogenesis

A. Inhibition of Spontaneous, Transplanted, or Induced Tumors

The first systematic investigation into effects of under-feeding on carcinogenesis was begun by Tannenbaum[8] who showed that reduced food intake could inhibit the development of spontaneous mammary tumors in mice (Table 1). Tannenbaum later instituted a type of caloric restriction and showed that this modality, too, could inhibit both spontaneous (mammary or lung) or induced tumors in several strains of mice.[9] Tannenbaum used a diet that consisted of dog or fox chow, skim milk powder, and corn starch and deleted the corn starch to effect caloric restriction. The first study using a scientifically prepared semi-purified diet was carried out by Boutwell et al.[10] who confirmed the effects of caloric restriction.

David Kritchevsky ● The Wistar Institute, 3601 Spruce Street, Philadelphia, Pennsylvania

Exercise, Calories, Fat, and Cancer, Edited by M.M. Jacobs
Plenum Press, New York, 1992

Table 1. Effects of Under-feeding on Carcinogenesis[a]

Mouse strain	Carcinogen	Site	Duration (weeks)	No. of tumors Full fed	No. of tumors Under-fed
ABC	BP	Skin	67	22	7
Swiss	BP	Skin	26	24	6
C57	BP	Subq.	34	36	22
DBA[b]	Spont.	Breast	64	13	3
DBA[c]	Spont.	Breast	56	20	1

[a] After Tannenbaum.[8]
[b] 12 virgin, 32 parous females.
[c] 50 virgin females.

B. Combined Effects of Dietary Fat and Caloric Restriction on Carcinogenesis

Lavik and Baumann[11] compared the separate effects of calories and fat on methylcholanthrene-induced skin tumors in mice. They found (Table 2) that a diet low in fat but high in calories led to almost twice the incidence of skin tumors as did a diet high in fat but low in calories. Albanes[12] analyzed the data relating to caloric intake and incidence of both induced and spontaneous tumors in 82 experiments in mice. His findings (Table 3) are remarkably similar to those of Lavik and Baumann.[11] On the average caloric intake was 29% lower and tumor incidence was 42% less than in *ad libitum* groups. At the lowest level of caloric intake ($\leq$ 8 kcal/day) incidence of mammary tumors was reduced by about 79% and that of skin tumors by 46%. A number of reviews have demonstrated thoroughly that caloric restriction will reduce the incidence of spontaneous, transplanted, or induced tumors in mice and rats.[12-15] Two studies merit mention. Giovanella *et al.*[16] have shown that caloric restriction inhibits growth of transplanted human tumors in nude mice and Ohno and Cardullo[17] have reported that caloric restriction inhibits the effects of Rauscher leukemia virus in mice.

Our own work has concentrated on the effects of 7,12-dimethylbenz(a)anthracene (DMBA)-induced mammary tumors in female Sprague-Dawley rats and on 1,2-dimethylhydrazine (DMH)-induced colon tumors in male F344 rats. We found that 40% caloric restriction inhibited both types of tumor[18,19] and confirmed the observation of Carroll and

Table 2. Influence of Calories and Fat on Methylcholanthrene-Induced Skin Tumors in Mice[a]

Regimen Calories	Regimen Fat	Tumor incidence (%)
Low	Low	0
Low	High	28
High	Low	54
High	High	66

[a] After Lavik and Baumann.[11]

Table 3. Caloric Intake and Tumor Incidence in Mice (82 Experimental Groups)[a]

| Regimen | | Experiments (no.) | Tumor incidence (%) |
Calories (kcal/day)	Fat (g/day)		
7.1 ± 0.3	0.08 ± 0.02	23	34.4 ± 4.3
8.1 ± 0.3	0.19 ± 0.02	19	23.1 ± 4.7
10.8 ± 0.3	0.04 ± 0.02	18	52.4 ± 4.7
12.0 ± 0.2	0.19 ± 0.02	22	54.4 ± 3.4

[a] After Albanes.[12]

Khor[20] that unsaturated fat was more co-carcinogenic than saturated fat. Boissonneault *et al.*[21] compared dietary effects in three groups of DMBA-treated rats. One group was fed a high-fat diet (30% corn oil) *ad libitum*. They ingested 7.9 ± 0.6 g of diet daily (40.7 kcal/day) and exhibited a tumor incidence of 73%. A second group was fed a low-fat diet (5% corn oil) *ad libitum*. This group ingested 11.0 ± 0.9 g of food daily (42.5 kcal/day) and had a tumor incidence of 43%. The third group was fed the high-fat diet but their intake was restricted to 6.8 ± 0.7 g/day (34.8 kcal/day) and their tumor incidence was only 7%.

In order to determine the limits of our system we examined the degree of energy restriction required for effective suppression of DMBA-induced tumorigenesis.[22] We compared the effects of 10, 20, 30, and 40% caloric restriction using a diet providing 5% corn oil (12.3, 40.0, 16.0, 18.4, and 22.0% of calories in *ad libitum* or 10, 20, 30, or 40% energy-restricted diets, respectively). The results (Table 4) show that 10% caloric restriction did not affect tumor incidence, but reduced tumor multiplicity and tumor burden by 36 and 47%, respectively. Energy restriction by 20% led to a significant reduction in tumor incidence, and tumor multiplicity and burden were reduced by 40 and 53% compared to the *ad libitum*-fed group. At 30% restriction, tumor incidence was 42% below that of the control group, tumor multiplicity was 72% lower, and tumor burden was 91% lower.

The effects of caloric restriction in DMBA-treated rats fed high-fat diets was also tested.[23] Rats were fed diets containing 5, 15, or 20% fat *ad libitum* or were energy restricted by 25% and fed diets containing 20 or 26.7% fat. Thus the two restricted groups received exactly as much fat daily as the *ad libitum*-fed rats given 15 or 20% fat. Despite their fat intake the restricted groups showed lower tumor incidence and tumor burden than

Table 4. Degree of Energy Restriction and DMBA-Induced Mammary Tumorigenesis[a]

Group	Incidence (%)	Multiplicity[b]	Tumor burden (g)
Ad lib	60	4.7 ± 1.3	10.1 ± 3.3
10% Restricted	60	3.0 ± 0.8	5.4 ± 3.0
20% Restricted	40	2.8 ± 0.7	4.7 ± 1.9
30% Restricted	35	1.3 ± 0.3	0.9 ± 0.8
40% Restricted	5	1.0	–
p	<0.005	NS	<0.05

[a] After Klurfield *et al.*[22]
[b] Tumors/tumor-bearing rat.

Table 5. Inhibition of DMBA-Induced Mammary Tumorigenesis in Rats Fed High-fat Diets[a]

Group	Incidence (%)	Multiplicity[b]	Tumor burden (g)
Ad libitum			
5% corn oil	65	1.9 ± 0.3	4.2 ± 1.9
15% corn oil	85	3.0 ± 0.6	6.6 ± 2.7
20% corn oil	80	4.1 ± 0.6	11.8 ± 3.2
Restricted (25%)			
20% corn oil	60	1.9 ± 0.4	1.5 ± 0.5
26.7 corn oil	30	1.5 ± 0.3	2.3 ± 1.6

[a]After Klurfield *et al.*[22]
[b]Tumors/tumor-bearing rat.

the rats ingesting 5% fat *ad libitum* (Table 5). Beth *et al.*[24] have also found that energy restriction inhibits tumorigenesis independently of dietary fat level.

Must caloric restriction be imposed early in life? Weindruch and Walford[25] showed that caloric restriction instituted in 1-year-old mice retarded development of spontaneous tumors. Tannenbaum[26] showed that energy restriction inhibited spontaneous tumorigenesis in mice when instituted at 2, 5, or 9 months of age (Table 6). We[27] tested effects of caloric restriction for different periods during the promotion phase of DMBA-induced mammary tumorigenesis and found varying effects with tumor incidence being significantly correlated with weight gain, total caloric intake, and feed efficiency (Table 7). Ross and Bras[28] studied rats fed *ad libitum* or 33% calorically restricted and a third group that was subjected to restriction for only 7 weeks post-weaning. The severely restricted rats lived about 40% longer than the other groups and had 90% fewer tumors, which would be expected. The very short-term post-weaning restriction resulted in an almost 40% decrease in incidence of benign tumors (Table 8).

C. Exercise, Caloric Restriction, and Carcinogenesis

Another means of increasing caloric flux is exercise. Rusch and Kline[29] showed that exercise (cage rotation) could decrease the weight of a transplanted tumor by about 30%.

Table 6. Effect of Age at which Caloric Restriction Was Instituted on Spontaneous Mammary Tumors in DMBA Mice[a]

Age at which restriction commenced (months)	Incidence (%) at 20 months	
	Restricted	*Ad libitum*
2	0	38
5	2	40
9	5	25

[a] After Tannenbaum.[26]

Table 7. DMBA-Induced Mammary Tumor Incidence in Rats Subjected to Variable Caloric Restriction[a]

Regimen[b]	Incidence (%)	Weight gain (g)	Caloric intake	FE x 10^{2c}
A-A-A-A	50	156	7508	2.08
R-R-R-R	20	76	5624	1.35
R-A-A-A	60	152	7401	2.05
R-R-A-A	40	126	6746	1.87
A-R-R-A	45	126	6691	1.88
A-A-R-R	30	99	6958	1.42
Correlation with incidence, r		0.96	0.83	0.94

[a] After Kritchevsky et al.[27]
[b] A = *ad libitum*; R = restricted. Each letter = 1 month.
[c] FE = feed efficiency (weight gain/caloric intake).

Table 8. Early Caloric Restriction and Tumor Risk in Rats[a]

	Group[b]		
	L	R	R-AL
Last survivor (days)	<1000	<1500	<1000
Avg. food intake (g)[c]	18.2 ± 0.42	5.5 ± 0.30	15.6 ± 0.86
Tumor incidence[d]			
Benign	100	6.0	50.9
Malignant 100	100	6.5	84.1

[a] After Ross and Bras.[28]
[b] AL = *ad libitum*; R = restricted; R-AL = restricted from day 21 of life to day 70, then *ad lib*.
[c] After day 70.
[d] AL taken as 100%.

Cohen et al.[30] found that voluntary exercise reduced the incidence of N-methylnitrosourea-induced mammary tumors in rats but the extent of inhibition was not correlated with the number of cage rotations. We[31] compared effects of vigorous treadmill exercise with caloric restriction incidence of colon cancer in DMH-treated rats. Exercise halved tumor incidence in *ad libitum*-fed rats and was equivalent to 25% caloric restriction (Table 9). Others[32, 33] have also found exercise to inhibit experimentally induced carcinogenesis. However, Thompson et al.[34,35] have found treadmill exercise to enhance DMBA-induced mammary tumorigenesis. Energy restriction and exercise may not be of equal value. Goodrick et al.[36] compared the two means of reducing energy availability and concluded that insofar as longevity of rats is concerned intermittent feeding had a positive effect even when instituted in mature rats but voluntary exercise had an early effect beyond which no increases in longevity were observed.

Table 9.   Influence of Caloric Restriction ± Treadmill Exercise on DMH-Induced Colon
Tumors in Male F344 Rats[a]

Regimen[b]		Tumor incidence	Multiplicity[c]
Diet	Exercise[d]	(%)	
AL	−	75	2.1 ± 0.4
AL	+	36	1.3 ± 0.2
CR (25%)	−	35	1.3 ± 0.2
CR (25%)	+	29	1.1 ± 0.1
CR (40%)	−	21	1.2 ± 0.2

[a] After Klurfield et al.[31]
[b] AL = *ad libitum*; CR = calorically restricted.
[c] Tumors/tumor-bearing rat.
[d] Treadmill 20 meters/min at 7° incline, 60 min/day, 5 day/week.

III. Proposed Mechanisms for Inhibition of Tumorigenesis by Caloric Restriction

There are several mechanisms by which energy restriction could influence tumorigenesis and these are not mutually exclusive. Boutwell et al.[37] suggested that the pituitary-adreno-corticotropic axis was stimulated by caloric restriction resulting in adrenal hypertrophy and reduced uterine and ovarian size in female rats (pseudohypophysectomy). Caloric restriction reduces cellular proliferation and mitotic activity[38,39] and prolongs cell-mediated immuni-ty.[40,41] Energy restriction may influence levels of circulating mammotrophic hormones and thus influence mammary tumorigenesis.[42-44] Energy restriction can also lead to enhanced DNA repair[45] and has been shown to reduce oncogene expression.[46,47]

Ross et al.[48] have suggested that among the nutritional factors that could enhance spontaneous tumorigenesis in rats were high levels of food intake, rapid growth in early post-natal life, and high feed efficiency at puberty. Limited nutrient availability can limit progression of neoplastic cells.[49,50]

The specific effects of insulin and its deprivation on tumor growth and cell division are well documented.[51-53] In our studies (Table 10) plasma insulin levels were shown to decrease significantly under energy restriction regimens that led to significant reduction in mammary tumor incidence.[22,23] This effect was also demonstrable in genetically obese rats.[54] Levels of plasma insulin in rats declined almost immediately after institution of caloric restriction[55] and did not rebound over the duration of the study (4 months).

How does any of this relate to man? Early menarche and tall stature, both of which are influenced by nutritional status, have been correlated with increased risk of breast and other cancers.[56-61] In 1975 Berg[62] suggested that the cancers prevalent in developed countries might be due, in part, to overnutrition and suggested the term "cancers of affluence." Weindruch et al.[63] reviewed seven case-control studies in which the connection between caloric intake and risk of cancer were addressed. Five of the studies found a positive association[64-68] and two[69,70] found negligible differences.

Colon cancer risk has been shown to be enhanced significantly in men in sedentary occupations.[71-77] Participation in college athletics has been found to carry the benefit of reduced cancer risk by some authors[78] but not by others.[79,80] It is of interest that men who were letter winners in major varsity sports were found to have shorter lives than their non-athlete classmates, but men who participated in minor sports or who had not won letters in

Table 10. Effect of Caloric Restriction on Plasma Insulin Levels

Experimental groups	Insulin (mU/ml)	Reference
Ad libitum (5% fat)	122 ± 16	22
30% restricted	42 ± 5	
40% restricted	41 ± 8	
Ad libitum		23
5% fat	143 ± 16	
15% fat	164 ± 15	
20% fat	158 ± 11	
Restricted (25%)		
20% fat	100 ± 12	
26.7% fat	117 ± 13	
Ad libitum (obese)	1003 ± 193	54
40% restricted (obese)	328 ± 41	

major sports had the longest lives.[81] Lew and Garfinkel[82] examined the relationship between mortality and body weight in 750,000 men and women and found over-weight people to be at greatly increased risk of death. Cancer mortality was elevated in those probands who were 40% or more overweight.[83] A more recent study (in 868,620 persons) again shows risk of death to be elevated in obese subjects but also finds standard mortality ratios to be decreased by exercise.[84] In 1945 Potter[85] suggested reduced caloric intake and exercise as possible means of preventing cancer. It would appear as if moderation in diet as well as in exercise is the appropriate suggestion.

Acknowledgment

Supported, in part, by a Research Career Award (HL 00734) and a grant (CA 43856) from the National Institutes of Health and by funds from the Commonwealth of Pennsylvania.

References

1. F.L. Hoffman, "Cancer and Civilization," Prudential Insurance Co., Newark, NJ (1923).
2. F.L. Hoffman, "Cancer Increase and Overnutrition," Prudential Insurance Co, Newark, NJ (1927).
3. C. Moreschi, Beziehungen zwischen ernährung und tumorwachstum, *Z Immunitätsforsch* 2:651 (1909).
4. P. Rous, The influence of diet on transplanted and spontaneous mouse tumors, *J Exp Med.* 20:433 (1914).
5. K. Sugiura and S.R. Benedict, The influence of insufficient diets upon tumor recurrence and growth in mice, *Am J Cancer.* 10:309 (1926).
6. F. Bischoff, M.L. Long, and L.C. Maxwell, Influence of caloric intake upon the growth of Sarcoma 180, *Am J Cancer.* 24:549 (1935).
7. F. Bischoff and M.L. Long, The influence of calories *per se* upon the growth of Sarcoma 180, *Am J Cancer.* 32:418 (1938).

8. A. Tannenbaum, The initiation and growth of tumors. Introduction I. Effects of under-feeding, *Am J Cancer*. 38:335 (1940).

9. A. Tannenbaum, The genesis and growth of tumors II. Effects of caloric restriction *per se*, *Cancer Res*. 2:460 (1942).

10. R.K. Boutwell, M.K. Brush, and H.P. Rusch, The stimulating effect of dietary fat on carcinogenesis, *Cancer Res*. 9:741 (1949).

11. P.S. Lavik and C.A. Baumann, Further studies on tumor-promoting action of fat, *Cancer Res*. 3:749 (1943).

12. D. Albanes, Total calories, body weight and tumor incidence in mice, *Cancer Res*. 47:1987 (1987).

13. D. Kritchevsky and D.M. Klurfeld, Influence of caloric intake on experimental carcinogenesis. A review, *Adv Exp Med Biol*. 206:55 (1986).

14. M.W. Pariza, Caloric restriction, *ad libitum* feeding and cancer, *Proc Soc Exp Biol Med*. 183:293 (1986).

15. D. Kritchevsky and D.M. Klurfeld, Caloric effects on experimental mammary tumorigenesis, *Am J Clin Nutr*. 45:236 (1987).

16. B.C. Giovanella, R.C. Shepard, J.S. Stehlin, J.M. Venditti, and B.J. Abbott, Caloric restriction: Effect on growth of human tumors heterotransplanted in nude mice, *J Nat Cancer Inst*. 68:249 (1982) .

17. T. Ohno and A.C. Cardullo, Effect of caloric restriction on neoplasm growth, *Mt Sinai J Med*. 50:338 (1983).

18. D. Kritchevsky, M.M. Weber, and D.M. Klurfeld, Dietary fat versus caloric content in initiation and promotion of 7,12-dimethylbenz(a)anthracene-induced mammary tumorigenesis in rats, *Cancer Res*. 44:3174 (1984).

19. D.M. Klurfeld, M.M. Weber, and D. Kritchevsky, Inhibition of chemically-induced mammary and colon tumor promotion by caloric restriction in rats fed increased dietary fat, *Cancer Res*. 47:2759 (1987).

20. K.K. Carroll and H.T. Khor, Effect of level and type of dietary fat on incidence of mammary tumors induced in female Sprague-Dawley rats by 7,12-dimethylbenz(a)anthracene, *Lipids*. 6:415 (1971).

21. G.A. Boissonneault, C.E. Elson, and M.W. Pariza, Net energy effects of dietary fat on chemically induced mammary carcinogenesis in F344 rats, *J Nat Cancer Inst*. 76:335 (1986).

22. D.M. Klurfeld, C.B. Welch, M.J. Davis, and D. Kritchevsky, Determination of degree of energy restriction necessary to reduce DMBA-induced mammary tumorigenesis in rats during the promotion phase, *J Nutr*. 119:286 (1989).

23. D.M. Klurfeld, C.B. Welch, L.M. Lloyd, and D. Kritchevsky, Inhibition of DMBA-induced mammary tumorigenesis by caloric restriction in rats fed high-fat diets, *Int J Cancer*. 43:922 (1989).

24. M. Beth, M.R. Berger, M. Aksoy, and D. Schmähl, Comparison between the effects of dietary fat level and of caloric intake on methylnitrosourea- induced mammary carcinogenesis in female SD rats, *Int J Cancer*. 39:737 (1987).

25. R. Weindruch and R.L. Walford, Dietary restriction in mice beginning at 1 year of age: Effect on life-span and spontaneous cancer incidence, *Science*. 215:1415 (1982).

26. A. Tannenbaum, Effects of varying caloric intake upon tumor incidence and tumor growth, *Ann NY Acad Sci*. 49:5 (1947).

27. D. Kritchevsky, C.B. Welch, and D.M. Klurfeld, Response of mammary tumors to caloric restriction for different time periods during the promotion phase, *Nutr Cancer*. 12:259 (1989).

28. M.H. Ross and G. Bras, Lasting influence of early caloric restriction on prevalence of neoplasms in the rat, *J Nat Cancer Inst*. 47:1095 (1971) .

29. H.P. Rusch and B.E. Kline, The effect of exercise on the growth of a mouse tumor, *Cancer Res*. 4:116 (1944).

30. L.A. Cohen, K. Choi, and C-X. Wang, Influence of dietary fat, caloric restriction, and voluntary exercise on N-Nitrosomethylurea-induced mammary tumorigenesis in rats, *Cancer Res*. 48:4276 (1988).

31. D.M. Klurfeld, C.B. Welch, E. Einhorn, and D. Kritchevsky, Inhibition of colon tumor promotion by caloric restriction or exercise in rats, *FASEB J.* 2:A433 (1988)

32. C. Moore and P.W. Tittle, Muscle activity, body fat, and induced rat mammary tumors, *Surgery.* 73:329 (1973).

33. B.D. Roebuck, J. McCaffrey, and K.J. Baumgartner, Protective effects of voluntary exercise during the postinitiation phase of pancreatic carcinogenesis in the rat, *Cancer Res.* 50:6811 (1990).

34. H.J. Thompson, A.M. Ronan, K.A. Ritacco, A.R. Tagliaferro, and L.D. Meeker, Effect of exercise on the induction of mammary carcinogenesis, *Cancer Res.* 48:2720 (1988).

35. H.J. Thompson, A.M. Ronan, K.A. Ritacco, and A.R. Tagliaferro, Effect of type and amount of dietary fat on the enhancement of rat mammary tumorigenesis by exercise, *Cancer Res.* 49:1904 (1989).

36. C.L. Goodrick, D.K. Ingram, M.A. Reynolds, J.R. Freeman, and N.L. Cider, Differential effects of intermittent feeding and voluntary exercise on body weight and lifespan in adult rats, *J Gerontol.* 38:36 (1983).

37. R.K. Boutwell, M.K. Brush, and H.P. Rusch, Some physiological effects associated with chronic caloric restriction, *Am J Physiol.* 154:517 (1949).

38. A. Koga and S. Kimura, Influence of restricted diet on the cell renewal of the mouse small intestine, *J Nutr Sci Vitaminol.* 25:265 (1979).

39. A. Koga and S. Kimura, Influence of restricted diet on the cell cycle in the crypt of mouse small intestine, *J Nutr Sci Vitaminol.* 26:33 (1980).

40. D.G. Jose and R.A. Good, Quantitative effects of nutritional protein and caloric deficiency upon immune responses to tumors in mice, *Cancer Res.* 33:807 (1973).

41. R.H. Weindruch, B.H. Devens, H.V. Raff, and R.L. Walford, Influence of dietary restriction on aging and natural killer cell activity in mice, *J Immunol.* 130:933 (1983).

42. P.W. Sylvester, C.F. Aylsworth, and J. Meites, Relationship of hormones to inhibition of mammary tumor development by under-feeding during the "critical period" after carcinogen administration, *Cancer Res.* 41:1383 (1981).

43. P.W. Sylvester, C.F. Aylsworth, D.A. van Vogt, and J. Meites, Influence of under-feeding during the "critical period" or thereafter on carcinogen-induced mammary tumors in rats, *Cancer Res.* 42:4943 (1982).

44. N.H. Sarkar, G. Fernandes, N.T. Telang, I.A. Kourides, and R.A. Good, Low calorie diet prevents the development of mammary tumors in C3H mice and reduces circulating prolactin levels, murine mammary tumor virus expression and proliferation of mammary alveolar cells, *Proc Nat Acad Sci (USA).* 79:7758 (1982).

45. J.M. Lipman, A. Turturro, and R.W. Hart, The influence of dietary restriction on DNA repair in rodents: A preliminary study, *Mech Aging Dev.* 48:135 (1989).

46. G. Fernandes, A. Khare, S. Langamere, B. Yu, L. Sandberg, and B. Fredericks, Effect of food restriction and aging on immune cell fatty acids, functions and oncogene expression in SPF Fischer 344 rats, *Fed Proc.* 46:567 (1987).

47. K.D. Nakamura, P.H. Duffy, M-S. Lu, A. Turturro, and R.W. Hart, The effect of dietary restriction on MYC protooncogene expression in mice: A preliminary study, *Mech Aging Dev.* 48:199 (1989).

48. M.H. Ross, E.D. Lustbader, and G. Bras, Body weight, dietary practices and tumor susceptibility in the rat, *J Nat Cancer Inst.* 71:1041 (1983).

49. L. Lagopoulos and R. Stalder, The influence of food intake on the development of diethylnitrosamine-induced liver tumors in mice, *Carcinogenesis.* 8:33 (1987).

50. B.A. Ruggeri, D.M. Klurfeld, and D. Kritchevsky, Biochemical alterations in 7,12-dimethylbenz(a)anthracene-induced mammary tumors from rats subjected to caloric restriction, *Biochim Biophys Acta.* 929:239 (1987).

51. J-C. Henson and N. Legros, Influence of insulin deprivation on growth of the 7,12-dimethylbenz(a)anthracene-induced mammary carcinoma in rats subjected to alloxan diabetes and food restriction, *Cancer Res.* 32:226 (1972).

52. N.D. Cohen and R. Hilf, Influence of insulin on growth and metabolism of 7,12-dimethylbenz(a)anthracene-induced mammary tumors, *Cancer Res.* 34:3245 (1974).

53. R. Taub, A. Roy, R. Dieter, and J. Koontz, Insulin as a growth factor in rat hepatoma cells, *J Biol Chem.* 262:10893 (1987).

54. D.M. Klurfeld, L.M. Lloyd, C.B. Welch, M.J. Davis, O.L. Tulp, and D. Kritchevsky, Reduction of enhanced mammary carcinogenesis in LA/N-cp (Corpulent) rats by energy restriction, *Proc Soc Exp Biol Med.* 196:381 (1991).

55. B.A. Ruggeri, D.M. Klurfeld, D. Kritchevsky, and R.W. Furlanetto, Caloric restriction and 7,12-dimethylbenz(a)anthracene-induced mammary tumor growth in rats: Alterations in circulating insulin, insulin-like growth factors I and II, and epidermal growth factor, *Cancer Res.* 49:4130 (1989).

56. J. Staszewski, Age at menarche and breast cancer, *J Nat Cancer Inst.* 47:935 (1971).

57. F. DeWaard, Breast cancer incidence and nutritional status with particular reference to body weight and height, *Cancer Res.* 35:3351 (1975).

58. D. Apter and R. Vihko, Early menarche, a risk factor for breast cancer indicates early onset of ovulatory cycles, *J Clin Endocrinol Metab.* 57:82 (1983).

59. D. Albanes, D.Y. Jones, A. Schatzkin, M.S. Micozzi, and P.R. Taylor, Adult stature and risk of cancer, *Cancer Res.* 48:1658 (1988).

60. C.A. Swanson, D.Y. Jones, A. Schatzkin, L.A. Brinton, and R.G. Ziegler, Breast cancer risk assessed by anthropometry in the NHANES I epidemiological follow up study, *Cancer Res.* 48:5363 (1988).

61. D. Albanes and P.R. Taylor, International differences in body height and weight and their relationship to cancer incidence, *Nutr Cancer.* 14:69 (1990).

62. J.W. Berg, Can nutrition explain the pattern of international epidemiology of hormone-dependent cancer, *Cancer Res.* 35:3345 (1975).

63. R. Weindruch, D. Albanes, and D. Kritchevsky, The role of calories and caloric restriction in carcinogenesis, *Hematol/Oncol Clinics of No America.* 5:79 (1991).

64. A.B. Miller, A. Kelly, N.W. Choi, V. Mathews, R.W. Morgan, L. Munan, J.D. Burch, J. Feather, G.R. Howe, and M. Jain, A study of diet and breast cancer, *Am J Epidemiol.* 107:499 (1978).

65. M. Jain, G.M. Cook, F.G. Davis, M.G. Grace, G.R. Howe, and A.B. Miller, A case-control study of diet and colorectal cancer, *Int J Cancer.* 26:757 (1980).

66. J.B. Bristol, P.M. Emmett, K.W. Heaton, and R.C. Williamson, Sugar, fat and the risk of colorectal cancer, *Br Med J.* 291:1467 (1985).

67. J.L. Lyon, A.W. Mahoney, D.W. West, J.W. Gardner, K.R. Smith, A.W. Sorenson, and W. Stanish, Energy intake: Its relationship to colon cancer risk, *J Nat Cancer Inst.* 78:853 (1987).

68. S. Graham, B. Haughey, J. Marshall, J. Brasure, M. Zielezny, J. Freudenheim, D. West, J. Nolan, and G. Wilkinson, Diet in the epidemiology of gastric cancer, *Nutr Cancer.* 13:19 (1990).

69. G.N. Stemmermann, A.M.Y. Nomura, and L.K. Heilbrun, Dietary fat and the risk of colorectal cancer, *Cancer Res.* 44:4633 (1984).

70. S. Kune, G.A. Kune, and L.F. Watson, Case-control study of dietary etiological factors: The Melbourne colorectal cancer study, *Nutr Cancer.* 9:21 (1987).

71. D.H. Garabrant, J.M. Peters, T.M. Mack, and I. Bernstein, Job activity and colon cancer risk, *Am J Epidemiol* 119:1005 (1984).

72. J.E. Vena, S. Graham, M. Zielezny, M.K. Swanson, R.E. Barnes, and J. Nolan, Lifetime occupational exercise and colon cancer, *Am J Epidemiol.* 122:357 (1985).

73. M. Gerhardsson, S.E. Norell, H. Kiviranta, N.L. Pedersen, and A. Ahlbom, Sedentary jobs and colon cancer, *Am J Epidemiol.* 123:775 (1986).

74. M. Gerhardsson, B. Floderus, and S.E. Norell, Physical activity and colon cancer risk, *Int J Epidemiol.* 17:743 (1988).

75. M. Fredriksson, N-O. Bengtsson, L. Hardell, and O. Axelson, Colon cancer, physical activity and occupational exposures. A case-control study, *Cancer* 63:1838 (1989).

76. R. Ballard-Barbash, A. Schatzkin, D. Albanes, M.H. Schiffman, B.E. Kreger, W.B. Kannel, K.M. Anderson, and W.E. Helsel, Physical activity and risk of large bowel cancer in the Framingham study, *Cancer Res.* 50:3610 (1990).

77. R.S. Paffenbarger Jr., R.T. Hyde, A.L. Wing, and C-C. Hsieh, Physical activity, all-cause mortality and longevity of college alumni, *N Engl J Med.* 314:605 (1986).

78. R.E. Frisch, G. Wyshak, N.L. Albright, T.E. Albright, I. Schiff, K.P. Jones, J. Witschi, E. Shiang, E. Koff, and M. Marguglio, Lower prevalence of breast cancer and cancers of the reproductive system among former college athletes compared to non-athletes, *Br J Cancer.* 52:885 (1985).

79. H.J. Montoye, W.D. Van Huss, H. Olson, A. Hudee, and E. Mahoney, Study of the longevity and morbidity of college athletes, *J Am Med Assoc.* 162:1132 (1956).

80. A.P. Polednak, College athletics, body size and cancer mortality, *Cancer.* 38:382 (1976).

81. A.P. Polednak and A. Damon, College athletics, longevity and cause of death, *Human Biology.* 42:28 (1970).

82. E.A. Lew and L. Garfinkel, Variations in mortality by weight among 750,000 men and women, *J Chronic Dis.* 32:563 (1979).

83. L. Garfinkel, Overweight and cancer, *Ann Intern Med.* 103:1034 (1985).

84. L. Garfinkel and S.D. Stillman, Mortality by relative weight and exercise, *Cancer.* 62:1844 (1988).

85. V.R. Potter, The role of nutrition in cancer prevention, *Science.* 101:105 (1945).

Chapter 13

Breast Cancer — The Optimal Diet

ERNST L. WYNDER, EMANUELA TAIOLI and DAVID P. ROSE

I. Introduction

Epidemiologists are in general agreement that cancer is not an inevitable consequence of aging. Rather, as shown by the differences in incidence patterns and geographical distribution, many of the prevalent cancers relate to environmental causes associated with life-style and traditions. The same concept applies to the specific case of the epidemiology of cancer of the breast.

We have particularly focused on comparisons in cancer incidence and dietary habits between Japan and the U.S., since these populations have equally good vital statistics but show major differences in the incidence rate of hormone-related cancers (Figure 1).[1-3] Breast cancer incidence is much lower among Japanese women; the difference is most evident among post-menopausal women. It could be postulated that the Japanese are "genetically immune" against these cancers, but this argument does not hold since the incidence of these cancers increases rapidly among Japanese immigrants to the U.S.[4] Among the possible risk factors for breast cancer, reproductive variables have been suggested to have a major impact. As shown by various investigators[5] and confirmed by our own data base (Table 1), none of these factors alone can account for the difference in incidence between U.S. and Japanese women. Furthermore, because these factors are not readily modified, attention has to be focused on factors that are more amenable to change in order to be in a position to reduce risk based on key, intrinsic mechanisms.

Data on obesity show that for pre-menopausal women leanness is associated with a higher risk of breast cancer, while for post-menopausal women, the risk is slightly higher with increases in body weight.[6] Our data show the same results, after controlling for the possible confounding factors (Table 2). The occurrence of obesity could be a "marker" of excessive fat consumption because the energy density for fats is higher than it is for carbohydrates or proteins.

Ernst L. Wynder and Emanuela Taioli • American Health Foundation, Division of Epidemiology, 320 East 43 Street, New York, New York; David P. Rose • American Health Foundation, Division of Nutrition and Endocrinology, Valhalla, New York

Exercise, Calories, Fat, and Cancer, Edited by M.M. Jacobs
Plenum Press, New York, 1992

Table 1.   General Characteristics of the Study Population—Hospital Breast Cancer Cases and Matched Controls, American Health Foundation, 1988-1991

	Pre-menopausal women			Post-menopausal women		
	Cases	Controls	OR (95% CI)	Cases	Controls	OR (95% CI)
Education (years)	N	N		N	N	
≤ 12	35	50	1.0 (–)	199	148	1.0 (–)
13-16	91	88	1.5 (0.9–2.5)	138	125	0.8 (0.6–1.1)
≥ 17	70	53	1.9 (1.1–3.3)	83	66	0.9 (0.7–1.4)
Marital status						
Married	135	125	1.0 (–)	251	216	1.0 (–)
Single/divorced	51	52	0.9 (0.6–1.4)	75	54	1.2 (0.8–1.7)
Separated/widowed	10	14	0.7 (0.3–1.6)	94	69	1.2 (0.8–1.6)
Age at menarche (years)						
≤ 12	95	93	1.0 (–)	181	158	1.0 (–)
13	67	64	1.0 (0.7–1.6)	133	90	1.3 (0.9–1.8)
≥ 14	34	34	1.0 (0.6–1.7)	102	89	1.0 (0.7–1.4)
Age at first birth (years)						
< 22	30	31	1.0 (–)	64	58	1.0 (–)
22-25	49	37	1.4 (0.7–2.6)	109	90	1.1 (0.7–1.7)
≥ 26	61	60	1.1 (0.6–1.9)	157	138	1.0 (0.7–1.6)
Parity						
Yes	156	145		349	297	
No	39	46	0.2 (0.5–1.3)	70	41	1.5 (1.0–2.2)
Abortion						
Yes	73	73		122	112	
No	83	73	1.1 (0.7–1.8)	227	186	1.1 (0.8–1.6)

Source: American Health Foundation, 1991

II. The Evidence

The question then is: What is the evidence that a Western level of dietary fat increases the risk of breast cancer, particularly in post-menopausal women?   In part, the evidence stems from the correlation between the dietary fat intake and disappearance data and the geographic distribution of breast cancer.   This is particularly noteworthy in the Japanese data that show a very low intake of fat in the 1940s and 1950s and a corresponding low incidence of breast cancer compared with the United States.   Total fat intake in Japan as well as intake of foods rich in fats has risen progressively, but even today, it is significantly lower in Japan than in the U.S. (Figure 2; Table 3).[7-14]   Such ecologic comparisons do not allow any causal inference on individual risk, but they do contribute significantly to the generation of etiologic hypotheses.   The concept that dietary fat intake relates to breast cancer is supported by a large number of animal studies that record an effect not only of total fat but also of specific kinds of fat both in the promotion and progression of breast cancer.[15,16]

Table 2. Risk of Breast Cancer with Height, Weight and Body Mass by Menopausal Status

	Pre-menopausal			Post-menopausal		
	Cases (196)	Controls (191)	Adjusted RO* (95%CL)	Cases (421)	Controls (340)	Adjusted RO* (95%CL)
Height (cm)						
< 160	47	42	1.0	146	102	1.0
160–162.5	24	26	0.8 (0.4–1.7)	64	38	1.2 (0.8–1.8)
162.6–167.6	80	75	1.0 (0.6–1.6)	149	148	0.7 (0.5–1.0)
≥ 167.7	45	48	0.8 (0.5–1.5)	62	52	0.8 (0.5–1.3)
Weight (kg) 1 year before						
< 57.2	69	46	1.0	102	85	1.0
57.3–63.5	47	39	0.8 (0.4–1.3)	78	71	1.0 (0.6–1.5)
63.6–72.6	41	39	0.7 (0.4–1.2)	118	86	1.2 (0.8–1.8)
≥ 72.7	39	67	0.4 (0.2–0.7)	123	98	1.1 (0.7–1.6)
BMI (kg/m^2) 1 year before						
< 21	54	39	1.0	59	56	1.0
21–23	72	59	0.8 (0.5–1.4)	127	101	1.2 (0.8–2.0)
24-26	35	23	1.1 (0.5–2.1)	94	93	1.0 (0.6–1.6)
≥ 27	35	70	0.4 (0.2–0.6)	141	90	1.5 (1.0–2.3)
Change in weight after the age of 18						
Lost or inv.	51	40	1.0	86	74	1.0
+1–9 kg	61	65	0.7 (0.4–1.3)	1.7	94	1.0 (0.6–1.6)
+10–19 kg	57	45	1.1 (0.7–1.9)	136	100	0.8 (0.6–1.8)
+20+ kg	27	41	0.5 (0.3–1.0)	92	72	1.2 (0.8–2.0)

* Adjusted for age (cont), education (≤ 12, 13–16, 17+), age at menopause (≤ 12, 13, ≥ 14), pregnancies (Y/N), physical activity at the age 15–22 (Y/N).

Source: American Health Foundation, 1991.

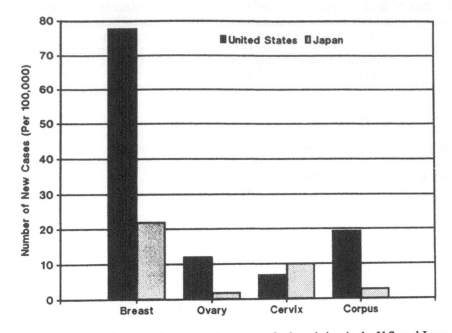

Figure 1. Age-standardized incidence rates for cancer of selected sites in the U.S. and Japan, 1980. Source: Reference 3.

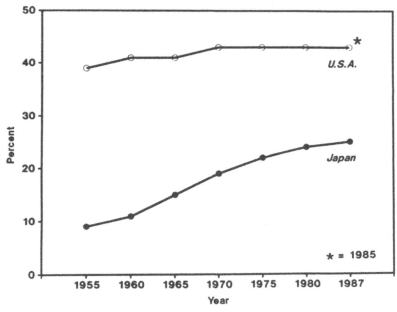

Figure 2. Percentage of total calories attributable to fat, by year, in the U.S. and Japan, 1955-1987. Sources: References 7, 8.

In general, it has been shown that the polyunsaturated fats, rich in linoleic acid (an omega-6 fatty acid), enhance the promotional stage of carcinogenesis and subsequent progression of experimental mammary cancer, whereas omega-3 fatty acid-containing fish oils exert a protective effect.[15,17-22]

Table 3. Net Per Capita Food Supply (g/day), 1934-1985

Food item		1934-1938	1951-1953	1955-1959	1960-1964	1965-1969	1970-1974	1975-1979	1982	1985
Cereal	U.S.	247	207	186	182	178	174	198	161	189
	Japan	444	430	422	410	380	346	325	305	297
Sugar &	U.S.	120	127	131	135	140	150	165	174	192
sweets	Japan	38	27	36	45	58	75	71	62	58
Potatoes &	U.S.	175	137	128	130	126	123	90	88	85
starches	Japan	173	155	121	92	75	66	71	83	90
Vegetables	U.S.	——	312	269	268	270	273	259	260	270
	Japan	——	190	229	281	322	318	356	358	298
Fruits	U.S.	——	289	210	195	194	196	201	190	191
	Japan	——	34	48	68	93	113	157	152	102
Red meat	U.S.	195	231	254	268	291	310	314	307	322
	Japan	11	8	14	26	42	63	84	97	105
Fats & oils	U.S.	55	52	57	57	66	66	82	85	91
	Japan	5	5	9	15	23	30	35	42	40
Eggs	U.S.	44	60	57	51	50	48	44	43	42
	Japan	8	7	12	24	33	40	44	46	41
Milk	U.S.	——	——	532	502	490	484	476[a]	——	——
products	Japan	——	——	25	44	67	82	87[a]	——	——
Fish	U.S.	14	14	17	17	17	19	20	19	20
	Japan	49	53	124	101	83	97	102	96	102

[a]1975 data only.
Source: References 7-14.

Saturated fats act as promoters only if a "threshold" amount of omega-6 fatty acid is present.[19] Cohen et al.[22] showed that there is also a threshold requirement for the level of corn oil (a dietary source of linoleic acid) when this is the sole source of fat in the diet. Using a chemically induced rat mammary carcinoma model, they found that isocaloric diets with 30% or 40% of the total calories coming from corn oil were equally effective in tumor promotion; in contrast, diets with 10% or 20% fat calories were equally ineffective.

Recent studies by Rose and co-workers have shown that the different types of fatty acids also influence human breast cancer cell growth and the expression of their metastatic potential. Experiments in vitro using culture in serum-free medium demonstrated a dose-dependent stimulatory effect of linoleic acid, whereas two omega-3 fatty acids inhibited tumor cell growth.[23, 24] In the nude mouse, the growth rate of breast cancer cells at the mammary fat pad inoculation site was stimulated by feeding a high-fat, linoleic acid-rich diet (23% corn oil) compared with a low-fat (5% corn oil) diet.[25] Moreover, the metastatic spread of these human cancer cells to the lymph nodes and lungs occurred more frequently, and was more extensive, in mice fed the high-fat diet. It should be stressed that the two diets used in this study were isocaloric, and that the body weight gains were similar in the two groups.

There is currently considerable interest in the relationship between dietary fiber intake and breast cancer risk.[16,26-30] Cohen et al.,[31] again using a chemically induced rat mammary tumor model, found that the addition of a wheat bran supplement to a 23% corn oil diet had a profound inhibitory effect on the tumor-promoting activity of the fat.

As we consider these large-scale animal studies, recently well reviewed by Galli and Butrum[32] we are surprised that when experimental studies show megadoses of a certain chemical to be carcinogenic in animals, our scientific peers and the media often regard such substance as a "probable" human carcinogen. But somehow when it concerns the effects of different types of fat and fiber, of which human intake can be equivalent in dosage to that used in animals to promote or protect against cancer, the animal data tend to be minimized or even ignored.

The question that needs to be addressed is whether the same relationships hold for dietary fat and human breast cancer in both its promotional and metastatic stages. The ongoing experiments using human breast cancer cells support this belief because of their consistency relative to the data from promotional studies in animal models. Similar support comes from a combination of epidemiologic and experimental studies. For example, the breast cancer incidence in southern Italy is relatively low despite a high intake of fat in the form of olive oil,[33] and this oil, rich in oleic acid, an omega-9 fatty acid, does not affect the promotional stage of mammary carcinogenesis in animal models.[15]

From an epidemiologic point of view, we note that there is an increase in the incidence of post-menopausal breast cancer and prostatic cancer in the United States, and question the extent to which this is due to improved early detection and/or increased use of unsaturated fatty acids in the U.S. diet and the relative contributions of these two factors.

While we have considerable data relative to the promotion and progression of breast cancer both from laboratory studies and descriptive and metabolic epidemiologic investigations, we are uncertain about factors that lead to the initiation of breast cancer. Petrakis has suggested a role for cholesterol epoxide,[34] whereas recent work by Sugimura, Weisburger, Felton, and Adamson[35-38] suggests a role for heterocyclic amines. In these instances, the contribution of epidemiology is limited, particularly as far as heterocyclic amines are concerned. These mainly result from frying and broiling of meat, but in the Western world any independent effect of frying and broiling is difficult to assess because of the confounding effect of fat intake.

The potential benefit of a low-fat diet on human breast cancer growth may involve several pathways. Although dietary fat does not appear to have a significant effect on blood estrogens in the rat[39,40] a 50% reduction in total fat intake does cause a significant decrease in serum estradiol and estrone in women[41-43] as does also a dietary wheat bran supplement such that the total daily intake is approximately doubled to 30 g/day.[44] But, the results of the data on nude mouse experiments, referred to earlier, also demonstrate that dietary fat, and specifically omega-6 polyunsaturated fatty acids, can also affect metastatic growth by mechanisms other than those involving the estrogens. Thus, the human breast cancer cells used in this study are estrogen independent and, moreover, the nude mouse is deficient in estrogens.

In conflict with the experimental and animal data are several case-control studies, as well as the prospective study by Willett,[6] that show no correlation between dietary intake and breast cancer. However, in these cases, the lowest fat intake of American women was about 30% of calories, a level at which animal tests likewise displayed an incidence of breast cancer similar to that observed with an intake of fat at 40% of total calories. However, with dietary fat at a level of 20% of calories, the incidence of mammary cancer in the rat model was sharply lower.[22] Thus, the human and laboratory observations suggest that 30% fat calories, so far the official recommendation of a number of bodies, will not serve to lower breast cancer risk. We think, in agreement with the view expressed by Hegsted, that nutritional assessment in a homogenous population such as the U.S. are unlikely to make significant contributions to understanding whether and how diet relates to cancer.[45] It is important to recognize that a control group sampled from such a population is necessarily "exposed" and at high risk since virtually everyone is on a high-fat diet.[46] Other problems that have to be considered are the numerous measurement errors inherent in nutritional assessment, such as recall problems, errors in estimating and reporting portion sizes, and the individual variability in diet over lifetime. We believe, therefore, that carrying out nutritional assessments in homogenous populations is a relatively useless exercise. A possibly more productive approach may be in determining so-called "indicator" foods.[47] For example, breakfast habits appear to be a good indicator of dietary fat consumption. Resnicow showed in children the influence of breakfast eating on cholesterol levels, with those who do not eat breakfast regularly having the highest values of cholesterol.[48] A study of over 11,000 adults from NHANES revealed that those who consumed cereals had a lower fat and cholesterol intake during the day than non-cereal eaters.[49,50] In a study on college students, those who ate a low-fat breakfast continued to eat less fat throughout the day compared with those who ate a high-fat breakfast.[51] Moreover, we have shown that among post-menopausal women the risk of breast cancer is 50% higher among women who either did not eat breakfast or who consume a high-fat breakfast compared with those consuming a low-fat breakfast (Taioli *et al.*, American Health Foundation, unpublished data, 1991). It may be possible that having no breakfast is associated with fewer meals being taken per day. Finally, a "nibbling" or "grazing" type of dietary pattern, when multiple small meals are consumed through the day, may have different, and beneficial, effects on metabolic parameters than does a bolus type of eating pattern.[52] The latter is likely to occur when only one or two meals per day are consumed.

III. The Optimal Diet and Its Implementation in Clinical Practice

The key question both from an epidemiologic and intervention point of view is to define the optimal diet. "Optimal" can be defined as a diet that can prevent disease and/or reduce its recurrence, yet is relatively acceptable to the population. McDougal has suggested a diet of less than 5% fat of total calories,[53] Pritikin recommended about 10% fat,[54] but an ideal diet in the sense that it would probably lead to the lowest risk of disease might not be acceptable to most persons. For this reason, we are proposing a diet for adjuvant therapy in post-menopausal breast cancer patients of about 15% fat of total calories and a diet for the population at large of about 20-25%. In terms of fiber intake, we suggest about 25 g/day with half of the fibers being insoluble, even though an optimal fiber intake in terms of disease prevention might be in excess of 40 g/day (Table 4). The question of the relative role of different types of fat in human breast cancer etiology and progression presents an as yet unanswered challenge to both the laboratory investigator and the epidemiologist.

It has been shown by Heber[55] that a 10% fat diet will reduce the plasma estradiol in post-menopausal women by about 50%. The data in the Women's Intervention Nutrition Study (WINS),[56] an intervention trial aimed at reducing the recurrence rate of Stage I and II breast cancer in post-menopausal women within 6 months after standard therapy, are showing an average reduction of the plasma estradiol of 20%, which has been sustained for over 18 months on a diet that has about 20-24% of its calories as fat (Rose *et al.*, American Health Foundation, unpublished observations, 1991). The data from this trial also show a reduction of 25% in plasma free fatty acids. The effect that diet has on post-menopausal breast cancer might be duplicated in pre-menopausal women who have undergone ovarian ablation. We have previously suggested that if the early studies testing the possible effect of such ablation on survival of pre-menopausal patients had been accompanied by a low-fat diet, the outcome might have been more favorable.[57] Clinical trials among these patients should be considered.

The WINS trial has demonstrated that breast cancer patients can be accrued to a low-fat diet. Our experience has taught us that the accrual rate depends largely on direct involvement by the principal investigators to the extent to which they have direct control of these

Table 4. The "25-25" Diet (calories from fat: 25%; total dietary fiber: 25g)

	kcal	Fat (g)	Fiber (g)
Breakfast			
2/3 cup bran flake cereal	90	0.4	5.0
1/2 cup low-fat (1%) milk	51	1.2	0
1 slice whole wheat toast	59	1.0	2.1
1 tsp soft margarine	34	3.8	0
1 banana	105	0.5	4.1
1 cup coffee	8	0.2	0
Snack			
2 fig bars	106	1.9	2.0
1 cup coffee	8	0.2	0
Lunch			
1 cup minestrone soup	83	2.5	1.7
1 tuna sandwich:			
water-packed tuna	116	2.0	0
on rye bread w/	131	1.8	2.4
1 tsp low calorie mayonnaise	7	0.7	0
tomatoes and lettuce	5	0	0.6
1/2 cup low-fat (1%) milk	51	1.2	0
1/2 cup melon	28	2.0	0.8
Snack			
1 cup ice milk			
Dinner			
3 oz skinless turkey breast	223	4.6	0
1/4 cup gravy-fat skimmed			
1 baked potato w/	115	0.6	0
1 tbsp soft margarine	2	0	0
1 green salad w/	115	0	3.1
1 tbsp olive oil/vinegar	101	11.0	0
1 cup stir fried vegetables w/	32	0	0.8
2 tsp olive oil	59	6.7	0
1 slice angel food cake w/	46	0.4	0.6
sliced peaches (1 peach)	80	9.0	0
Total (approximate values)	142	0.1	—
	37	0.1	1.4
	1834	52	25

Source: American Health Foundation, 1991

patients. We have demonstrated that the majority of patients will comply with the diet. As to be expected, the greater the intervention by the nutritionist the more likely the patient will comply. In this case as in therapy in general, it is the effective dose that makes for the success. We would certainly like to determine the survival outcome, particularly among post-menopausal breast cancer patients, in medical practices that are able to maintain these patients on a 5-10% fat diet although in such a multicenter, national trial this goal is unlikely to be attained with uniformity. Now that we have completed the feasibility phase of the WINS study, we expect to go into the outcome phase, which has been designed to determine whether a 15% fat diet as an adjuvant to surgery additional to chemotherapy and endocrine therapy will improve the recurrence rate and survival of patients on such a regimen. In subsequent trials, the addition to a low-fat diet of wheat fiber supplements should also be considered.

IV. Summary

In summary, the evidence based upon global and metabolic epidemiology, and animal studies supported by biologic understanding of the various mechanisms in which dietary fat can affect promotion and progression of breast cancer supports the concept that dietary fat, in particular, certain types of fat, and dietary fiber affect the causation, promotion, and progression of breast cancer. The epidemiologic evidence of the link between breast cancer and dietary fat is still controversial due to methodological problems in designing a valid test. Also a number of studies dealt with the question of fat intake in pre-menopausal women, where admittedly the association is weak. What now needs to be done is to verify the effect of a low-fat diet in post-menopausal breast cancer patients. We suggest that a similar trial on pre-menopausal breast cancer patients in conjunction with ovarian ablation should be conducted. The question to be considered is what in terms of dose, type, and duration of fat and fiber will be required to obtain a measureable effect on the recurrence rate and survival of breast cancer patients.

Acknowledgments

Research described herein was supported in part by U.S.P.H.S., National Cancer Institute grants CA-32617 and CA-45504, and American Cancer Society Special Institutional Grant (SIG-8).

References

1. E.L. Wynder, Y. Fujita, R.E. Harris, T. Hirayama, and T. Hiyama, Comparative epidemiology of cancer between the United States and Japan: a second look, *Cancer.* 67:746 (1991).
2. E.L. Wynder and T. Hirayama, Comparative epidemiology of cancers in the United States and Japan, *Prev Med.* 6:567 (1977).
3. World Health Organization (WHO), "Cancer Incidence in Five Continents, vol. IV," International Agency for Research on Cancer (IARC), Lyon, France (1982).
4. T. Hirohata, Shifts in cancer mortality from 1920 to 1970 among various ethnic groups in Hawaii, *in*: "Genetic and Environmental Factors in Experimental and Human Cancer," H.V. Gelboin, M. MacMahon, T. Matsushima, and T. Sugimura, eds., Japan Sci. Soc. Press, Tokyo, Japan (1980).
5. J. Kelsey and M. Gammon, Epidemiology of breast cancer, *Epidemiol Rev.* 12:228 (1990).
6. W.C. Willett, M.J. Stampfer, G.A. Colditz, B.A. Rosner, C.H. Hennekens, and F.E. Speizer, Dietary fat and the risk of breast cancer, *New Engl J Med.* 316:22 (1987).
7. U.S. Bureau of Census: Statistical Abstract of the United States, U.S. Govt. Printing Office, Washington, DC (1988).
8. Ministry of Health and Welfare of Japan: Vital Statistics, Tokyo Ministry of Health and Welfare of Japan, Tokyo, Japan (1986).
9. Japan National Bureau of Tax. The Annual Report of Statistics, Japan National Bureau of Tax, Tokyo, Japan (1986).
10. Food and Agriculture Organization of the United Nations: Production Year Book, 1955. United Nations Publication, Rome (1956).
11. Food and Agriculture Organization of the United Nations: Production Year Book, 1981. United Nations Publication, Rome (1982).
12. Food and Agriculture Organization of the United Nations: Production Year Book, 1987. United Nations Publication, Rome (1988).
13. Organization of Economic Cooperation and Development: Food Consumption Statistics, 1955-1973. Organization for Economic Cooperation and Development, Paris (1975).

14. E.L. Wynder, Y. Fujita, R.E. Harris, T. Hirayama, and T. Hiyama, Comparative epidemiology of cancer between the United States and Japan: a second look, *in*: "Epidemiology and Prevention of Cancer," R. Sasaki and K. Aoki, eds., The University of Nagoya Press, Nagoya, Japan, (1990).

15. L.A. Cohen, D.O. Thompson, Y. Maeura, K. Choi, and M.E. Blank, Dietary fat and mammary cancer. Promoting effects of different dietary fats on N-nitrosomethylurea-induced mammary tumorigenesis, *J Natl Cancer Inst*. 77:33 (1986).

16. L.A. Cohen, M.E. Kendall, E. Zang, C. Meschter, and D.P. Rose, Modulation of N-nitrosomethylurea-induced mammary tumor promotion by dietary fiber and fat, *J Natl Cancer Inst*. 83:497 (1991).

17. K.K. Carroll and H.T. Khor, Dietary fat in relation to tumorigenesis, *Progr Biochem Pharmacol*. 10:308 (1975).

18. K.K. Carroll and L.M. Braden, Dietary fat and mammary carcinogenesis, *Nutr Cancer*. 6:254 (1985).

19. C. Ip, C.A. Carter, and M.M. Ip, Requirement of essential fatty acid for mammary tumorigenesis in the rat, *Cancer Res*. 45:1997 (1985).

20. L.A. Hillyard and S. Abraham, Effect of dietary polyunsaturated fatty acids on growth of mammary adenocarcinomas in mice and rats, *Cancer Res*. 39:4430 (1979).

21. J.J. Jurkowski and W.T. Cave, Jr., Dietary effects of menhaden oil on the growth and membrande lipid composition of rat mammary tumors, *J Natl Cancer Inst*. 74:1145 (1985).

22. L.A. Cohen, K. Choi, J.H. Weisburger, and D.P. Rose, Effect of varying proportions of dietary fat on the development of *N*-nitrosomethylurea-induced rat mammary tumors, *Anticancer Res*. 6:215 (1986).

23. D.P. Rose and J.M. Connolly, Stimulation of growth of human breast cancer cell lines in culture by linoleic acid, *Biochem Biophys Res Commun*. 164:277 (1989).

24. D.P. Rose and J.M. Connolly, Effects of fatty acids and inhibitors of eicosanoid synthesis on the growth of a human breast cancer cell line in culture, *Cancer Res*. 50:7139 (1990).

25. D.P. Rose, J.M. Connolly, and C.L. Meschter, Effect of dietary fat on human breast cancer growth and lung metastasis in nude mice, *J Natl Cancer Inst*. 83:1491 (1991)

26. H. Adlercreutz, T. Fotsis, R. Heikkinen, J.T. Dwyer, M. Woods, B.A. Goldin, and S.L. Gorbach, Excretion of the lignans entrolactone and enterodiol and of equol in omnivorous and vegetarian postmenopausal women and in women with breast cancer, *Lancet*. ii:1295 (1982).

27. S.L. Gorbach, Estrogens, breast cancer and intestinal flora, *Rev Infect Dis*. 6 (suppl 1):S85 (1984).

28. S.L. Gorbach and B.R. Goldin, Diet and the excretion and enterohepatic cycling of estrogens, *Prev Med*. 16:525 (1987).

29. D.P. Rose, Dietary fiber and breast cancer, *Nutr Cancer*. 13:1 (1990).

30. D.P. Rose, Dietary fiber, phytoestrogens and breast cancer, *Nutrition*. 8:47 (1992).

31. L.A. Cohen, M.E. Kendall, E. Zang, C. Meschter, and D.P. Rose, Modulation of NMU-induced mammary tumor promotion by dietary fiber and fat, *J Natl Cancer Inst*. 83:496 (1991).

32. C. Galli and R. Butrum, Dietary omega-3 fatty acids and cancer, an overview, *World Rev Nutr Diet*. 66:446 (1991).

33. E. Taioli, A. Nicolosi, and E.L. Wynder, Dietary habits and breast cancer: a comparative study of United States and Italian data, *Nutr Cancer*. 16:259 (1991).

34. N.L. Petrakis, L.D. Gruenke, and J.C. Craig, Cholesterol and cholesterol epoxides in nipple aspirates of human breast fluid, *Cancer Res*. 41:2563 (1981).

35. H. Ohgaki, S. Takayama, and T. Sugimura, Carcinogencities of heterocyclic amines in cooked food, *Mutation Res*. 259:399 (1991).

36. T. Tanaka, W.S. Barnes, G.M. Williams, and J.H. Weisburger, Multipotential carcinogenicity of the fried food mutagen 2-amino-3-methylimidazo[4,5-f]quinoline in rats, *Jpn J Cancer Res*. 76:570 (1985).

37. J.S. Felton and M.G. Knize, Occurrence, identification, and bacterial mutagenicity of hetrocyclic amines in cooked food, *Mutation Res*. 259:205 (1991).

38. R.H. Adamson, Mutagens and carcinogens formed during cooking of foods and methods to minimize their formation, *in:* "Cancer Prevention." V. DeVita, Jr., S. Hellman, S.A. Rosenberg, eds., J.B. Lippincott, Philadelphia (1990).

39. C.F. Aylsworth, D.A. Van Vingt, P.W. Sylvester, and J. Meites, Role of estrogen and pro- lactin in stimulation of carcinogen-induced mammary tumor development by a high-fat diet, *Cancer Res.* 44:2835 (1984).

40. C. Ip and M.M. Ip, Serum estrogens and estrogen responsiveness in 7,12-dimethylbenz(a)- anthracene-induced mammary tumors as influenced by dietary fat, *J Natl Cancer Inst.* 66:291 (1981).

41. D.P. Rose, A.P. Boyar, C. Cohen, and L.E. Strong, Effect of a low-fat diet on hormone levels in women with cystic breast disease. I. Serum steroids and gonadotropins, *J Natl Cancer Inst.* 78:623 (1987).

42. A.P. Boyar, D.P. Rose, J.R. Loughridge, A. Engle, A. Palgi, K. Laakso, D. Kinne, and E.L. Wynder, Response to a diet low in total fat in women with postmenopausal breast cancer: a pilot study, *Nutr Cancer.* 11:93 (1988).

43. R. Prentice, D. Thompson, C. Clifford, S. Gorbach, B. Goldin, and D. Byar, Dietary fat reduction and plasma estradiol concentration in healthy postmenopausal women, *J Natl Cancer Inst.* 82:129 (1990).

44. D.P. Rose, M. Goldman, J.M. Connolly, and L.E. Strong, A high-fiber-supplemented diet reduces serum estrogen levels in premenopausal women, *Am J Clin Nutr.* 54:520 (1991).

45. D.M. Hegsted, Errors of measurement, *Nutr Cancer.* 12:105 (1989).

46. E.L. Wynder, J.H. Weisburger, and S.K. Ng, Nutrition: the need to define "optimal" intake as a basis for public policy decisions, *Am J Publ Health.* 82:346 (1992).

47. B. D'Avanzo, E. Negri, C. Gramenzia, S. Franceshi, F. Parazzini, P. Boyle, and C. LaVecchia, Fats in seasoning and breast cancer risk: an Italian case-control study, *Eur J Cancer.* 27:420 (1991).

48. K. Resnicow, The relationship between breakfast habits and plasma cholesterol levels in school children, *J Sch Health.* 2:81 (1991).

49. G. Block, C. Dresser, A. Hartman, and M. Carrol, Nutrient sources in the American diet: quantitative data from the NHANES II survey, *Amer J Epidemiol.* 122:27 (1985).

50. J.L. Stanton and D. Rose Keast, Serum cholesterol, fat intake, and breakfast consumption in the United States adult population, *J Am Coll Nutr.* 8:1 (1989).

51. R.C. Ellison, "Second International conference on preventive cardiology," Washington, D.C., (1989).

52. D.J.A. Jenkins, T.M.S. Wolever, and V. Vuksam, Nibbling versus gorging: Metabolic advan- tages of increased meal frequency, *N Engl J Med.* 321:929 (1989).

53. J.A. McDougal, The McDougal Program, NAL Books Publ., Penguin Books, New York (1990).

54. M.B. Rosenthal, R.J. Barnard, D.P. Rose, S. Inkeles, J. Hall, and N. Pritikin, Effects of a high-complex-carbohydrate, low-fat, low-cholesterol diet on levels of serum lipids and estradiol, *Am J Med.* 78:23 (1985).

55. D. Heber, J.M. Ashley, D.A. Leaf, and J. Barnard, Reduction of serum estradiol in postmen- opausal women given free access to low-fat high carboydrate diet, *Nutrition.* 7:137 (1991).

56. E.L. Wynder, A. Morabia, D.P. Rose, and L.A. Cohen, Clinical trials of dietary interven- tions to enhance cancer survival, *Prog in Clin and Biol Res.* 346:217 (1990).

57. T. Hirayama and E.L. Wynder, A study of the epidemiology of cancer of the breast. II. The influence of hysterectomy, *Cancer.* 15:28 (1962).

Chapter 14

Dietary Fat and Breast Cancer: Testing Interventions to Reduce Risks

JOHANNA T. DWYER

I. Introduction

The presentation discusses the issue of testing dietary interventions in post-menopausal breast cancer prevention. The many dietary hypotheses that might be tested are very briefly summarized. For illustrative purposes, the progress made in feasibility studies of the Women's Health Trial, a low-fat intervention study to decrease incidence of breast cancer in post-menopausal women at increased risk of cancer of the breast is used. Results of several other similar interventions to test the fat hypothesis are also reviewed, including the Nutrition Adjuvant Study, the WINS study, the Swedish breast cancer trial, a Canadian study conducted at the Ludwig Institute, and a possible study by the American Cancer Society. Some research questions that arise in testing dietary interventions are discussed. These include underlying assumptions about mechanisms, and controlling errors, particularly response errors. Practical issues such as how to measure adherence in the absence of a good biologic marker are also addressed. The review concludes with a section on future research and action directions.

Breast cancer remains among the major cancer killers of post-menopausal women today. Progress continues in breast cancer treatment, although the pace is not as rapid as we would like. It has long been clear that steroid receptors are important determinants of response to treatment and survival. This finding opened the door to considerable progress using hormonal treatments during the 1980s.[1] When both estrogen and progestin receptors are present, response is best to treatment, when estrogen receptors are present but progestin receptors are absent, results are less positive, and when both are absent, outcomes are very much poorer. Over 70% of all women have estrogen-positive tumors at diagnosis, and at least one-third to one-half of these appear to respond to hormone treatments. Both tamoxifen and cytotoxic therapy can reduce 5-year mortality from breast cancer.[2] Recent results indicate that tamoxifen, one adjuvant hormonal therapy for primary breast cancer, reduces

Johanna T. Dwyer • Frances Stern Nutrition Center, New England Medical Center Hospitals, 750 Washington Street, Boston, Massachusetts

Exercise, Calories, Fat, and Cancer, Edited by M.M. Jacobs
Plenum Press, New York, 1992

incidence of cancer in the contralateral breast by 45% at 5 years.[3] Some have also called for prophylactic trials of tamoxifen or other hormonal therapies in post-menopausal women at high risk for breast cancer.[4] However, even if such hormone prevention trials are mounted, there will be a great deal of disease left to prevent and to treat. Therefore the role of nutrition both in primary prevention and control of breast cancer remains of interest.

II. Possible Diet-Related Hypotheses

Table 1 provides some of the current theories involving diet and their hypothesized modes of action. These are only a few of the many possible diet-related factors.

A. Fat

Other papers in this volume and elsewhere describe the ecologic, experimental animal, analytical epidemiologic and other evidence supporting the hypothesis that amount of dietary fat is associated with increased incidence of breast and other cancers.

Evidence supporting the fat hypothesis also continues to accumulate in studies of experimental animals.[5] The combination of high fat and low dietary fiber appears to be particularly pernicious.[6] The effects of fat and calories on metastasis are also being elucidated.

The arguments and counterarguments with respect to human epidemiologic data are well summarized in a recent symposium on the topic.[7-11]

Table 1 summarizes current views of the associations of total fat and different fatty acids with risk of breast cancer. The amount of fat is thought to influence hormone status.

Type of fat is thought to influence the production of different prostaglandins and also immune response. Different fatty acids may increase or decrease risks. Both metabolic overloads or a contribution to increased body weight may also increase risks.

The omega-6 polyunsaturated fatty acids (PUFAs) form the prostaglandins PGE_2 and PGF_2 alpha. In animal experiments some studies suggest that PUFAs are associated with increased risk of breast cancer.[5] In some human studies low fat and low PUFA (omega 6) fatty acids are associated with enhanced natural killer cytotoxicity for tumor cells *in vitro*, and effects are especially pronounced, but the results are not entirely clear; although the low-fat (25% or 30% of calories) diet did have such an effect, alterations in P:S ratios did not.[12,13] Thus at present the role of PUFA is not clear; one recent report suggested that the data were mixed.[14,15]

Investigators have studied the role of the omega-3 fish oils in animal models and have concluded that many effects operate through prostaglandin metabolism. Because the omega-3 and omega-6 PUFAs are metabolized to prostaglandins of different types and different activities, their effects may be quite different. The omega-3 fatty acids give rise to prostaglandins PGD_3, PGE_3, and PGF_3, that appear to have lower biologic activity than those formed from the omega-6 fatty acids, not only on natural killer cell activity, but on other mediators such as the lymphokines, leukotrienes, and thromboxanes.[16] Although the mechanisms are not yet clear, immunosurveillance is thought to be involved. Studies in humans are now being completed.

B. Caloric Excess and Body Weight, Effects of Physical Activity

These variables are discussed in several chapters in this volume. Excessive body weight increases risk of breast cancer in post-, but not pre-menopausal women (see Table 1).[17] The many difficulties in measurement of energy intake and output present formidable challenges to exploring the effects of long-term positive and negative energy balance in human be-

Table 1. Possible Dietary Effects on Breast Cancer

Factor	Possible mechanism
Total fat (increase risk)	Via endocrine effects as by affecting free to bound estrogens,[69] estrogen binding globulin, estrogen metabolism,[73] pituitary and thyroid hormone production, etc., or possibly by other means, such as altered membranes and intracellular metabolism
Saturated fat (increase risk)	Unknown; possibly entrohepatic circulation of estrogens affected by altered metabolism of bile and fatty acids, or production of cholesterol epoxides associated with high intakes of saturated fat and cholesterol.[74] Other causes of lipid peroxidation also might be involved.
Omega-6 PUFAs (increase risk)	Possibly membrane-related effects,[75] specifically on membrane composition and fluidity or lipid peroxidation
Monounsaturated fats (decrease risk)	Lesser endocrine effects than other fats, at least in animal models[76]
Omega-3 PUFAs (decrease risk)	Positive endocrine effects via prostaglandin biosynthesis and metabolism and thus on intracellular metabolism and control systems in animal models
Medium-chain triglycerides (decrease risk)	Lesser endocrine effects because metabolism is more like carbohydrate than fat, at least with C8:0,C10:0 MCT in experimental animals?
Excess calories and overweight (pre-menopausal)	Fat cells convert androgens to estrogens, especially estrone; breast adipose tissue converts estrone to estradiol, more in heavier women (estradiol biologically active form of estrogen)
	Reduced plasma sex hormone-binding globulin for binding and transport of estradiol in obesity so increased free and albumin-bound estrogens, enhancing biologic activity in breast tissue in obesity
	Possible increase in estrogen receptors in obesity and increased rates of estrogen receptor-positive tumors
	Altered immune system?
(post-menopausal)	Increased amenorrhea in obese women so lesser exposure to estrogens and progesterone, decreasing risk.
	Lower progesterone secretion in obese in luteal phase of menstrual cycle causing increased mitotic activity in later part of menstrual cycle under influence of estrogens and progesterone.[77]
	Increased cell proliferation among epithelial cells that have already undergone partial malignant transformation under influence of estrogens, especially if acinii are still in stage when they can proliferate.
	Altered immune system.[21]
Phytoestrogens and soya products	Lignans such as enterolactone and enterodiol and equol, produced in gut by plant precursors, may have protective effects.[78-80]
Alcohol	Effects on membrane fluidity?
Dietary fiber	Possible effects on enterohepatic circulation of estrogens and some direct effects of fiber-associated phytoestrogens
Protein	Prolactin and possibly other hormones altered by diet.

Source: Adapted and expanded from Reference 5.

ings.[18-20] Physical activity appears to have a protective effect in some studies and therefore it is important to continue to explore these relationships.

Body weight is somewhat easier to measure, and deserves attention. In one recent study, using weights above 73 kg or a BMI over 28, risk of recurrence was found among heavier women.[21]

Height is also positively associated with breast cancer risk, at least among North American and European women who had reached puberty during the Great Depression or World War II. Some recent studies suggest that the associations with height perhaps are due in part to caloric deprivation during the pubertal growth spurt, and presumably, increased numbers of anovulatory menses or delayed menarche.[22]

C. Phytoestrogens and Soya Products

Another hypothesis that is currently receiving much interest is that various plant foods, containing phytoestrogens like isoflavonoids, lignans, and the like may have estrogenic activity in humans. Recent studies suggest that among post-menopausal women temporary effects on vaginal cytology can be observed with feeding of various foods high in phyto-estrogens.[23] Among Chinese women living in Singapore the consumption of soya products, high in phytoestrogens, appeared to exert protective effects on breast cancer risk in a case-control study, whereas animal protein and red meat consumption appeared to increase risks, perhaps because diets high in them tended to be low in these phytoestrogen compounds.[15] Soya products also contain protease inhibitors that appear to have cancer-preventive activity although not seemingly for breast cancer.[24] Saponins and phytoesterols are also present in plants such as soybeans. Phytoesterols are similar structurally to cholesterol but they have cholesterol-lowering, not -raising effects. They are high in plant food diets; vegetarians usually consume about 400 mg/day vs. about 80 mg/day among omnivores.[25,26] Their effects on sex hormone metabolism need further investigation.

D. Alcohol

Some cohort studies in humans suggest that alcohol consumption is associated with breast cancer.[27-29] Alcohol intakes appear to be easier to measure at moderate levels of consumption than fat intakes, and these items discriminate well on food-frequency question-naires.[30] In some studies, fat and alcohol intakes appear to be positively correlated, so it is important to control for these associations.[31] For example, Schatzkin et al.[27] found that compared to not drinking at all, the relative risk of about 5 g/day (the equivalent of 3 drinks a week) was about 1.6, even after adjusting for other factors known to influence incidence. The relative risk of any amount of drinking vs. nondrinking was about 1.5. However, food-frequency questionnaires are not always accurate in determining the absolute amounts of intakes. In the NHANES follow-up study, less than 10% of the women drank more than a drink a day on average. Willett's nurses also reported intakes that were very much lower than other studies of American women. But data from other sources on very large or population-based samples of Americans indicate that intakes range from about 6 g ethanol per day from self-reports of adult females who drink, and this is thought to be an under-estimate.[32] Apparent consumption from liquor sales or taxes gives much higher estimates of alcohol consumption, of over an ounce a day (30 g) per person.[32] How much alcohol is being drunk among those experiencing the increased risk, and the mechanisms whereby these effects come about deserve more study.

E. Dietary Fiber

There is also a considerable body of epidemiologic studies, some animal experiments, and some limited human work that suggests that dietary fiber may have a protective effect on breast cancer risk.[33]

F. Protein

Most of the interest in protein as a possible enhancer of breast cancer risk is the observation that prolactin levels are often increased in advanced and aggressive breast cancers, and increased prolactin levels seem to be associated with increased cell proliferation and poor prognosis regardless of estrogen receptor status.[34] Some early studies suggested that low-fat intakes were associated with decreased prolactin levels,[35] but later studies did not.[36] The effects do not appear to be due to fat, but rather to protein levels of diets, prolactin declining when protein levels decline.[37,38] It is thought that protein alters prolactin release, and that prolactin promotes breast cancer growth. However, this hormone acts in league with other hormones, such as estrogen and escort steroid hormones like progestins and possibly androgens. Lately, studies in humans suggest that there may be an effect of dietary protein in altering both prolactin and various gut hormone levels.[34]

III. Progress in Prospective Feasibility Studies to Date Testing the Fat Hypothesis

Table 2 summarizes several recent feasibility studies testing the hypothesis that low-fat diets are achievable among women living in various Western countries.

A. Women's Health Trial Vanguard Group Study

The Women's Health Trial Vanguard Group study was a feasibility study of the effects of low-fat diets on adherence and biochemical parameters among women 45 to 69 years at increased risk of breast cancer. The rationale for the study has been well described.[39,40] In three clinical study units, 303 women were randomized into a low-fat (20% of calories) or a customary (control) diet group.[70] By 6 months, they had reduced energy intakes from 39 to 21% of calories from fat in the low-fat group, and from 39 to 38% of calories in the control group. By 12 and 24 months, and after completing intervention sessions, reduced energy from fat was also sustained to a greater degree in the treatment than the control group.

The major ways in which the low-fat group reduced their fat intakes were by decreasing their intakes from milk products, red meats, and fats and oils. They cut back on cheddar cheese, American cheese, whole milk, butter, mayonnaise, salad dressing, bacon, and ate hamburgers less frequently, and used diet American cheese, low-fat cottage cheese, and skim milk more frequently. Also they consumed less fat in their vegetable dishes. Total caloric intakes from fruit increased slightly. Overall, quality of diet improved; energy-adjusted intakes of vitamins and minerals from food sources increased by 20 to 50%, depending on the nutrient.[83]

Also gratifying were changes in favorable directions in both serum cholesterol levels and in serum estradiol levels.[7,8]

The investigators concluded that such an intervention was possible and feasible.

Table 2. Characteristics of Selected Feasibility Studies for Reducing Dietary Fat

Characteristic	NAS	WINS	WHT	
			Study[a]	
Group size		220	220	
Treatment	17			
Control	11			
Dietary assessment methods	4 DDR at at B, 3 months		B, 6, 12, 24 months SQFF, 24-hour recall to compare to 4DDR, fat score used to measure adherence	
Duration (months)	3	12	12	
Calories			Intervention	Control
Baseline	1840 (419)		7258KJ (122)	7148KJ (168)
Follow-up at 3 months	1365 (291)			
Decrease	25%			
Follow-up at 12 months			5460 (112)	6619 (158)
Decrease			− 24%	−7%
Follow-up at 24 months			5691	6675
Decrease from B			− 22%	−5%
Decrease from 12 months			+2%	+2%
Fat, % calories				
Baseline	38% (4.3)		39%	39%
Follow-up at 3 months	23% (7.8)		22%	
Decrease	56%			
Follow up at 12 months			22%	37%
Decrease			−17%	−2%
Follow up at 24 months			23%	37%
Decrease			+1%	0%
Weight loss, g/day				
Actual	31 g			
Predicted from calorie deficit	65 g			
reported			40 (3 months) 53 (3 months)	

Table 2. (Continued)

	Study[a]			
Characteristic	Swedish Breast Cancer Study[81]		AHF Study[82]	
Group size				
Treatment	121 randomized, 63 completed (52%)		19 breast cancer 16 fibrocystic disease	
Control	119 randomized, 106 completed (89%)			
Diet assessment methods	Diet histories (all) Food records (treatment only)		4DDR	
Duration (months)	24		3	
Calories	Intervention	Control	Cancer	Cystic disease
Baseline	7.7 MJ	8.2MJ	1504	1743
Follow-up at 24 months	6.8	7.6	1347[b]	1344
Decrease	−11.6%	−7.3%	−10.4%	−22.8%
Fat, % calories				
Baseline	36.9%	37.2%	33.5%	35.6%
Follow-up at 24 months	24.0	34.1	20.7[b]	21.4
Decrease	−12.9%	−3.1%	−12.8%	−14.2%
Weight loss, g/day Actual	Not reported precisely, but intervention group decreased slightly (most in first year) then increased but not to baseline; but controls increased		22.6 g 66.33 64.29	15.5 g/day 59.3 57.9
Predicted from calorie deficit reported	Should have decreased in both groups almost equally if reporting were equally erroneous		20.4 g	51.9 g

[a] DDR = 4-Day Diet Record; B = Baseline; SQFF = Semiquantitative Food-Frequency Questionnaire; KJ = Kilojoules; MJ = Megajoules.
[b] 3 months.

B. Future National Cancer Institute Studies

In the early fall of 1991, the National Cancer Institute launched a new study in three clinical centers to determine the feasibility of changing diets of minority and under-served populations to low-fat (20% of calories from fat) patterns that may be associated with decreased risks of breast, colon, and other cancers. Of particular interest are methods that permit black, Hispanic, and low-income populations to change their current eating patterns. Currently, like other Americans, they eat diets that are high in fat. At present we have little data on the impact of social customs, culture, or economics on achieving and maintaining low-fat patterns. The Women's Health Trial second study will involve one center with half or more of the population from blacks, another predominantly with Hispanics, and a third with other key minorities as well as women representative of the general U.S. population. The National Heart, Lung and Blood Institute will join in this effort and provide funding for examining the effects of the low-fat eating pattern on cholesterol, triglycerides, and other lipids in the women's blood.

The trial complements and provides a prelude to the larger Women's Health Initiative of the National Institutes of Health. The Women's Health Initiative is a larger, longer term, and broader study that is Institute-wide. It will involve dietary changes, including a low-fat dietary pattern, supplementation with vitamins and minerals, hormone replacement therapy, exercise, and smoking cessation to reduce risks of cancer, heart disease, and osteoporosis. All WHT women are eligible to participate in the NIH-wide study.

C. Nutrition Adjuvant Study (NAS) and the Women's Intervention and Nutrition Study (WINS)

These two studies are considered together since they both involved the same investigators. The NAS was a randomized multicenter clinical trial pilot study with the goal of reducing dietary fat intakes in post-menopausal women with stage II breast cancer to 15% of calories. Women were also receiving chemotherapy or hormonal treatment. They were given individual and group guidance to reduce fat intakes. At 3 months of follow-up, of 32 individuals initially studied, those 17 in the low-fat treatment group experienced large decreases in their fat intake. But controls also decreased their fat intakes and lost weight, although to a lesser degree.[41] Complete data were collected on 17 patients on the low-fat diet. They finally achieved a diet of 23% of calories from fat, down from 38% of calories at baseline. This was a reduction of about 56% in fat calories. However, energy intakes also decreased from 1840 to 1365 after 3 months (about a 25% reduction), and weight loss of 2.8 kg also ensued. If such weight were all adipose tissue weight, the caloric deficit per day should have been about 219 calories; in actuality decreases from baseline to 3 months into treatment were reported to be 475 calories, suggesting considerable under-reporting of energy intakes and of food intakes in general. Thus it is possible that fat intakes did not drop as much as reported. However, they did drop somewhat since serum cholesterols as well as weight and food records all suggested that intakes were very much reduced. On a more positive note, intakes of vitamins and minerals exceeded two-thirds of the RDA for most nutrients even in the low-fat diet group, suggesting that diet quality remained high.[42,43]

After many delays the NAS study was cancelled.[44] The investigators in eight of the ten participating centers successfully submitted a revised proposal as an investigator-initiated grant, and the study was renamed the Women's Intervention and Nutrition Study (WINS). The preliminary results of that study are now about to be published and are generally positive; the low-fat intervention was achieved and sustained at 1-year follow-up in the intervention group at a level of about 22% of calories.[45]

Another smaller study of very-low-fat (20% of calories) diets was also conducted on 19-resected post-menopausal breast cancer patients after mastectomy and 16 pre-menopausal women with cystic breast disease and cyclical mastalgia by the group at the American Health Foundation that led the NAS clinical center there.[46] After 3 months of intervention, intakes, as measured by 4-day food records, had fallen from 1504 to 1347 calories in the post-menopausal group, with a reduction in fat from 56 to 31 g/day, and a decline of 2 kg in weight. Among the pre-menopausal women, intakes also fell and so did weights. Serum cholesterols declined significantly. Total serum estrogens, estrone, and estradiol rose, although nonsignificantly, among the post-menopausal women. In contrast, serum estrogens fell in the pre-menopausal women, and these differences, but not those in serum cholesterol, were significant. It was again concluded that these women were able to follow fat-modified diets successfully, at least over the short run, and that at least some biochemical indices were positive.

D. Canadian (Ludwig Institute) Studies

The group at the Ludwig Institute in Toronto, Canada studied dietary compliance in 57 women, who had participated for a year in a randomized trial of dietary fat reduction.[47] A larger feasibility study involving 230 women has also been published.[48] The smaller study is helpful for assessing possible errors in dietary assessment methods because duplicate meals were analyzed. Both food records and meal duplicates over 4 days showed that fat intake was significantly reduced in the experimental (low-fat) group from 36% to 23% calories. Also, serum cholesterol levels dropped by 7% and weight by about 1 kg at 6 months, but returned to baseline values by 12 months. None of the differences were statistically significant.

The Canadian National Breast Screening study involves a cohort of 56,837 women who are being followed. They completed a dietary questionnaire before the occurrence of their breast cancer. The questionnaire has been described in several publications.[49-51] At baseline, the intakes of the women ranged from about 31% (for the lowest quartile) to 47% of calories from fat for the highest quartile.

Between 1982 and 1987, 519 new, histologically confirmed cases of breast cancer were identified. In a recent analysis of these data, Howe et al.[52] reported a positive association between breast cancer and total fat intake, with relative risks of 1.35 per 77 g per day, and with some evidence of a dose-response relationship.[52] Howe adjusts for energy by putting each nutrient with calories from other sources into a regression model. Even after adjusting for other sources of calories, and scaling estimates by the differences in mean intakes between the highest and lowest quintiles (40 g in the cohort study) and adjusting for nondietary risk factors, risks were 1.3 in the post-menopausal women for saturated fats, and approximately 1.4 for pre-menopausal women. In a meta-analysis of 12 case-control studies, this group also reported a positive and consistent association between breast cancer and saturated and monounsaturated, but not polyunsaturated fat intakes primarily in post-menopausal women.[53] Concerns about the small number of cases in the cohort study which limited the power to detect differential effects among fats or among women of different menopausal status were such that initially the group did not report findings from the cohort study. But subsequently estimates were provided, such as 1.34 for the cohort data.[54] The women in the lowest quintile were suspected to include some individuals who were systematically under-reporting dietary intakes; it was also possible that they were at increased risk of breast cancer for some other reason. For example, frequent dieting would give rise to very low intakes if the dieting days were averaged out in the semiquantitative food-frequency questionnaire. Thus it is important to determine if and how systematic errors in response to dietary questionnaires occur.

E. Scandinavian Studies

The Swedes have published the results of a dietary intervention study among 240 women who were 50-65 years old at the time of operation for stage I or II breast cancer. Post-surgery they were assigned randomly to an intervention group that received individual dietary counseling supplemented by group support (nearly biweekly for the first 2 months and quarterly thereafter, with extra group meetings with families invited every 6-8 weeks). The aims were to provide assistance to reduce dietary fat intakes to 20-25% of calories and increase carbohydrate intake to substitute for calories lost. Those in the control group received no dietary counseling.

The dietary-assessment interview was a diet history. Diet histories were repeated at baseline and once a year for 2 years thereafter in the intervention group and at baseline and year 2 in the control group. In addition, those in the intervention group kept food records quarterly in year 1 of the study and once in year 2, and these records were used in the intervention to provide additional information for individual counseling.

Baseline intakes of nutrients were similar, except controls had slightly higher energy intakes. Follow-up at 2 years was achieved in over 79% of the women; among 63 (52% follow-up) of the intervention group, and among 106 (89% follow-up) of the control group. At 2 years, energy intake had decreased in both groups, but the differences in energy intakes remained. The intervention group's fat intakes had declined by 13% to 23% of calories from a baseline measure of 36% of calories at 2 years, compared to a 3% decrease from 37% to 34% of calories in the control group.

Intakes of minerals and vitamins generally rose in the intervention group, suggesting that quality of diet increased rather than decreased. Protein intakes also rose slightly.

However, differential reporting bias was considered likely, since both the intervention and control group women reported later energy intakes below their first intakes, yet only the intervention group showed any decreases in weight, whereas the control group actually increased in weight. Also, the investigators had previously noted a tendency for women to exaggerate their reporting in line with desirable dietary behavior, and this was thought to have affected results. No weight changes or changes in biochemical measures were reported in the study.

The Finns recently completed an observational study of a cohort of 3998 initially cancer-free Finnish women 20-69 years old.[55] Their fat intakes, like those of American women, are about 38% of calories on average. Follow-up is now over 20 years, and 54 breast cancer cases have been diagnosed. These are significantly and inversely related to energy intake. Unfortunately data on physical activity and energy outputs are unavailable. Absolute fat intake is not associated with risk, but when fat intakes are adjusted for energy, there is a weak positive association between energy-adjusted fat intake and risk. The relative risk in the highest tertile is 1.7 for total fat, 1.4 for saturated fat, 2.7 for monounsaturated fat, 1.2 for PUFAs, and 2.2 for dietary cholesterol intakes, and these differences hold even after adjusting for potential confounders.

F. Possible American Cancer Society Initiative

The American Cancer Society is currently considering an initiative that will involve a very-low-fat diet (15%) and calorie control or the American Cancer Society Diet Recommendations (30% calories) to be administered in a randomized study to post-menopausal women at least 105% of ideal body weight who have had surgery for adenocarcinoma of the breast and who are no more than 6 months post-operative. Either mastectomy or breast-sparing procedures, with or without radiotherapy, tamoxifen, or chemotherapy are acceptable. Thus the goal is to achieve ideal weight in the very-low-fat diet group in addition to consumption of a very-low-fat diet, by a combination of diet and exercise. Progress will be measured by 4-day diet diaries, the Block version of the National Cancer Institute's semi-quantitative food-frequency questionnaire, 24-hour recalls by phone on a subsample of subjects, changes in serum estradiols and serum fatty acids, and weight checks.

IV. Unsettled Research Issues

Some of the major criticisms of these feasibility studies were that long-term (e.g., 2-10 year) adherence might be poor, that diet would change in many ways, including weight loss, (which might have potent metabolic effects in itself), that there was no adequate way to evaluate adherence to low-fat regimens, that recruitment would be a problem, and that sample sizes might be too low. Some of these points have already been discussed by Prentice,[7] Willett[9] and others[10,13] elsewhere.

A. Nutritional Homogeneity

Under particular dispute is the interpretation of negative results linking fat intake to breast cancer in two cohort studies, and whether the negative results are due to the power of the cohort study analyses, or are actually evidence of nonassociation between this dietary variable and disease. The Nurses Health Study analyzed results from 601 cases of breast cancer, using semiquantitative food-frequency questionnaires on nurses whose reported spread in quintiles of intake from fat were from 31% to 47%. There was no evidence of any positive association between fat intake and increased breast cancer risk after adjusting for energy intakes.[28] Also, the follow-up of the National Health and Nutrition Examination Study, which involved use of a 24-hour recall and 99 cases of breast cancer did not find any risk with increased fat consumption. In fact if anything there was a decreased risk.[27] Finally, among 20,341 Seventh Day Adventist women followed for 6 years, among whom 215 cases of histologically confirmed primary breast cancer developed, with a mean age of diagnosis of 66 years, neither increased consumption of high-fat animal products nor childhood and teenage dietary habits (e.g., vegetarian vs. nonvegetarian) were associated with breast cancer. Neither was a derived index of the percent of calories from animal fat during adult life found to be associated.[56] Seventh Day Adventist women consume fewer calories from fat (about a mean of 36% vs. 42% in the population at large) and from animal fat (8% from animal fat vs. 24% in the population at large) than do omnivores.

Hebert and Kabat[57] and Prentice et al.[7] argue that the cohort studies covered too little a range in fat intakes to detect differences in risk by fat intake, and thus that nutritional homogeneity was a problem. Hebert uses smoking data to illustrate the point; if very low intakes are excluded, even an association as powerful as that between smoking and lung cancer is seriously weakened. The methods they use for adjusting energy intakes are also matters of dispute, although all agree such adjustments are necessary.[10,58,59] It is also possible that changes in hormone background on very-low-fat intakes, especially when they are associated with periodic dieting, are associated with differences in risk.

Hebert and Kabat[57] have shown that when the usual ranges of intakes for fat in this country are examined, there is a tendency to under-estimate relative risks of associations between diet or any other exposure variable (in this case the example used was smoking and lung cancer) and disease.

Other investigators, working in Singapore, in the study mentioned earlier, have shown that there is considerable dietary heterogeneity between older Chinese women (who have very-low-fat intakes, even after adjusting for energy intakes) and younger Chinese women, and that these differences may account for the varying associations between diet and breast cancer in their study.

B. Indirect Measures of Adherence

The studies reviewed here attempted to assess dietary adherence by different measures: comparisons of predicted and actual body weight loss (as a check on energy intakes), serum cholesterol lowering (as a marker of adherence to low-saturated fat diets), by duplicate weighing, or use of several dietary assessment techniques. Each of these methods has limitations. None are totally satisfactory.

The problems with using actual body weight losses to check or correct for possible reporting bias are many. First, on very-low-fat diets (e.g., 20% of calories from fat), even when they are supposedly corrected to maintain weight, on the order of 2 kg was lost by normal subjects under metabolic ward conditions over a 6-month period.[60] The problem may reside in preliminary estimates of energy intake being too low, diets actually being less well absorbed than is assumed when standard absorption values are assumed, or true differences in efficiency of metabolism.

Second, using comparisons of baseline energy intake values to intakes at some point later in intervention is problematic. Energy intakes are seriously and perhaps systematically under-reported when dietary records are used. Also, weight-loss and -gain predictions mean little without information on body composition changes.

If future studies can obtain estimates of energy intakes directly, it should be possible to get a better estimate of possible differential reporting bias with respect to energy intakes between control and experimental groups in future intervention studies, particularly by quintile of intake. This should permit examination of adjustments in fat intakes by energy adjustment.

There is no easy-to-measure, valid, and objective biochemical marker or dietary assessment tool for assessing adherence to low-fat diets.[9] The need to develop such a marker is urgent.

Until the advent of doubly labeled water, it was not possible to assess the validity of energy intakes directly. Now it is possible to check long-term energy intakes quite precisely.[20] It is to be hoped that in future studies, doubly labeled water will be used to assess the degree of under-reporting of energy intakes and response bias present, especially in intervention groups.

C. Reliability and Validity of Dietary Assessment Methods

Lee-Han and others[47] recently reviewed the various methods used to ascertain validity and reliability in studies of diet and cancer. The most usual way of assessing validity was similar to that employed in the studies cited here—concurrent validity, by comparison of one dietary method to another, and assessment of their agreement. Reliability was most frequently determined by test-retest reliability.

D. The Limitations of Dietary Assessment Methods

Dietary assessment has been done for many years in research studies. By the mid-twentieth century, scientific advances had identified the major sources of nutrients and other constituents found in foods and most of the major dietary assessment methods had been developed.

However, the development of dietary assessment methods that were suitable for large scale epidemiologic and clinical studies lagged behind until recently. The development of semiquantitative food-frequency questionnaires derived from population-based dietary surveys and their availability in a form that could be analyzed readily with computerized dietary analysis software made it possible to include dietary assessment in many studies, opening new vistas for exploration.[9,61]

Table 3 summarizes basic questions to be asked in studies of diet and breast cancer using dietary methods. Table 4 summarizes some possible uses of dietary information. The limitations of dietary methods, including their ability to ascertain intakes of dietary fat, calories, and other difficult to measure food constituents, such as phytoestrogens, have often been disregarded in the applications to which they are put. In the past few years there has been growing disillusionment and recognition of their inadequacies. This has led some investigators to abandon them entirely and to search for other indicators that can be used in their stead. However, alternative methods and proxies for the direct assessment of fat, alcohol, and phytoestrogen intakes also have severe limitations for many purposes.[62] No

Table 3.   Basic Questions To Be Considered in Choosing a Dietary Assessment Method

Why is the dietary assessment to be carried out?	What is the respondent burden?
	What other constraints are present?
What is to be assessed?	
	How much will it cost?
Who is to be assessed?	
	How well must the factor of interest be measured?
What is the time frame of interest?	

Table 4. Uses of Dietary Assessment Tools in Studies of Diet and Breast Cancer

Screening of subjects for possible participation on intakes of fat, saturated fat, alcohol, etc.

Assessment of adequacy of dietary intakes during study

Assessment of diet for clinical evaluation in conjunction with other indices of health risk, nutritional status, incidence of pre-malignant disease or breast cancer

Monitoring or surveillance of intakes both as adherence aids and to ensure intervention is being applied

Evaluation of intervention effects

Description of population studied

Consumption of specific food or foods suspected to have biologic effects, such as phytoestrogens, and estimation of their average intakes and range of intakes

single biochemical indicator provides evidence of long-term fat or alcohol intakes. Energy outputs ascertained by doubly labeled water are now available for measuring energy intakes, although presently the supplies of the substance and its expense hinder its use. Weight loss or gain can provide some information on overall energy balance or the lack thereof, but without simultaneous measures of body composition and energy output it is not very sensitive.   Therefore in assessing and monitoring dietary status for the aspects of food consumption of interest in nutrition and breast cancer studies, a combination of dietary, biochemical, and anthropometric methods are usually needed.

In the studies of diet and breast cancer, the purpose of the studies is to clarify the associations of diet with metabolic changes thought to be indicators of disease, to clarify associations between diet or dietary constituents and later disease, and, in prospective studies, to test the strength of purposeful changes in diet and disease progression. The specific purpose of the study influences the type of data that must be collected, the number of observations necessary, and the best methods to use. Many monographs on dietary assessment methods have recently been published.[9,63-68]

The characteristics of intakes of interest in studies of diet and breast cancer may include nutrients or other food constituents, foods, food groups, dietary patterns and characteristics.

Studies may also include additional information on dietary characteristics, such as use of weight reduction diets, physical activity, alcohol consumption patterns, and the like that are helpful for descriptive purposes, even if they are not necessary for the major purpose of the analysis. For specific purposes, combinations of one or all of these types of information may be needed.

The target group selected is important for three reasons: generalization of results, choice of most appropriate assessment methods, and period of observation likely to be necessary.

The capabilities of those who are being assessed impose limitations on the choice of methods. Fortunately, in studies of diet and breast cancer, women, who often are the food buyers, preparers, and cooks and therefore knowledgeable about food preparation, are the subjects. They are usually quite interested in diet.

Table 5 presents a brief summary of the advantages and disadvantages of each method of dietary assessment. Some errors of particular concern are mentioned below.

Neither prospective nor retrospective dietary assessment methods can be assumed to be totally free of response bias, such as the desire on the part of some individuals to portray their diets as "healthy." Likewise, bias from systematic under-estimation or over-estimation by some individuals cannot necessarily be avoided by using two methods and assuming that if they agree the method is valid. For example, it has recently been shown that using doubly-labeled water techniques, weighed records, records in household portions, and recalls, all under-estimate true energy intakes. Some data are also available using urinary nitrogen appearance, a biochemical measure, to validate protein intakes, which suggest that protein intakes are also commonly underestimated.[63] Unfortunately there is no valid biochemical measure for fat intake, but there is no reason to assume that systematic, nonrandom errors inherent in the individual do not apply to assessments of its intake as well. Adjustments for differences in energy intakes may help to reduce these errors, but they are not likely to do away with them entirely, since it cannot be assumed that all individuals who under-report their fat intakes under-report energy intakes to the same degree. This is a particularly vexing problem today because public perceptions that fat intake is harmful to health are prevalent, making the selective under-reporting of fatty foods perhaps even more likely than under-reporting of over-all food intakes, so many estimate. Only long-term studies in which actual fat intakes can be assessed by truly objective means as well as by subjective measures are

Table 5. Advantages and Disadvantages of Different Dietary Assessment Methods

Methods and advantages	Disadvantages
24-hour recall	
Easy to administer.	Does not provide adequate quantitative data on nutrient intakes.
Time required to administer is short.	
Inexpensive.	Individual diets vary daily, so that a single day's intake may not be representative.
Respondent burden is low.	
Useful in clinical settings.	An experienced interviewer is required.
More objective than diet history.	Relies heavily on memory, making it unsuitable for certain groups, such as the elderly.
Serial 24-hour recalls can provide estimates of usual intakes on individuals.	
Data obtained can be repeated with reasonable accuracy.	Selective forgetting of foods such as liquids, high-calorie snacks, alcohol, and fat occurs.
Good reliability between interviewers.	

Table 5. (Continued)

Methods and advantages	Disadvantages

24-hour recall (continued)

	Reported intake may not be actual intake, but rather what the interviewer wants to hear.

Reported intake may not be actual intake, but rather what the interviewer wants to hear.

Does not reflect differences in intake for weekday vs. weekend, season to season, or shift to shift.

Data may not accurately reflect nutrient intakes for populations due to variations in food consumption from day to day.

May be a tendency to over-report intake at low level and under-report intake at high levels of consumption, leading to "flat-slope syndrome" with reports of group intakes.

Food-frequency questionnaire

May be either self-administered or interviewer-administered.

Inexpensive.

Quick to administer.

Good at describing food intake patterns for diet and meal planning.

No observer bias.

Can be used for large population studies.

Useful when purpose is to study association of a specific food or a small number of foods and diseases such as alcoholism and birth defects.

Specific information about nutrients can be obtained if food sources of nutrients are confined to a few sources.

Can be analyzed rapidly for nutrients or food groups using a computer.

Foods can be ranked in relation to intakes of certain food items or groups of foods.

Response rates may be lower if questionnaire is self-administered.

Incomplete responses may be given.

Lists compiled for the general population are not useful for obtaining information on groups with different eating patterns (food inappropriate).

Total consumption is difficult to obtain because not all foods can be included in lists; under-estimation can occur.

Respondent burden rises as the number of food items queried increases.

Analysis is difficult without use of computers and special programs.

Reliability is lower for individual foods than for food groups.

Foods differ in extent to which they are over- and under-reported (errors are not random).

Each questionnaire must be validated.

Translation from intakes of food groups to nutrient intakes requires that many assumptions be made.

For assessing single nutrients, longer lists are acceptable.

Table 5. (Continued)

Methods and advantages	Disadvantages

Semiquantitative questionnaires

Inexpensive.

May be self-administered.

Rapid.

Usual diets are not altered.

Can rank or categorize individuals by rank of nutrient intakes rather than measuring group means.

Precoding and direct data entry to computer available to speed up analysis of some versions.

Correlations between this and other methods are satisfactory for food items and targeted nutrients when groups are the focus of the analysis.

Sufficiently simple to obtain dietary information in large epidemiologic studies that would not be possible with other methods.

Inexpensive.

Can provide useful information on intake of a wide variety of nutrients.

Validation studies are proceeding rapidly.

Respondent burden varies.

Good only for the general population, not necessarily for specific groups.

Culture-specific, i.e., assessment of intake in a culturally distinct group would require the creation and validation of another instrument.

Has not been validated for individual dietary assessments.

Needs to be constantly updated.

Most questionnaires available are to be used only on adults.

Specific nutrients are measured, rather than all nutrients or food constituents.

Not yet validated for those who eat modified or unusual diets (frequency and amount of intake from food groups may differ).

Ability to monitor short-term changes (weeks or months) in food intake is not known.

Correlations for individual nutrient intakes obtained with semiquantitative food-frequency questionnaires are poor when compared to diet histories and food records in household measures.

May be reliable and invalid in some cases.

Default codes may influence results unduly.

May only reflect "core diets" of a few weeks' duration.

Burke-type dietary history

Produces a more complete and detailed description of both qualitative and quantitative aspects of food intake than do food records, 24-hour recalls, or food-frequency questionnaires.

Eliminates individual day-to-day variations.

Takes into consideration seasonal variations.

Good for longitudinal studies.

Provides good description of usual intake.

Provides some description of previous diet before beginning prospective studies.

Highly trained nutritionists are required to administer dietary histories.

Difficult to standardize due to considerable variability among interviewers.

Dependent upon subjects' memory.

Time-consuming (takes about 1-2 hours to administer).

Diet histories over-estimate intakes compared to food records collected over the same time period due to bigger portion sizes, greater frequencies reported, and does not account for missed meals or sick days.

Table 5. (Continued)

Methods and advantages	Disadvantages
<u>Burke-type dietary history</u> (continued)	
	Time frame actually used by subject for reporting intake history is uncertain, probably no longer than a few weeks.
	Costs of analysis are high because records must be checked, coded, and entered appropriately.
<u>Food diary</u>	
What is eaten is recorded (or should be recorded) at time of consumption.	Food intake may be altered.
Recording error can be minimized if subjects are given proper directions.	Respondent burden is great.
Does not rely heavily on memory, and thus may be good for the elderly.	Individual must be literate and physically able to write.
	Respondent may not record intakes on assigned days.
	Difficult to estimate portion sizes; food models or pictures may help.
	Under-reporting is common.
	Number of sampled days must be sufficient to provide usual intake.
	Records must be checked and coded in standardized ways.
	Measured food intakes are more valid than records above.
	Costs of coding and analysis are high.
	Sex difference exists, i.e., women are more competent than men in recording.
	Number of days surveyed is dependent on the nutrient being studied.
	The very act of recording may change what is eaten.
	Can be obtrusive.
<u>Weighed-food diary</u>	
Increased accuracy of portion sizes over food diaries (errors are substantial—up to 40% for foods and 25% for nutrients).	Respondent burden great, and may increase dropout rates.
	Consumption may be altered during recording days.
	Expensive.
	May restrict choice of food.
	Subjects must be highly motivated.
	Other disadvantages similar to food diary.
	Not highly portable.
	Obtrusive.
	Time consuming.
	Scales may break.

Table 5. (Continued)

Methods and advantages	Disadvantages
Telephone interviews	
Some anonymity is maintained.	Makes assumptions that portion sizes reported are actually eaten.
Respondent burden is low.	Validation studies are incomplete.
Validity is good.	
Respondent acceptance is good.	
Effects of forgetfulness is minimum.	
Outreach is greater.	
May be easier to carry out after a face-to-face interview and instruction.	
Duplicate portion collection and analysis	
Highly accurate in metabolic research.	Intakes may be altered.
Duplicate portion permits direct chemical analysis.	High respondent burden.
	Expensive.
Helpful for validating other methods for constituents on which food composition data are incomplete.	Time-consuming and messy.
	Differences between duplicate portions and weighed records large (7% for energy, larger for other nutrients).
Good for individuals consuming unusual foods.	
By trained observers	
Low respondent burden.	Expensive and time-consuming for observer.
Overt or covert observation is possible.	Not ideal for large studies.
Precise measurements may be obtained.	Intakes may or may not be altered, depending upon whether individual is aware of observation.
	Details may be overlooked.

Adapted from Reference 68.

likely to provide appropriate validity data in this regard. The problem is that, when those who eat the least or the most are not truly doing so, misclassification will be considerable. Systematic response errors may be greater among those who are seemingly at the extremes of the distribution of intakes. Thus, efforts to compare relative risks between tertiles or quintiles may be fraught with error.

Table 6 shows the various sources of error in different assessment methods. Note that no method is perfect.

E. Semiquantitative Food-Frequency Questionnaires: Uses and Need for Further Study

Because these methods are now so popular, special attention is given to them. Until the late 1970s, food-frequency questionnaires were used chiefly in epidemiologic studies of specific groups or in abbreviated versions based on food groups in clinical situations. Now

Table 6. Sources of Error in Dietary Assessment Methods

Source of error	Duplicate portion	Weighed record	Diary	24-hour recall	Diet history	SQFF[a]
Response bias						
Response errors						
Omitting foods	−	?	?	+	+	+
Adding foods	−	−	−	+	+	+
Estimate of weight of foods	−	−	+	+	+	+
Estimation of servings	−	−	−	−	+	+
Estimate of food consumption frequency	−	−	−	−	+	+
Day to day variation	+	+	+	+	−	−
Changes in diet	+	+	?	−	−	−
Coding errors	−	+	+	+	+	+
Errors in conversion of Foods to nutrients						
Food composition tables	−	+	+	+	+	+
Nutrient data base values used for groups of foods	−	−	−	−	−	+
Sampling errors						
Direct analysis	+	−	−	−	−	−
Population sampling bias	+	−	−	−	−	−
	+	+	+	+	+	+

[a] SQFF = Semiquantitative Food-Frequency Questionnaire.
Source: Adapted and modified from References 63 and 72.

more sophisticated methods have been developed using data on the foods that are the most common sources of nutrients in the general population which permit semiquantitative estimates of nutrient intakes of groups.

The food-frequency technique employs a list of various food items and inquires about usual intakes in terms of the frequency with which they are (or were) consumed per day, per week, or per month. Semiquantitative versions also obtain some information about portion size, and number of servings eaten to get an estimate of the total amount of a particular food or food group that is eaten. Data are categorized by frequency of consumption of various food items by themselves or by various food groups that have been included on the inventory. The number of food items that are specified varies, depending upon the purpose of the study, but never includes all items that would possibly be eaten. Presently available food-frequency questionnaires also vary as to whether they are self-administered or given in a face-to-face interview situation, whether portion size is assumed or asked for, what time unit is used as reference, and in many other ways.

Semiquantitative food-frequency questionnaires differ from earlier food-frequency recall questionnaires in that they have longer lists of foods, the lists are derived from national surveys of representative samples of the American adult population, vitamin and mineral intakes from supplements are included, and some estimates of portion size are provided.

Table 5 represents the strengths and limitations of the existing method. The two semi-quantitative food-frequency questionnaires presently in widespread use that have been tested most extensively are the instrument developed by Willett and colleagues at Harvard University and that developed by Block and co-workers at the National Cancer Institute. They differ in their method of construction, the reference populations used to select foods, the extent to which they have been validated, the reference portion sizes used, the number of foods they contain, the nutrient intakes they are designed to assess, the extent to which they account for over-all intakes of these nutrients and of other constituents, the questions they ask on vitamin, mineral and other dietary constituents, the nutrient data bases which have been used for translating findings from them into nutrient intakes, and probably in other respects as well. The extent to which they yield similar results, how they compare to each other in their performance, how they behave with populations who consume modified diets and among ethnic subgroups in the population whose dieting patterns differ markedly from the general population, and their ability to monitor changes in food intake over relatively short periods of time (e.g., weeks or months) are now being assessed.

Semiquantitative food-frequency recalls have serious limitations for making statements about the nutrient intakes of individuals. Time is saved by focusing on the frequency with which a limited number of specific foods or groups of food are eaten, but information on other foods consumed may be lost. Total dietary intakes of nutrients cannot be estimated unless the list of food items is very extensive, and information of portion size and number of servings per eating occasion are also obtained.

Frequencies of consumption are precoded and therefore possible ranges of intakes are somewhat constrained.

It is difficult to measure portion size. The use of "average" or usual portion sizes (which differ between men, women, and children) as reference standards may introduce further complications. Since total nutrient intakes are derived from both the frequency and amount and servings of foods consumed, unless portion size standards are relevant and estimation is appropriate, error is introduced.

People also often have difficulties in responding to the questionnaires in distinguishing between the number of servings they eat and frequency of consumption.

When questionnaires focus only on intakes of food groups or food exchange lists the assumptions involved in using estimates of "average" nutrient contributions from these groups further increase errors. Means for the nutrient contributions of food groups are based upon the usual mixture of foods eaten in a particular category by the population used to develop the food grouping system. If the individual surveyed has very different food choices from these, the nutrient contribution of the food category to the individual's diet may be markedly different than the value that is assigned to it. This is often true when food-frequency recalls based on healthy populations with "usual" eating habits are used to survey individuals who have unusual or markedly different diets. It also applies when interventions to lower the fat or calorie intakes of diets are instituted among the intervention group.

To illustrate, let us assume that the averages derived for the exchange lists or some similar list for the "starch" group are based on averages for bread, rice, and other commonly eaten starch foods, each food given an equal weight in the average. But what if one is dealing with a rural southern black population that eats mostly grits, or a Chinese-American population eating mostly rice? These are obviously quite different and while their frequency estimates for starchy foods might be similar, the nutrient contributions of the starchy foods to that category in their diets would be quite different. If one simply applies average values to these frequency estimates, the nutrient values obtained are likely to be false. The correct procedure is to "weight" the various foods contributing nutrients and develop averages for groups of foods for each population being studied. If there is any likelihood that the study population's "food choice mix" or portion size selected differs from that used for generating nutrient average values for the food groups, validity may be compromised in estimating nutrient intakes from such data.

It is important to evaluate the utility and performance of these questionnaires in the dietary assessment of individuals since they are now being widely used for this purpose.

It is vital that semiquantitative food-frequency questionnaires be frequently updated. The food supply and dietary habits are constantly changing, and such changes have large effects on both what foods are consumed and the nutrient composition of foods that are eaten. Therefore, if such questionnaires are to continue to include the major food contributors of nutrients or other constituents of interest, they must be periodically updated, as must the nutrient data bases that are used when nutrient intakes are calculated from them.

F. Response Errors and Bias with Dietary Assessment Methods

Most people are only vaguely aware of what they eat. Without training, food records and food recalls will lack sufficient detail to be useful for most purposes. Some instruction is also needed with semiquantitative food-frequency questionnaires if they are to be filled out correctly. The quality of reporting and dietary data that is obtained can be greatly improved by training respondents to become more aware of what they are eating.

Reporting errors of a random type are common. They include failures of memory that lead to omissions and additions of foods; recalls of past diet tend to be simple and stereotypical. The use of probes, memory aids, and cross checks on reports of intakes minimizes these errors, but still the errors in estimating the portion size or weight of foods when they are not actually weighed are very large; as high as 50% for foods and 20% for nutrients.[63] For fat they may be especially large.

Mistakes in the number of servings, and in food consumption frequency also contribute to error. It is important to obtain enough days of observation so that the report covers usual day to day, weekday to weekend, and other fluctuations in dietary habits. This is a problem in 1-day or several-day recalls and in prospective studies unless designs are used that help to sample for these variations. In recalls covering a longer interval, the problem may be that people have difficulties in describing their overall typical diet.

Response bias, or systematic errors in a single direction also may occur. These threaten validity. With prospective record keeping the individual consciously eats differently on reporting days either to make recording easier or to conform to what he perceives is an appropriate food intake. The person who is reporting may actually unconsciously change his diet during days on which the diet is being recorded or measured. This is called collection day bias. It is most common in prospective methods. This type of bias is one that is common in clinical trials among dietary intervention groups; the individual "eats to the study objectives" on recording days. Some individuals in studies also deliberately fabricate and report distorted diets that are not what they actually ate. Such bias may be present with both prospective and retrospective records.

In retrospective studies recalls of previous diet are also often inaccurate. This may occur inadvertently due to faulty memory since current diet exerts a very strong influence on recollection of past diet, or it may be that the respondent wishes to provide intakes that emphasize what they regard as "good" eating habits.

Table 7 provides information on methods for obtaining information for groups and individuals using various dietary assessment methods. Table 8 gives some examples of appropriate statistics to collect when the focus is on individuals and groups.

G. Converting Foods into Nutrients or Other Constituents: Errors Involved in these Procedures

All dietary assessment methods involve conversion of foods into nutrients or other constituents. The process of converting foods to nutrients involves many problems and assumptions that can lead to substantial errors in estimating intakes of which users may be unaware.

1. Completeness and Use of Imputed Values

Methods for determining many nutrients and other constituents in foods are still being developed, and data are still sparse for many items of interest, such as phytoestrogens and specific fatty acids.

One major difficulty with food tables for dietary assessment purposes is missing values, especially for certain nutrients, including naturally occurring compounds such as phytoestrogens.[15] When data are lacking, imputed values or "best estimates" of nutrients in similar foods can be used, but these are only approximations, introducing additional assumptions and errors.

2. Nutrient Data Bases Used for Semiquantitative Food-Frequency Questionnaires

The nutrient data bases used in computer programs to analyze semiquantitative food-frequency questionnaires consist of average values for different categories or groups of foods rather than individual food items. Ideally these averages are based on the frequency of usual

Table 7. Possible Approaches for Obtaining Different Types of Dietary Information

Information	Method						
	Duplicate portion	Weighed record	Estimated	24-hour recall	Diet history	Food frequency	SQFF[a]
Group mean intake	+	+	+	+			
Group mean and distribution of intake	+(2)	+(2)	+(2)	+(2)	+	+	+
Individual's ranking by tertile or fifth in distribution of intakes	+(many)	+(many)	+(many)	+(many)	+	+	+

[a] SQFF = Semiquantitative Food-Frequency Questionaire.
Adapted and modified from Reference 72.

Table 8. Examples of Types of Information Desired

Focus of interest	Examples
Individuals	
Description of intake	Mean intake of group of individuals Absolute magnitude (means) of usual intakes of individual
Adequacy of intake	Mean and distribution of intakes in a group to determine percent at risk due to low intakes
Relationship of diet to nutritional status or development of disease	Relative magnitude (ranks) of individual's intakes within distribution of intakes for determining associations with nutritional status or disease
Case control or prospective analytic epidemiology studies	Categorization of intakes of individuals into exposed or unexposed groups
Cross-sectional studies of relationships between diet and nutritional status or behavior	
Groups	
Description of intakes at baseline or after intervention	Mean of group
Exploratory studies of relationship of diet to health or disease	Mean of group

Source: Reference 84.

consumption of the mix of individual foods in each category, which are derived from some other data collected on a reference population similar to that which will be studied. However, if an individual's food choices within these food groups are atypical, his actual nutrient intakes may be quite different from results generated by the software program.

Existing nutrient data bases for semiquantitative food-frequency questionnaires and other programs based on food groups use average or median values based on consumption within these categories which date from the late 1970s and early 1980s or even earlier. They are vulnerable to errors due not only to changes in the nutrient composition of individual foods but also to changes in the portion size and frequency of consumption of various foods within the food groups or categories that are selected. Since the food supply and consumption patterns are constantly changing even within categories, errors will arise if they are not periodically updated.

H. The Biologic Effects of Dietary Fat Intake at Various Levels of Energy Balance

The substrates reaching bodily cells vary not only with dietary intake but with the energy state. In a hypocaloric state, the metabolic mix reaching target tissues of women who consume high- and low-fat diets is influenced by several factors: hormone status, other nutrient levels (e.g., protein and fat), and the extent of the energy deficit. In a hypocaloric state the cells will be nourished primarily by fatty acids. Thus the situation is somewhat different in the hypocaloric state than what the expected effects of high- and low-fat diets are when they are consumed by individuals in energy balance. These differences deserve exploration. Hormone levels, estrogen and progesterone receptors, and other variables may alter effects of the same dietary intake in hypocaloric and eucaloric states.

I. Errors in Interpretation of Dietary Intake Data and Inferences about Risk of Disease

The complexities of interpretation of dietary intake data are beyond the scope of this review. However, dietary assessment only imperfectly measures exposure to the chemicals of interest in studies of diet and cancer.

The correlation (concurrent validity) of dietary measures with other single indices of nutritional status such as a biochemical, clinical, or anthropometric measurements and sometimes even with multiple indices is also often low. There are several reasons for these discrepancies.

First, dietary intakes may not represent a wide enough range of exposure to be in the range at which effects are observable.[31] Second, that level of intake at which dietary risk from a constituent is apparent and that at which metabolic, pathological, or clinically apparent changes in indices are likely probably differ. Also it may be that intakes of some constituent, such as fat, that is associated with decreases in risk in some parameters, such as blood lipid levels, are apparent at one level, and that very much lower levels are necessary if intakes are to be associated with other parameters, such as changes in serum hormones and breast cancer risk. This has been our experience with dietary fat intakes, for example.[69-71] The levels of alcohol necessary to be associated with risk of breast cancer may also be lower than those associated with fetal alcohol effects.

Also similar centiles of the distribution of current intakes may represent very different points in the progress toward clinically apparent disease for different dietary constituents. Consider, for example, alcohol. Deviations in dietary intakes of some constituents may represent an earlier stage in the onset of pathology than biochemical, behavioral, anthropometric, or clinical indices. A considerable length of time may elapse before pathology actually becomes apparent at these other levels.

The association between dietary intakes and individual risk of breast cancer is influenced by factors other than intake itself, such as the individual's unique nutritional needs, which are never known precisely, genetics, environmental risk factors such as possibly exogenous hormones, body weight or weight fluctuations, distribution of body fat tissue, physical activity, the presence of nutrient imbalances or other aspects of dietary patterns, diseases or environmental stresses.

Finally, measurement of dietary intake is always imprecise. It is highly dependent on the food constituent being assessed; the content of the constituent (such as phytoestrogens) in the food supply may only be partially known. The time frame assessed may not be reflective of usual intakes. Interpretation is further complicated because, among individuals eating *ad libitum*, many aspects of intake may change simultaneously. All methods are partly subjective. As such they are highly dependent upon the capability and willingness of the respondent, and the skill of the interviewer (which varies greatly, even among professionals) to a greater extent than more objective methods.

In the next decade the uses of dietary assessment methods to study patterns of dietary intake and both nutrients and other substances in diets and their links to indices of health and disease will continue to expand. It is to be hoped that valid dietary assessment methods that are suitable for epidemiologic investigations will be perfected. Food composition data bases will become more complete for all of the many constituents we wish to study. Differences between methods and the sources of error they generate in apparent intakes will be elucidated. More attention will be paid to distinguishing between methods suitable for groups and for individuals. Better methods for analyzing information for specific purposes will be developed.

V. Future Directions

Is the evidence on an association between dietary fat and breast cancer good enough to proceed with a large-scale trial? Are other leads more promising? It seems to this observer that prudent haste is justified, and that it makes sense for the Women's Health Trial feasibility study and the American Cancer Society efforts to go forward. At the same time, additional data from the very large cohort studies here and abroad should be examined. Thus, we should certainly not do nothing. The cohort studies need continuation. Diet feasibility studies need continuation and expansion. Diet methodologies need to be validated and refined. If a prophylactic trial of hormone therapy for those at risk is considered, diet should be altered or controlled to minimize doses.

Acknowledgment

Partial support for the preparation of this manuscript was furnished by grant MCJ 9120 to Dr. Dwyer from the Maternal and Child Health Service, U.S. Department of Health and Human Services, through subcontracts to Dr. Dwyer and New England Medical Center, on a grant from the National Cancer Institute, 5R25-CA 49612-02 and another grant, Diet and Phytoestrogens, B. Goldin, Principal Investigator, from the National Institutes of Health. This paper has been funded at least in part from Federal funds from the United States Department of Agriculture, Agricultural Research Service, under contract 533K065-10. The contents of this publication do not necessarily reflect the views or policies of USDA.

References

1. U.S. Department of Health and Human Services, "Steroid Receptors in Breast Cancer: Information for Physicians," NIH Pub. No 83:1853 National Cancer Institute, Bethesda, August (1983).
2. Early breast cancer trialists collaborative group effects of adjuvant tamoxifen and of cytotoxic therapy on mortality in early breast cancer: an overview of 61 randomized trials among 38,896 women, *N Engl J Med*. 319: 1681 (1988).
3. T. Fornander, B. Cedarmark, A. Mattsson, L. Skoog, T. Theve, J. Askergrein, L.E. Rutqvist, U. Glas, C. Silversward, A. Somell, N. Wilking, and M.L. Hjalmar, Adjuvant tamoxifen in early breast cancer: occurrence of new primary cancers, *Lancet*. 1:117 (1989).
4. D.T. Kiang, Chemoprevention for breast cancer: are we ready?, *J Natl Cancer Inst*. 83:462 (1991).

5. J.W. Weisburger and E.L. Wynder, Dietary fat intake and cancer, *Hematology/Oncology Clinics of North America.* 5:7 (1991).
6. L.A. Cohen, M.E. Kendall, E. Zang, C. Meschter, and D.P. Rose, Modulation of N-Nitroso-methylurea induced mammary tumor promotion by dietary fiber and fat, *J Natl Cancer Inst.* 83: 496 (1991).
7. R.L. Prentice and L. Sheppard, Dietary fat and cancer: consistency of the epidemiologic data and disease prevention that may follow from a practical reduction in fat consumption, *Cancer Causes and Control.* 1:81 (1990).
8. R.L. Prentice and L. Sheppard, Dietary fat and cancer: rejoinder and discussion of research strategies, *Cancer Causes and Control.* 2:53 (1990).
9. W.C. Willett and M. Stampfer, Dietary fat and cancer: another view, *Cancer Causes and Control.* 1:103 (1990).
10. G.R. Howe, Dietary fat and cancer, *Cancer Causes and Control.* 1:99 (1990).
11. J.E. Hiller, and A.J. McMichael, Dietary fat and cancer: a comeback for etiological studies? *Cancer Causes and Control.* 1:101 (1990).
12. J.R. Hebert, J. Barone, M.M. Reddy, and J.Y. Backlund, Natural killer cell activity in a longitudinal dietary fat intervention trial, *Clin Immunol Immunopathol.* 54:103 (1989).
13. J. Barone, J.R. Hebert, and M.M. Reddy, Dietary fat and natural killer cell activity, *Am J Clin Nutr.* 50: 861 (1989).
14. Subcommittee on Nutritional Surveillance, Committee on Medical Aspect of Food Policy, The diets of British schoolchildren, *Rep Health Soc Subj.* (Lond) 36:1-293 (1989).
15. H.P. Lee, L. Gouley, S.W. Duffy, J. Esteve, J. Lee, and N.E. Day, Dietary effects on breast cancer risk in Singapore, *Lancet.* 337:1197 (1991).
16. L.D. Byham, Dietary fat and natural killer cell function, *Nutrition Today.* Jan/Feb 31 (1991).
17. E.L. Wynder, L.A. Cohen, and D.P. Rose, Etiology of breast cancer: dietary fat and weight, *Nutrition.* 5:361 (1989).
18. K.J. Acheson, I.T. Campbell, O.G.H. Edholm, D.S. Miller, and M.J. Stock, The measurement of daily energy expenditure: an evaluation of some techniques, *Am J Clin Nutr.* 33: 1155 (1980).
19. J.S. Stern, L. Grivetti, and T.W. Castonguay, Energy intake: uses and misuses, *In J Obes.* 8: 535 (1984).
20. M.B.E. Livingstone, A.M. Prentice, J.J. Strain, W.A. Coward, A.E. Black, M.E. Barker, P.G. McKenna, and R.G. Whitehead, Accuracy of weighed dietary records in studies of diet and health, *Brit Med J.* 300:708 (1990).
21. J.R. Hebert, A. Augustin, J. Barone, G.C. Kabat, D.W. Kinne, and E.L. Wynder, Weight, height, and body mass index in the prognosis of breast cancer: early results of a prospective study, *Int J Cancer.* 42:315 (1988).
22. L.J. Vattan and L. Kvinnsland, Body height and risk for breast cancer: a prospective study of 23,831 Norwegian women, *Br J Cancer.* 61:881 (1990).
23. G. Wilcox, M.L. Wahlquist, H.G. Burger and G. Medley, Oestrogenic effects of plant foods in postmenopausal women, *Br Med J.* 301:905 (1990).
24. M. Messina and S. Barnes, The role of soy products in reducing risk of cancer, *J Natl Cancer Inst.* 83:541 (1991).
25. P.P. Nair, N. Turjman, G. Kessie, B. Calkins, G.T. Goodman, H. Davidovitz, and G. Nimmagadda, Diet, nutrition intake, and metabolism in populations at high and low risk for colon cancer: dietary cholesterol, beta sitosterol, and stigmasterol, *Am J Clin Nutr.* 40:927 (1984).
26. K Hirai, C. Shimazu, R. Takazoe, Y. Ozek, Cholesterol, phytosterol, and polyunsaturated fatty acid levels in 1982 and 1957 Japanese diets, *J Nutr Sci Vitaminol.* 32:363 (1986).
27. A. Shatzkin, Y. Jones, R.N. Hoover, P.R. Taylor, L.A. Brinton, R.G. Ziegler, E.B. Harvey, C.L. Carter, L.M. Licitra, M.C. Dufour, and D.B. Larson, Alcohol consumption and breast cancer in the epidemiologic follow up study of the first National Health and Nutrition Examination Survey, *N Engl J Med.* 316:1169 (1987).

28. W.C. Willett, M.J. Stampfer, G.A. Colditz, B.A. Rosner, C.H. Hennedens, and F.E. Speizer, Moderate alcohol consumption and risk of breast cancer, *N Engl J Med.* 316:1174 (1987).

29. M.P. Longenecker, J.A. Berlin, M.J. Orza, and T.C. Chalmers, A metaanalysis of alcohol consumption in relation to risk of breast cancer, *J Amer Med Assoc.* 260:652 (1988).

30. J.W.G. Yarnell, A.M. Fehily, J.E. Milbank, P.M. Sweetnam, and C.L. Walker, A short dietary questionnaire for use in an epidemiological survey: comparison with weighed dietary records, *Hum Nutr Appl Nutr.* 37A:103 (1983).

31. J.R. Hebert and G.C. Kabat, Distribution of smoking and its association with lung cancer: implications for studies on the association of fat with cancer, *J Natl Cancer Inst.* 83:872 (1991).

32. C.T. Windham, B.W. Wyse, and R.G. Hansen, Alcohol consumption and nutrient density of diets in the Nationwide Food Consumption Survey, *J Am Diet Assoc.* 82:364 (1983).

33. D.P. Rose, A.P. Boyar, and E.L. Wynder, International comparisons of mortality rates for cancer of the breast, ovary, prostate, and colon, and per capita food consumption, *Cancer.* 58:2363 (1986).

34. D.M. Goettler, L. Levin, and W.Y. Chey, Postprandial levels of prolactin and gut hormones in breast cancer patients: association with stage of disease, but not dietary fat, *J Natl Cancer Inst.* 82:22 (1990).

35. P. Hill, E.L. Wynder, and P. Helman, Plasma hormone levels in premenopausal and postmenopausal vegetarian women fed a Western diet, *Fed Proc.* 38:865 (1979).

36. P. Hill, J.H. Thijssen, L. Garbaczewski, P.F. Koppeschaar, and F. De Waard, VIP and prolactin release in response to meals, *Scand J Gastroenteral.* 21:958 (1986).

37. M.A. Hagerty, B. Howie, S. Tan, and T.D. Shultz, Effect of low and high fat intakes on hormone levels in premenopausal women: a controlled metabolic feeding study, *Fed Proc.* 47:653 (1988).

38. D.M. Ingram, P.C. Bennett, D. Willcox, and N. De Klerk, Effect of low fat diet on female sex hormone levels, *J Natl Cancer Inst.* (1987).

39. R.L. Prentice, F. Kakar, S. Hursting, L. Sheppard, R. Klein, and L.H. Kushi, Aspects of the rationale for the Women's Health Trial, *J Natl Cancer Inst.* 80:802 (1988).

40. R.L. Prentice and L. Sheppard, Validity of international, time trend, and migrant studies of dietary factors and disease risk, *Prev Med.* 18:167 (1989).

41. R.T. Chlebowski, D.W. Nixon, G.L. Blackburn, P. Jochimsen, E.F. Scanlon, W. Insull, I.M. Buzzard, R. Elashoff, R. Butrum, and E.L. Wynder, Breast cancer nutrition adjuvant study (NAS): protocol design and initial patient adherence, *Breast Cancer Res Treat.* 10:21 (1987).

42. I.M. Buzzard, E.H. Asp, R.T. Chlebowski, A.P. Boyar, R.W. Jeffrey, D.W. Nixon, G.L. Blackburn, P.R. Jochimsen, E.F. Scanlon, W. Insull, R.M. Elashoff, R. Butrum, and E.L. Wynder, Diet intervention methods to reduce fat intake: nutrient and food group composition of self selected low fat diets, *J Am Diet Assoc.* 90:42 (1990).

43. R.T. Chlebowski, G.L. Blackburn, and I.M. Buzzard. Current status: Evaluation of dietary fat reduction as secondary breast cancer prevention, *in:* "Advances in cancer control: Screening and Prevention Research," Wiley Liss, Inc. (1990).

44. R.T. Chlebowski, G.L. Blackburn, and D.W. Nixon, P. Jochimsen, E.F. Scanlon, W. Insull, I.M. Buzzard, E.L. Wynder, and R. Elashoff, The nutrition adjuvant study experience and commentary, *Controlled Clinical Trials.* 10:368 (1989).

45. R.T. Chlebowski and D. Rose, Adjuvant dietary fat intake reduction in postmenopausal breast cancer management (1991).

46. A.P. Boyar, D.P. Rose, and E.L. Wynder, Recommendations for the prevention of chronic disease: the application for breast disease, *Am J Clin Nutr.* 48:896 (1988).

47. H. Lee-Han, M. Cousins, M. Beaton, V. McGuire, Y. Driudov, M. Chipman, and N. Boyd, Compliance in a randomized clinical trial of dietary fat reduction in patients with breast dysplasia, *Am J Clin Nutr.* 48:575 (1988).

48. N.F. Boyd, M.L. Cousins, S.E. Bayliss, E.D. Fishell, and W.R. Bruce, Diet & Breast Disease: evidence for the feasibility of a clinical trial involving a major reduction in dietary

fat, *in:* "Cancer Nutrient Eating Behavior," T.G. Burish, S.M. Levy, and B.E. Meyerowitz, eds., Lawrence Earlbaum Associates, Inc., New York (1984).

49. M.G. Jain, G.R. Howe, K.C. Johnson, and A.B. Miller, Evaluation of a diet history questionnaire for epidemiologic studies, *Am J Epidemiol.* 111:2112 (1980).

50. M.J. Jain, L. Harrison, G.R. Howe, and A.B. Miller, Evaluation of a self administered dietary questionnaire for use in a cohort study, *Am J Clin Nutr.* 36:931 (1982).

51. R.W. Morgan, M. Jain, A.B. Miller, N.W. Choi, W. Matthews, L. Munan, J.D. Burch, J. Feather, G.R. Howe, and A. Kelly, Comparison of dietary methods in an epidemiologic study, *Am J Epidemiol.* 107:488 (1978).

52. G.R. Howe, C.M. Friedenreich, M. Jain, and A.B. Miller, A cohort study of fat intake and risk factors of breast cancer, *J Natl Cancer Inst.* 83:336 (1991).

53. G.R. Howe, T. Hirohata, T.G. Hislap J.M. Iscovich, J.M. Yuan, K. Katsouyanni, F. Lubin, E. Marubini, B. Modan, T. Rohan, P. Toniolo, and Y. Shunzhang, Dietary factors and risk of breast cancer, *J Natl Cancer Inst.* 83:336 (1991).

54. G.R. Howe, Response, *J Natl Cancer Inst.* 83:1035 (1991).

55. P. Knekt, D. Albanes, R. Seppanen, A. Aromaa, R. Jarvinen, L. Hyvonen, L. Teppo, and E. Pukkala, Dietary fat and risk of breast cancer, *Am J Clin Nutr.* 52: 903 (1990).

56. P.K. Mills, W.L. Beeson, R.L. Philips, and G.E. Fraser, Dietary habits and breast cancer incidence among Seventh day Adventists, *Cancer.* 64:582 (1989).

57. J.R. Hebert and G.C. Kabat, Implications for cancer epidemiology of differences in dietary intake associated with alcohol consumption, *Nutrition and Cancer.* 15:107 (1991).

58. W. Willett and M.J. Stampfer, Total energy intake: implications for epidemiologic analyses, *Am J Epidemiol.* 124:17 (1986).

59. M.C. Pike, L. Bernstein, and R.K. Feters, Letter to the editor, *Am J Epidemiol.* 129:1312 (1989).

60. T.E. Prewitt, D. Schmeisser, P.E. Bowen, P. Aye, T.A. Dolecek, T. Langenberg, T. Cole, and L. Brace, Changes in body weight, body composition, and energy intake in women fed high and low fat diets, *Am J Clin Nutr.* 54:304 (1991).

61. G. Block, A.M. Hartman, C.M. Dresser, M.D. Carroll, J. Cannon, and L. Gardner, A data based approach to diet questionnaire design and testing, *Am J Epidemiol.* 124:453 (1986).

62. R.S. Gibson, "Principles of Nutritional Assessment" Oxford University Press, New York (1990).

63. S. Bingham, The dietary assessment of individuals: methods, accuracy, new techniques, and recommendations, *Nut Abst and Rev.* 57:707 (1987).

64. E.M. Pao and Y.S. Cypel, Estimation of dietary intake, *in:* "Present Knowledge in Nutrition: M.L. Brown, ed., International Life Sciences Institute, Washington, (1990).

65. E.M. Pao, K.E. Sykes, and Y.S. Cypel, USDA Methodological Research for Large Scale Dietary Intake Surveys, 1975-88 Washington United States Department of Agriculture, Human Nutrition Information Service, Home Economics Research Report Number 49 (1989).

66. G. Block and A.M. Hartman, Dietary Methods, *in:* "Nutrition and Cancer Prevention," T.E. Moon and M.S. Micozzi, eds. Marcel Dekkar, New York (1989).

67. D. Mackerras, Interpreting Dietary Data, Sydney Department of Public Health, University of Sydney (1990).

68. J.T. Dwyer, Assessment of dietary intake, *in:* "Modern Nutrition in Health and Disease" M.E. Shils and V.R. Young, eds. Philadelphia (1988).

69. M.N. Woods, S.L. Gorbach, C. Longscope, B.R. Goldin, J.T. Dwyer, and A. Morrill-LaBrode, Low fat high fiber and serum estrone sulfate in premenopausal women, *Am J Clin Nutr.* 49:1179 (1989).

70. W. Insull, M.M. Henderson, R.L. Prentice, D.J. Thompson, C. Clifford, S. Goldman, S. Gorbach, M. Moskowitz, R. Thompson, and M. Woods, Results of a randomized feasibility study of a low fat diet, *Arch Intern Med.* 150:421 (1990).

71. R.L. Prentice, D.J. Thompson, C. Clifford, S.L. Gorbach, B. Goldin, and D. Byar, Dietary fat reduction and plasma estradiol concentration in healthy postmenopausal women, *J Natl Cancer Inst.* 82:129 (1990).

72. S.A. Bingham, M. Nelson, and A.A. Paul, Methods for data collection at the individual level, *in*: "Manual on Methodology For Food Consumption Studies," M. Cameron and V. Staveren, eds.. Oxford University Press, Oxford (1988).

73. J.J. Michnovicz and H.L. Bradlow, Induction of estradiol metabolism by dietary indole 3-carbinol in humans, *J Natl Cancer Inst.* 82:947 (1990).

74. N.L. Petrakis, L.D. Gruenke, and J.C. Craig, Cholesterol and cholesterol epoxides in nipple aspirates on human breast fluid, *Cancer Res.* 41:2563 (1981).

75. L.A. Cohen, K. Choi, J.H. Weisburger, and D.P. Rose, Effect of varying dietary fat on the development of N-nitrosoethylurea induced in rat mammary tumors, *Anticancer Res.* 6:215 (1986).

76. L.A. Cohen and E.L. Wynder, Do dietary monosaturated fatty acids play a protective role in carcinogenesis and cardiovascular disease?, *Med Hypothesis.* 31:83 (1990).

77. A. Morabia and E.L. Wynder, Epidemiology and natural history of breast cancer: implications for the body weight-breast cancer controversy, *Surgical Clinics of North America.* 70:739 (1991).

78. H. Aldercreutz, T. Fotsis, R. Heikkinen, J.T. Dwyer, B.R. Goldin, S.L. Gorbach, A.M. Lawson, and K.D.R. Setchell, Diet and urinary excretion of lignan in female subjects, *Med Biol.* 59: 259 (1981).

79. H. Aldercreutz, T. Fotsis, R. Heikkinen, J.T. Dwyer, M. Woods, B.R. Goldin, and S.L. Gorbach, Excretion of the lignans anterolectone and enterodiol and of equol in omnivorous and vegetarian postmenopausal women with breast cancer, *Lancet.* ii:1295 (1982).

80. H. Adlercreutz, T. Fotsis, C. Bannwart, K. Wahala, T. Makela, G. Brunow, and T. Hase, Determination of urinary lignans and phytoestrogen metabolites, potential antiestrogens and anticarcinogens in urine of women on various habitual diets, *J Steroid Biochem.* 25:791, (1986).

81. E. Nordevang, E. Ikkala, E. Callmer, L. Hallstrom, and L.E. Holm, Dietary intervention in breast cancer patients: effects on dietary habits and nutrient intake, *European J Clin Nutr.* 44:681 (1990).

82. A.P. Boyar, D.P. Rose, J. Loughridge, A. Engle, A. Palgi, K. Laakso, D. Kinne, and E.L. Wynder, Response to a diet low in total fat in women with postmenopausal breast cancer, *Nutr Cancer.* 11:93 (1988).

83. S.L. Gorbach, A. Morrill-LaBrode, M.N. Woods, J.T. Dwyer, W.D. Selles, M. Henderson, W. Insull, S. Goldman, D. Thompson, C. Clifford, and L. Sheppard, Changes in food patterns during a low fat dietary intervention in women, *J Am Diet Assoc.* 90:802 (1990).

84. M.E. Cameron and W.A Van Stavaran, eds., "Manual on Methodology for Food Consumption Studies" Oxford University Press, Oxford, (1988).

Chapter 15

Possible Mechanisms through which Dietary Lipids, Calorie Restriction, and Exercise Modulate Breast Cancer

GABRIEL FERNANDES and JAYA T. VENKATRAMAN

I. Introduction

Though the exact cause of breast cancer still remains a mystery, years of investigations have suggested that several dietary and endocrine-related factors may induce and/or could modulate the growth of breast cancer. Epidemiologic and experimental evidence have indicated a close association between high-fat diets and increased incidence of breast cancer.[1-3] Furthermore, several immunologic functions, including the levels of growth factors, cytokines, and sex steroid hormones, may be altered or regulated by dietary lipids.[4,5] Excessive fat in the diet has been reported to enhance the growth of both spontaneously occurring and chemically induced colon and mammary tumors, as well as accelerated growth of transplantable carcinomas.[6-8] Diets containing high levels of ω-6 fatty acids derived from vegetable fats appear to enhance tumorigenesis, while ω-3-containing lipids, either from vegetable or marine origin, or low levels of fat in the diet can diminish tumorigenesis. Recently, a number of mechanisms have been proposed to explain the modulation of mammary tumorigenesis in experimental animals by increasing the levels of dietary fats.[9,10] Initiation and promotion have been linked to immune suppression,[11] prostaglandin production,[12,13] free radical formation,[14] membrane fluidity changes,[15] intracellular transport system modulation,[16] increased caloric utilization,[17] increased mammotrophic hormone secretion,[18] and cytokine changes.[19,20] Over-expression of oncogenes and certain growth factors are other mechanisms that have been linked to dietary changes that may influence mammary tumorigenesis.

Gabriel Fernandes and Jaya T. Venkatraman • Department of Medicine, University of Texas Health Science Center, 7703 Floyd Curl Drive, San Antonio, Texas

Exercise, Calories, Fat, and Cancer, Edited by M.M. Jacobs
Plenum Press, New York, 1992

II. Dietary Lipids and Tumor Growth

Most cancer-related deaths in humans are caused by metastasis, which is indeed a complex, multistep, progressive process, and dietary fats may influence specific events like survival and proliferation of tumor cells. When rodents are fed high-fat diets, the incidence of mammary tumors sharply increases and the latency of tumor appearance is greatly diminished when compared to animals fed diets containing low levels of fat. It appears high dietary fats may selectively influence the formation and development of metastasis.[21] Immunogenic or multidrug properties of the tumor cell may determine the nature and degree of the influence of the immune system on forming metastasis. It is possible dietary fats may change the microenvironment of the tumor cell or the host cell, particularly microviscosity[22] and the rigidity of membranes, which are linked to an increased rate of metastatic potential.[23] For instance, dietary fat may influence metastasis through the loss of cytotoxic ability of T cells and natural killer (NK) cells.[24,25]

Changes in intracellular communication include changes in cellular adhesion, hormone responsiveness, and alterations in the production of growth factors and cytokines by the immune cells as well as by the tumor cells themselves.[21] Raising dietary soybean oil from 5 to 20% by weight is associated with increased mammary tumorigenesis, reduced T-cell blastogenesis, and low cytotoxicity.[26,27] Epidemiologic studies reporting a correlation between fat intake and breast cancer are primarily supported by studies in rodent models showing that increasing dietary fat consumption causes a higher incidence of mammary cancer induced by viruses, chemicals, radiation, and also a higher growth rate of transplantable mammary tumors.[28,29] Changes in the endocrine system, mammary tissue growth and development, absorption and metabolism of carcinogens, and the decline of immune system (e.g., loss of T and NK cell functions) have been postulated as possible mechanisms whereby dietary fat can influence mammary tumorigenesis. Both quantity and saturation of dietary fat have been reported to influence the function of the immune system. Several studies with diets high in polyunsaturated fatty acids (PUFAs) have been reported either to raise or reduce the response to T-cell mitogens when compared to animals fed low-fat diets. Further, the decreased rate of lipid peroxidation in tumor tissues has been explained by the decreased availability of PUFAs in tumor membranes.

A. ω-3 Fatty Acids and Cancer Protection

In recent years, consumption of saturated fat has declined significantly due to the fear of increasing cardiovascular disease. The reduction of saturated fat has now been replaced by the increase in consumption of polyunsaturated lipids, which are known to reduce the cholesterol levels.[2] Several experiments have suggested that ω-3 lipids can protect against the development of cardiovascular disease, possibly mammary tumor incidence,[30-32] and the severity of autoimmune disease.[33] Significant reductions in chemically induced as well as transplanted tumors by high levels of dietary ω-3 fatty acids containing fish oil have been recently reported by several investigators.[34-38]

In addition, antimetastatic effects of fish oil have been observed by us[39] and indicate the importance of studying the therapeutic potential of ω-3 lipids in humans. It is important to recognize the role of anti-oxidant supplements, which appear to be crucial for preventing free radical formation. The latter may have adverse effects on host cells. Recently, some observations have suggested that peroxidizable lipids may have a beneficial effect in reducing the growth of tumor cells.[40,41] The effect of anti-oxidant supplements alone on the immune cell and/or tumor cell needs to be clarified. We and other investigators have pointed out the need to supplement ω-3 lipids with increased vitamin E levels for increasing the anti-oxidant levels in the membrane to reduce malandialdehyde (MDA) production,[42,43] thereby increasing the cytotoxic potential of immune cells.[44,45] It appears additional studies are required for establishing the role of anti-oxidants in reducing the free radical formation in the host tissues.

B. ω-3 Lipids and Human Breast Cancer Cells

We are studying the effects of dietary lipids on the growth of well-characterized estrogen receptor-positive human breast cancer cells in a nude mouse model. The immune-deficient nude mouse model has been well accepted as a useful animal model for examining cell kinetics of human-origin tumor cells, particularly breast carcinoma cells.[46,47] Estrogen-dependent (MCF-7) as well as estrogen-independent (MDA-MB 231) cell lines have been studied extensively to determine the role of growth factors and estrogen and anti-estrogen therapy on growth rate of tumor cells.[48,49] To examine the role of dietary lipids, we fed 4-week-old female athymic nude mice (Balb/c-nu/nu) a semi-purified diet containing 20% corn oil or 20% fish oil (containing adequate and equal levels of anti-oxidants) for 4 weeks. MCF-7 cells were injected subcutaneously (5×10^6 cells) into each mouse. The MCF-7 tumor cell intake in nude mice fed diets containing corn oil was 17/24 (71%) compared to a fish oil-fed group that had much less tumor growth—5/22 (23%) (Figure 1). The mice fed corn oil and bearing transplanted tumors had higher levels of estrogen (378 pg/ml) and prolactin (11.6 ng/ml) in the serum compared to the group fed dietary fish oil (245 pg/ml estrogen; 7.3 ng/ml prolactin) suggesting that changes in serum pituitary hormone levels by dietary fat may have an important role in regulating the growth rate of transplanted tumor cells. However, these findings need further study to confirm the results of anti-oxidant effects, the growth of tumor cells, and the functional changes in the immune cells.

Dietary lipids also had a striking effect on the tissue prostaglandin E_2 (PGE_2) levels in nude mice. The level of PGE_2 production was found considerably higher in corn oil-fed animals (spleen 1.92 ng/mg per 30 min; tumor-0.22 ng/mg per 30 min.) as compared to the group fed fish oil diet both in tumor (0.58 ng/mg/per 30 min.) and spleen tissues (0.14 ng/mg/per 30 min). As dietary fats are known to alter tissue fatty acid composition and thereby alter PGE_2 production, we decided to analyze the fatty acid composition to relate changes in PGE_2 levels in the tumor tissue. The fatty acid composition of the dietary lipids

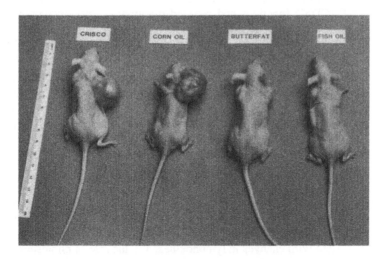

Figure 1. Effect of dietary lipids on growth of human breast cancer cells in nude mice.

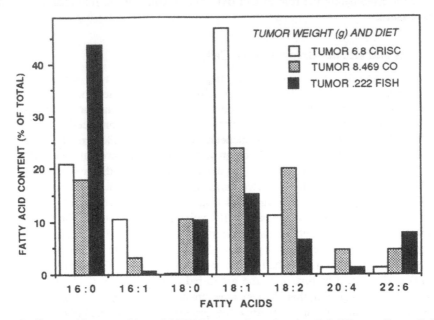

Figure 2. Fatty acid composition of MCF-7 tumors in nude mice fed different dietary lipids.

was closely related to changes in the fatty acid composition of tumor and spleen tissue of each dietary group. As expected, tumors from animals fed corn oil had higher incorporation of 18:2 and 20:4 fatty acids, while fish oil-fed animals had higher levels of ω-3 fatty acids (20:5 and 22:6) in their tumors (Figure 2). Experiments were carried out to measure changes in oncogene expression in tumor tissues obtained from animals fed various fats and revealed c-*myc* mRNA expression was high in the corn oil-fed group and was low in tumors from fish oil-fed mice.[32] The level of P21 proteins was also found higher in tumor lysate from corn oil-fed animals compared to the fish oil-fed group. This indicated that the increased *ras*-P21 protein level is closely linked to the rapid growth rate of tumor cells, which can be modulated by feeding diet containing ω-3 lipids (Figure 3).

We have also reported the beneficial effects of calorie/fat restriction on maintenance of high cytotoxic T-cell (CD8[+]) functions and reduced mammary tumor incidence.[50] Caloric restriction decreased prolactin and anti-MMTV antibody levels and decreased mammary tumor virus particles in C3H/Bi mice.[50,51] Several investigators have also found that diets based on fish oil containing high levels of ω-3 fatty acids, such as eicosapentanoic acid and docosahexaenoic acid, do show beneficial effects against breast cancer compared to corn oil. Although these ω-3 fatty acids differ from arachidonic acid (ω-6) and inhibit both the cyclooxygenase and lipooxygenase enzyme systems, the role of the immune system in modulating the tumor growth is not yet fully elucidated. More studies are required to confirm the role of the immune system in modulating the growth of tumor cells *in vivo*.

C. Membrane Lipids

Cellular functions of various immune cells, including cytotoxic cell-mediated immune parameters, may be directly affected by modifications in membrane lipid composition and lipid interaction with membrane proteins. Alterations in the lipid composition of plasma membranes are associated with changes in lymphokines, and the rate of cholesterol synthesis by leukemia cells has been reported to be 10 to 30 times that of normal lymphocytes. The

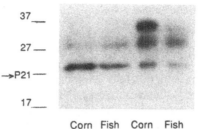

Figure 3. Western blot showing the effects of dietary lipids on the *ras*-P21 protein levels in tumor tissues of nude mice.

plasma membranes of leukemia cells may contain more cholesterol relative to membrane phospholipids than do normal lymphocytes. The modifications in lipids may alter physico-chemical characteristics of membranes and thereby alter cellular functions, including carrier-mediated transport, properties of certain membrane-bound glycoproteins and/or enzymes, binding of hormones to receptors, phagocytosis, endocytosis, cytotoxicity of NK cells and macrophages (Mφ), prostaglandin production, and cell growth and differentiation.[52] Membrane lipid structural changes affect bulk lipid fluidity or specific lipid domains. Transport-ers, receptors, and enzymes may be highly sensitive to changes in the structure of their lipid microenvironment, leading to changes in production of various cytokines and PGs, which act adversely on immune cells.[53,54]

Changes in lipids may have direct effects on protein kinase C (PK-C)[55-57] and thereby may alter tumor cell proliferation and/or the immune cell response to growth factors to increase the cytotoxic function. Whether the tumor-inhibiting properties of longer chain n-3 fatty acids in marine oils are shared by shorter chain linoleic acid (18:3) in linseed oil is not clear. Recently, Pritchard *et al.*[58] have reported that a 10-11% fish oil diet inhibited the development of human breast cancer MCF-7 cells injected into nude mice. The tumors in fish oil-fed groups seem to be more responsive to chemotherapy with mitomycin C and doxorubicin than those fed 10% corn oil.[59] The tumor cells in fish oil-fed groups may be more susceptible to chemotherapeutic agents due to alterations in fluidity of the mem-branes.[60]

Other studies, including the experiments carried out by Jurkowski and Cave[61] on carcinogen-induced mammary tumors, have suggested that menhaden oil increased tumor latency period and reduced tumor incidence and tumor mass. Their data as well as our data indicate that tumor tissue membranes from mice fed different lipids have a distinctive lipid composition.[32,62] Certain membrane fatty acid alterations may affect cellular responsiveness to external stimuli-like growth factors, hormones, and antibodies, as well as affecting membrane permeability and enhancing selective enzyme pathways, thereby influencing cellular metabolism of carcinogens or chemotherapeutic agents. Diets high in n-3 fatty acids reduce both cyclooxygenase and lipoxygenase activity in the tumors and thereby affect eicosanoid metabolism.[63] Recent evidence suggests that tumor necrosis factor (TNF), lymphotoxin, leukoregulin, interferons (IFNs) and certain PGs derived from *cis*-unsaturated fatty acids have selective tumoricidal actions.[64] Further, tumor cells are deficient in delta-6-desaturase[65] and secrete excess PGE_2.[66,67]

Low rates of lipid peroxidation and free radical generation in tumor cells may be attributed to low *cis*-unsaturated fatty acid content and decreased activity of NADPH cytochrome reductase and cytochrome P450.[68,69] Lymphokine (e.g., IFN and TNF)-induced free radical generation in neutrophils and tumor cells may be dependent on *cis*-unsaturated fatty acid release. An altered membrane composition may prevent adverse lymphokine production and action on host and tumor cells.

III. Energy Balance

The cachexia seen in cancer is not fully explained by inadequate energy intake and increased energy expenditure.[70] Studies in humans and animals suggest that depletion of body fat is out of proportion to protein loss and may account for the majority of weight loss seen with cancer. Studies in humans and animals have shown that total host lipids decrease as tumor growth increases, free fatty acids increase before marked losses of body weight occur, and that glucose fails to suppress fatty acid oxidation.

In one report, mice bearing even a nonmetastatic tumor (ESR 586) were found to have lipid depletion.[71] Abnormalities in insulin secretion or sensitivity could affect the rates of lipolysis and lipogenesis in patients with cancer. Insulin administered to tumor-bearing animals ameliorates the loss of fat that occurs, suggesting that insulin deficiency may play a role in the increased fat mobilization seen in patients with cancer. It appears diet therapy with specific lipid and carbohydrate intake may modify both cytokines and insulin levels in cancer patients.

IV. Endocrine System

Modulation of endocrine hormone production by diet appears to be a very attractive strategy for facilitation of drug therapy at the receptor level. Growth of human breast cancer cells *in vitro* is regulated by several growth factors, including estrogen, androgen, progesterone, glucocorticoids, insulin, insulin-like growth factors (IGFs I and II), cathepsin-D, platelet-derived growth factor (PDGF), epidermal growth factor (EGF-1), prolactin, and thyroid hormone.[72-75] About one-third of human breast cancers are hormone-dependent and require estrogen for maximal growth. Therapy designed to reduce the estrogen concentration or to inhibit the effects of estrogen by competitive blockade of the estrogen receptor results in regression of these tumors.[76,77] The mechanisms by which endocrine therapy inhibit tumor growth have not been completely defined. Studies on endocrine effects suggest that dietary lipids may alter estrogen, prolactin, and pituitary-derived hormones.

A. Estradiol

It is generally accepted that estradiol plays an important role in influencing proliferation of breast cancer. Considerable evidence is accumulating to suggest that neoplastic growth may be under autocrine control via secreted peptide growth factors. An autocrine system occurs in human breast cancer, since breast cancer cell lines secrete autostimulatory growth factors, either constitutively or under the positive control of estrogen. Furthermore, a paracrine influence of breast stromal fibroblasts also occurs in breast cancer.[78] Previous studies have demonstrated that cultured human breast fibroblasts secrete a high-molecular-weight polypeptide that stimulates the ability of human breast-cancer MCF-7 cells to convert estrone (E1) to the biologically more active 17β-estradiol (E2). This effect is mediated by an increase in reductive E2 oxidoreductase (EOR) activity, interleukin 6 (IL-6), or an immunologically related peptide.[78] A polyclonal neutralizing antibody to IL-6 completely abolished the reductive EOR-stimulating activity. Breast tissues can accumulate estrogens not only by uptake from plasma, but also by intra-tissue enzymatic conversion of precursors to E1 and E2 via the actions of aromatase and EOR.

B. Glucocorticoids, Progestins, and Androgens

Glucocorticoids are used in chemotherapeutic strategies for treatment of malignancies of lymphoreticular origin. Lipopolysaccharide (LPS)-responsive monoclonal leukemia cells differentiate to antibody-secreting cells in a manner resembling normal, nontransformed B cells. Murine B-cell leukemia (BCL1) cells respond to glucocorticoids by reducing the rate of DNA synthesis.[79] Glucocorticoid treatment rapidly increases membrane lipid mobility in both resting B cells and LPS-activated lymphoblasts.[80,81] Synthetic progestins and androgens have been used to treat human breast cancer and breast fibrocystic diseases. Their mechanism of action in human breast cells is not well understood. In the human breast cancer cell line T47D, the synthetic progestin R5020 and 5α-dihydrotestosterone significantly increase the number of lipid droplets per cell compared to control cells or estradiol- and dexamethasone-treated cells. The progestin antagonist, RU486, inhibits lipid accumulation. Progestins and androgens may increase lipid accumulation by interacting with their own receptor[82,83] and thereby induce triglyceride accumulation in T47D cells. This effect follows fatty acid synthase induction and precedes cell growth inhibition. In T47D cells, progestins inhibit estradiol-induced cell growth. An association of lipid accumulation and cell growth inhibition has been shown in receptor-positive breast cancer cell lines treated with human prolactin or growth hormone in the presence of hydrocortisone, or following treatment with sodium butyrate. This lipid accumulation may be involved in increasing the differentiation of lactating mammary gland cells. These observations suggest that progestin induces the commitment of cancer cells to terminal differentiation. In other studies, the mitotic index appears to be higher in the luteal phase of the menstrual cycle, suggesting a mitogenic activity of progesterone, whereas progesterone may serve as anti-proliferative in breast cancer cells. The above evidence suggests a close interaction among lipids, growth factors, and endocrine hormones in promoting the differentiation of breast cancer cells.

V. Cytokines, Growth Factors, and Prostaglandins

It is fairly well established that a rise in various age-associated diseases is linked to stem cell defects at the molecular level. Environmental factors, such as diet and smoking, can act as triggers to promote malignancy. Alteration in lymphokine production may increase proliferation of target cells that may eventually become malignant cells (Figure 4). Tumor-derived growth factors that regulate cell proliferation are hormones extracted from various malignant and nonmalignant cell lines. They are found to act synergistically.[84] These factors compete with normal growth factors for specific binding to receptors, thereby affecting the metabolic responses of target cells to circulating growth factors. Cytokines control both specific and nonspecific aspects of normal growth, inflammatory repair, and immune responses. Each cytokine acts through its own specific receptor situated on the surface of the target cell. A receptor that has been bound by cytokine transduces a signal into the cell, resulting in altered gene transcription, and protein synthesis and changes in the metabolic state of the cell. Given their pivotal role in the regulation of cell growth, it is not surprising that cytokines and their receptors have a profound oncogenic potential.[84]

A. Interleukin-2 and Interferon-γ

On the basis of several currently understood *in vitro* actions, cytokines are being used as supportive, cytotoxic or immunomodulatory factors. Two cytokines, IL-2 and IFN-γ, act through their ability to augment the host's normal immune response. During incubation with IL-2, lymphocytes develop greatly increased cytotoxic potential—so-called lymphokine activated killing (LAK)—and will kill any cancer cells that they make surface contact with. Recent reports have suggested that *in vivo* re-infused LAK cells may not directly interact

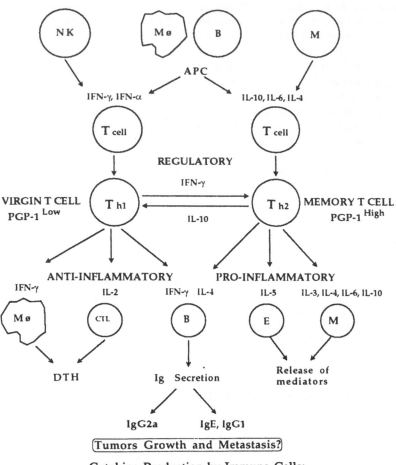

Cytokine Production by Immune Cells:
Influence by Genetic and Environmental Factors

Figure 4.   Effect of genetic and dietary factors on cytokine production and thereby on growth and
metastasis.

with the tumors that they destroy. IFN-γ has widespread effects throughout the immune
system, including activation of macrophages, T cells, B cells, and NK cells and the induction
of class II major histocompatibility complex molecules. Apart from its potential for antitu-
mor immunomodulation, IFN-γ acts in host defenses against microbial attack.

B. Interleukin-6

A number of observations suggest that IL-6 may be involved in tumor progression, and
increased serum IL-6 levels are found after induction of tumors in mice.[84]   Similarly,
elevated serum IL-6 levels are found in some patients with solid tumors and IL-6 immunore-
activity can be detected in a number of different types of neoplastic tissue.[84] IL-6 induces
some physiologic alterations often associated with cancerous states (e.g., cachexia), decreased
serum albumin, and increased acute-phase plasma proteins. IL-6 itself is mitogenic for some
types of tumor cells and its local production may result in an autocrine/paracrine alteration

of tumor proliferation. Human breast fibroblasts may have a paracrine role in controlling breast epithelial cell function exerted by IL-6, or a closely related polypeptide.[85]

C. Tumor Necrosis Factor

TNF is a cytokine derived from activated macrophages. This agent is cytostatic and cytolytic against transformed human cell lines *in vitro* and has *in vivo* activity against a variety of murine tumors. Activated macrophages produce TNF-α, whereas mitogen-stimulated lymphocytes produce TNF-β. Both cytokines have cytostatic and cytotoxic effects *in vitro* against a wide range of human tumor cells, but have no such effects against normal human fibroblasts. Although the exact mechanism by which TNF exerts its anti-tumor activity is still unknown, it has been hypothesized that TNF must first bind to a cell surface receptor, be internalized, and then perhaps trigger the release of lysosomal enzymes that lead to lysis of the target cell.[86]

D. TGF-β

TGF-β is a 25-kDa disulfide-linked homodimer originally found in transformed fibroblasts. It has either growth-stimulatory or -inhibitory properties depending upon the cell type. It has been hypothesized that the absence of TGF-β production is of pathogenic significance to the transformed state of T-MG-1.[87]

E. Prostaglandins

Tumor cell dissemination and metastasis can be regulated by the metabolic products of both tumor and host cells. PGE_2 is secreted by both tumor and host cells and has long been known to be important in facilitating tumor dissemination, although the mechanisms of action are unknown.[88,89] Metastasis can be decreased by reducing PG levels of tumor bearers with PG synthesis inhibitors or with eicosapentaenoic acid. The amount of PGE_2 produced by tumor cells does not reflect their capacity to metastasize. The level of PGE_2 production is directly associated with increased metastasis formation by malignant breast tissue and by B16 melanoma cells but is not correlated with metastatic capacities of Lewis lung carcinoma (LLC) variants or of human lung or breast cancers. The responsiveness of tumor cells to PGE_2 may be more important in regulating dissemination than is the amount of PGE_2 secreted. Metastatic 410.4 mammary tumor cells have a greater affinity and specificity for binding PGE_2 than do nonmetastatic 410 cells. While the importance of PGs in promoting tumor dissemination has long been suggested, the mechanisms are not well defined.

Our hypothesis is that initiation and promotion of normal and/or pre-neoplastic cells are triggered to a great extent by genetic and environmental factors, and these may determine the production and secretion of growth factors from immune cells and cells from different tissues. It is quite possible that imbalance between anti-inflammatory (IL-2, IFN-γ, TNF-β) and pro-inflammatory (IL-4, IL-6, TNF-α) cytokines may increase the differentiation and proliferation of tumor cells. Pro-inflammatory dietary lipids may increase several pro-inflammatory cytokines. An understanding of the mechanism(s) of maintaining an optimal balance between pro- and anti-inflammatory cytokines to create an optimal immune response to inhibit tumor growth needs more investigation.

VI. Oncogenes

Many cellular proto-oncogenes are expressed in human and other tumor cell lines.[90] Various oncogenes, their regulation, and their gene products are described in this section.[91,92]

A. c-*ras*

Increased expression of c-*ras* protein,[76] loss of a normal c-*ras* allele,[93] and acquisition of abnormal c-*ras* alleles[94] appear to correlate with progression of breast cancer to more aggressive forms. Two other oncogenes, c-*erb* B and *neu*, are both closely linked, are related to the EGF receptor, and have been detected in breast cancer cell lines and tumor biopsies.[95,96] In our studies we noted that both c-*myc* expression and the c-*ras* protein level are reduced in MCF-7 tumors in fish oil-fed mice. Others have also noted less formation of P21-*ras* protein in tumor cells cultured *in vitro* in the presence of ω-3 fatty acids.[97]

The activation of point mutations in *ras* genes has been reported in human tumors and in rat mammary carcinomas induced by a single dose of NMU. Nearly 86% of rat mammary carcinomas exhibit a G-to-A transition at codon 12 of H-*ras* gene.[98] Carcinogen-specific gene alterations produced at the time of initiation may affect the morphogenesis as well as the biologic properties of carcinoma cells.[99] The high incidence of the mutation suggests that the H-*ras* codon might be a very important genetic event for intra-ductal proliferation and for progression to frank carcinomas.

B. Her-2/*neu*

The HER-2/*neu* (*neu*) oncogene, which belongs to the tyrosine kinase oncogene family and codes for a 185-kDa glycoprotein, has been suggested to be involved in the pathogenesis of several human tumors. Overexpression of p185 has been found to be related to tumor size and has shown a negative impact upon survival in node-positive, but not in node-negative, patients.[100,101] The subcellular localization of a p185 protein that reacts with anti-p185 oncoprotein monoclonal antibodies is discussed by DePotter *et al.*[102] In rats the *neu* oncogene in tumor cells may undergo a mutation and code for a modified immunogenic p185. So far, no mutation of the *neu* oncogene has been reported in humans. *Neu* overexpression is induced by an early event in carcinogenesis and is then maintained at a constant level during tumor growth. Some report that activation of oncogenes appears to be linked to high fat consumption, whereas a reduction in calorie intake appears to reduce oncogene expression.[103]

VII. Modulation of Immune Function by Food Restriction and Physical Activity

Under-feeding of rodents is reported to prolong lifespan, increase *in vitro* T-lymphocyte proliferative responses, and retard T-lymphocyte-associated immune senescence.[104,105] Underfeeding also results in increased levels of physical activity.[106] Dietary calorie or fat restriction delays the development of autoimmune, renal, and cardiovascular diseases, inhibits involution of immunologic functions with aging, and inhibits both chemical carcinogen-induced and spontaneous cancers.[107-111] Long ago, Rusch and Kline[112] showed that regular exercise inhibited the development of certain tumors. In studying the influence of diet on immunologic involution occurring with age and on development of diseases of aging, including malignancies, we noted that mice on restricted dietary intake were regularly more active in their cages and appeared to get more exercise than controls fed diets higher in calories or fat. It thus seemed relevant to study the influence of regular exercise on the development of cancer and immunologic functions. We observed that treadmill exercise can inhibit growth of transplantable tumors in experimental animals, and further, that regular exercise influenced immune responses, such as NK cell function, and maintained reduced tumor growth.[113]

We also reported that either food restriction alone or regular treadmill exercise increased the T-cell proliferative response as well as prevented changes in T-cell subsets in normal and hypertensive rodents.[114,115] Others have reported that moderate to severe caloric restriction and exercise (with or without calorie restriction) profoundly affect the incidence, size, and multiplicity of DMH-induced colon tumors in F-344 rats.[116] As discussed elsewhere, cancer protection with calorie restriction and exercise appears to be mediated through reduced levels of glucose and insulin, increased levels of corticosteroids, increased anti-inflammatory cytokine levels, and insulin receptor expression in splenic T cells.[117-119] In addition, food restriction prevented a rise in 20:4 and 22:4 fatty acids and produced significantly low levels of PGE_2, increasing anti-inflammatory functions. Studies are now underway to compare the changes in various lymphokine mRNA expression and cytokine production in activated spleen cells both in food-restricted and/or treadmill-exercised rodents.[120,121] Clearly, more complete analyses of tumor immunity and immune suppressor cell functions need to be done in exercise regimens of varying duration and intensity.

In addition to influences on tumor growth and immune function, exercise decreases muscle glycogen and stimulates glycogen synthetase.[122] Exercise changes interferon production, blood pressure, serum lipids, functions of leukocytes, metabolism of ascorbic acid, and tissue cholesterol levels. Any one or several of these factors together might alter the resistance to the formation of tumors. It is possible that exercise deprives tumors of adequate nutrients because cessation of exercise accelerates tumor growth.[113] In a longevity study, *ad libitum*-fed exercising mice of the short-lived, autoimmune-prone MRL/1pr strain lived 15% longer than mice housed without access to running wheels.[123]

Cancer is a multifactorial disease, involving different etiologic, genetic, and environmental factors. It is clear from the foregoing discussion that in normal and malignant systems the influence of fat, energy metabolism, and physical activity on endocrine and immune function and nutrient metabolism is complex and open to considerable study.

Acknowledgment

This research was supported partially by grants from the NIH AG 03417, National Dairy Board, Robert J. Kleberg Jr. & Helen C. Kleberg Foundation and Amy Shelton McNutt Trust. Address correspondence to Gabriel Fernandes, Ph.D., Department of Medicine, The University of Texas Health Science Center, 7703 Floyd Curl Drive, San Antonio, Texas 78284-7874.

References

1. National Academy of Sciences Committee on Diet, Nutrition, and Cancer, "Diet, Nutrition, and Cancer," National Academic Press, Washington, D.C. (1982).
2. A. Irai, T. Terano, H. Saito, V. Tamura, and S. Yoshida, Clinical and epidemiological studies of eicosapentanoic acid in Japan, *in:* "Polyunsaturated Fatty Acids and Eicosanoids," W.E.M. Lands, ed., American Oil Chemists' Society, Champaign (1987).
3. R.K. Chandra, ed., "Health Effects of Fish and Fish Oils," ARTS Biomedical Publishers and Distributors Ltd., St. John's, Newfoundland, Canada (1989).
4. D.W. Golde, H.R. Herschman, and A.J. Lusis, Growth factors, *Ann Intern Med.* 92:650 (1980).
5. G. Fernandes and J.T. Venkatraman, "Human Nutrition: A Comprehensive Treatise," D. M. Klurfeld, ed., Plenum Publishing Corporation, New York (In press).
6. E.L. Wynder and T. Hirayama, Comparative epidemiology of cancers in United States and Japan, *Rev Med.* 6:567 (1977).
7. B.S. Reddy and Y. Maeura, Tumor promotion by dietary fat in azoxymethane-induced colon carcinogenesis in female Fischer 344 rats: Influence of amount and source of dietary fat, *J Natl Cancer Inst.* 72:745 (1984).

8. G.M. Kollmorgen, M.M. King, S.D. Kosanke, and C. Do, Influence of dietary fat and indo-methasin on the growth of transplantable mammary tumors in rats, *Cancer Res.* 43:4714 (1983).

9. P.F. McAndrew, Fat metabolism and cancer, *Surgical Clinics of North America.* 66:1003 (1986).

10. E.B. Katz and E.S. Boylan, Effects of reciprocal changes of diets differing in fat content on pulmonary metastasis from the 13762 rat mammary tumor, *Cancer Res.* 49:2477 (1989).

11. L.A. Hillyard and S. Abraham, Effect of dietary polyunsaturated fatty acids on growth of mammary adenocarcinomas in mice and rats, *Cancer Res.* 39:4430 (1979).

12. R.A. Karmali, S. Welt, H.T. Thaler, and F. Lefevre, Prostaglandins in breast cancer: Rela-tionship to disease stage and hormone, *Brit J Cancer.* 48:689 (1983).

13. J. Dupont, Essential fatty acids and prostaglandins, *Prev Med.* 16:485 (1987).

14. M.M. King, D.M. Bailey, D.D. Gibson, J.V. Pitha, and P.B. McCay, Incidence and growth of mammary tumors evidenced by 7,12-dimethylbenzanthracene as related to dietary con-tent of fat and anti-oxidant, *J Natl Cancer Inst.* 63:657 (1979).

15. C.D. Stubbs and A.D. Smith, The modification of mammalian membrane polyunsaturated fatty acids composition in relation to membrane fluidity and function, *Biochim Biophys Acta.* 779:89 (1984).

16. C.F. Aylsworth, C. Jones, J.E. Trosko, J. Meites, and C.W. Welsch, Promotion of 7,12-dimethylbenzanthracene induced mammary tumorigenesis by high dietary fat: Possible role of intracellular communication, *J Natl Cancer Inst.* 72:637 (1984).

17. G.A. Boissonneault, C.E. Elson, and M.W. Pariza, Net energy effects of dietary fat on chemically-induced mammary epithelial cells in vivo and in vitro, *J Cell Science.* (1986).

18. P.C. Chan, F. Didoto, and L. Cohen, High dietary fat, elevation of rat serum prolactin and mammary cancer, *Proc Soc Exptl Biol Med.* 149:133 (1975).

19. K.P. Windebank, The cytokines are coming, *Arch Disease in Childhood.* 65:1283 (1990).

20. A.S. Fauci, S.A. Rosenberg, S.A. Sherwin, C.A. Dinarello, D.L. Longo, and H.C. Lane, Immunomodulators in medicine, *Ann Intern Med.* 106:421 (1987).

21. K.L. Erickson, and N.E. Hubbard, Dietary fat and tumor metastasis, *Nutr Rev.* 48:6 (1990).

22. C.D. Stubbs and A.D. Smith, The modification of mammalian membrane polyunsaturated fatty acid composition in relation to membrane fluidity and function, *Biochim Biophys Acta.* 779:89 (1984).

23. L. Weiss, F.W. Orr, and K.V. Honn, Interaction between cancer cells and the microvascula-ture: a rate regulator for metastasis, *Clin Exp Metastasis.* 7:127 (1989).

24. R. Gill and W. Clark, Membrane structure function relationships in cell-mediated cytolysis. 1. Effect of exogenously incorporated fatty acids on effector cell function in cell-mediated cytolysis, *J Immunol.* 125:689 (1980).

25. K.L. Erickson, Dietary fat influences murine melanoma growth and lymphocyte-mediated cytotoxicity, *J Natl Cancer Inst.* 72:115 (1985).

26. L.M. Olson, S.K. Clinton, J.I. Everitt, P.V. Johnston, and W. J. Visek, Lymphocyte activa-tion, cell-mediated cytotoxicity and their relationship to dietary fat-enhanced mammary tumorigenesis in C3H/OUJ mice, *J Nutn.* 117:955 (1987).

27. G. Fernandes, J.T. Venkatraman, and N. Mohan, Effect of omega-3 lipids in delaying the growth of human breast cancer cells in nude mice, *in:* "Proc Internatl Conference in Nu-trition and Immunology," ARTS Biomedical Publishers and Distributors Ltd., St. John's, Newfoundland, Canada (1991).

28. K.K. Carroll, The role of dietary fat in carcinogenesis, *in:* "Dietary fats and health," E.P. Perkins and W.J. Visek, eds., American Oil Chemists Society, Champaign (1983).

29. S. Abraham and L.A. Hillyard, Lipids, lipogenesis and the effects of dietary fat on growth in mammary tumor model systems, *in:* "Dietary fats and health," E.P. Perkins and W.J. Visek, eds., American Oil Chemists Society, Champaign (1983).

30. L. Kaizer, N.F. Boyd, V. Kriukov, and D. Tritchler, Fish consumption and breast cancer risk: An ecological study, *Nutr Cancer.* 12:61 (1989).

31. R.A. Karmali, Do tissue culture and animal model studies relate to human diet and cancer? *Prog Lipid Res.* 25:533 (1986).

32. G. Fernandes and J.T. Venkatraman, Modulation of breast cancer growth in nude mice by ω-3 lipids, *World Rev Nutr Dietet.* 66:488 (1991).

33. G. Fernandes, Effect of dietary fish oil supplement on autoimmune disease: changes in lymphoid cell subsets, oncogene mRNA expression and neuroendocrine hormones, *in:* "Health Effects of Fish and Fish Oils," R.K. Chandra, ed., ARTS Biomedical Publishers and Distributors Ltd., St. John's, Newfoundland, Canada (1989).

34. G. Fernandes and J.T. Venkatraman, Micronutrient and lipid interactions in cancer, *Ann NY Acad Sci.* 587:78 (1990).

35. K.K. Carroll and L.M. Braden, Dietary fat and mammary carcinogenesis, *Nutr Cancer.* 6:254 (1985).

36. W.T. Cave, Jr. and J.J. Jurkowski, Comparative effects of omega-3 and omega-6 dietary lipids on rat mammary tumor development, *in:* "Proc. AOAC Short Course on Polyunsaturated Fatty Acids and Eicosanoids," American Oil Chemists' Society, Champaign (1987).

37. R.A. Karmali, J. Marsh, and C. Fuchs, Effect of omega-3 fatty acids on growth of rat mammary tumor, *J Natl Cancer Inst.* 73:457 (1984).

38. U.N. Das, Gamma-linolenic acid, arachidonic acid and eicosapentaenoic acid as potential anticancer drugs, *Nutrition.* 6:429 (1990).

39. G. Fernandes, Inhibition of MCF-7 estrogen-dependent human breast cancer cell growth in nude mice by omega-3 fatty acid diet, *Clin Res.* 37:466A (1989).

40. A. Bendich, E. Gabriel, and L.J. Machlin, Dietary vitamin E requirement for optimum immune responses in the rat, *J Nutr.* 116:675 (1986).

41. E. Seifter, G. Rettura, J. Padawer, F. Stratford, P. Goodwin, and S.M. Levenson, Regression of C3HBA mouse tumor due to x-ray therapy combined with supplemental beta carotene or vitamin A, *J Natl Cancer Inst.* 71:409 (1983).

42. S. Laganiere, B.P. Yu, and G. Fernandes, Studies on membrane lipid peroxidation in Omega-3 fatty acid fed autoimmune mice. Effects of vitamin E supplementation, *in:* "Antioxidant nutrients and immune functions," A. Bendich, M. Phillips, R.P. Tengerdy, eds., *Advances in Experimental Medicine and Biology* 262: Plenum press, New York (1988).

43. S.N. Meydani, S. Yogeeswaran, S. Liu, S. Baskar, and M. Meydani, Fish oil and tocopherol induced changes in natural killer cell-mediated cytotoxicity and PGE2 synthesis in young and old mice, *J Nutr.* 118:1245 (1988).

44. L.J. Jenski, Fish oil diets increase tumor cell sensitivity to cell-mediated lysis and alter tumor cell antigen expression, Nutrition and immunology conference, St. John's, Newfoundland, Canada, August (1991).

45. A. Coquette, B. Vray, and J. Vanderpas, Role of vitamin E in the protection of the resident macrophage membrane against oxidative damage, *Arch Int Physiol Biochem.* 94:S29 (1986).

46. "The Nude Mouse in Experimental and Clinical Research," J. Fogh and B.C. Giovanella, eds., vol. II, Academic Press, New York (1982).

47. K. Seibert and M.E. Lippman, Influence of tamoxifen treatment on heterotransplanted tumors in nude mice, *Clin Res.* 32:422 (1984).

48. I.W. Taylor, P.J. Hodson, M.D. Green, and R.L. Sutherland, Effects of tamoxifen on cell cycle progression of synchronous MCF-7 human mammary carcinoma cells, *Cancer Res.* 43:4007 (1983).

49. T. Pawson, Growth factors, oncogenes and breast cancer, *in:* "Fundamental Problems in Breast Cancer," A.H.G. Paterson and A.W. Lees, eds., Martinus Nijhoff Publishing, Boston (1987).

50. G. Fernandes, E.J. Yunis, and R.A. Good, Suppression of adenocarcinoma by the immunological consequences of caloric restriction, *Nature.* 263:504 (1976).

51. N. Sarkar, G. Fernandes, N.T. Telang, F.A. Kourides, and R.A. Good, Low calorie diet prevents the development of mammary tumors of C3H mice and reduces circulating prolactin level, murine mammary tumor virus expression, and proliferation of mammary alveolar cells, *Proc Natl Acad Sci.* 79:7758 (1982).

52. I.K. Thomas and K.L. Erickson, Lipid modulation of mammary tumor cell cytolysis: Direct influence of dietary fats on the effector component of cell-mediated cytotoxicity, *J Natl Cancer Inst.* 74:675 (1985).

53. M.G. Lewis, T.L. Kaduce, and A.A. Spector, Effect of essential polyunsaturated fatty acid modifications on prostaglandin production by MDCK canine kidney cells, *Prostaglandins.* 22:747 (1981).

54. B.R. Lokesh, B. German, and J.E. Kinsella, Differential effects of docosahexanenoic acid and eicosapentanoic acid on suppression of lipoxygenase pathway in peritoneal macrophages, *Biochim Biophys Acta.* 958 (1988).

55. V. Nishizuka, The role of protein kinase C in cell surface signal transduction and tumor promotion, *Nature.* 308:693 (1986).

56. C.W. Welsch, Enhancement of mammary tumorigenesis by dietary fat: Review of potential mechanisms, *Am J Clin Nutr.* 45:192 (1987).

57. C.W. Mahoney and A. Azzi, Vitamin E inhibits protein kinase C activity, *Biochem Biophys Res Commun.* 154:694 (1988).

58. G.A. Pritchard, D.L. Jones, and M.E. Mansel, Lipids in breast carcinogenesis, *Brit J Surg.* 76:1063 (1989).

59. C.E. Borgeston, L. Pardini, R.S. Pardini, and R.C. Reitz, Effects of dietary fish oil on human mammary carcinoma and on lipid-metabolizing enzymes, *Lipids.* 24:290 (1989).

60. M.E. Begin, G. Ells, and U.N. Das, Selected fatty acids as possible intermediates for selective cytotoxic activity of anticancer agents involving oxygen radicals, *Anticancer Res.* 6:291 (1986).

61. J.J. Jurkowski, and W.T. Cave, Dietary effects of menhaden oil on the growth and membrane lipid composition of rat mammary tumors, *J Natl Cancer Inst.* 74:1145 (1985).

62. W.T. Cave, Jr., Dietary n-3 (w-3) polyunsaturated fatty acid effects on animal tumorigenesis, *FASEB J.* 5:2160 (1991).

63. S. Abou-El-Ela, K.W. Prasse, R. Carroll, A.E. Wade, S. Dharwadkar, and O.R. Bruce, Eicosanoid synthesis in 7,12-dimethylbenz(a)anthracene-induced mammary carcinomas in Sprague Dawley rats fed primrose oil, menhaden oil or corn oil diet, *Lipids.* 23:948 (1988).

64. T. Sakai, N. Yamaguchi, and Y. Shiroko, Prostaglandin D2 inhibits the proliferation of human malignant tumor cells, *Prostaglandins.* 27:17 (1984).

65. L.M. Dunbar and J.M. Bailey, Enzyme deletions and essential fatty acid metabolism in cultured cells, *J Biol Chem.* 250:1152 (1975).

66. G.R. Devi, U.N. Das, and K.P. Rao, Prostaglandins and mutagenesis: modification of phenytoin-induced genetic damage by prostaglandins in lymphocyte cultures, *Prostaglan Leuko Med.* 15:109 (1984).

67. J.A. Badway, J.T. Curnutte, and M.L. Karnovsky, Cis-polyunsaturated fatty acids induce high levels of superoxide production by human neutrophils, *J Biol Chem.* 265:12640 (1981).

68. T. Galeotti, G.M. Bartoli, and S. Bartoli, Superoxide radicals and lipid peroxidation in tumor microsomal membrane, *in:* "Biological and clinical aspects of superoxide and superoxide dismutase," W.H. Bannister and J.V. Bannister, eds., *Proc Fed Eur Biochem Soc Symp.* No 62:106 (1982).

69. M.E. Begin, G. Ells, and U.N. Das, Differential killing of human carcinoma cells supplemented with n-3 and n-6 polyunsaturated fatty acids, *J Natl Cancer Inst.* 77:1053 (1986).

70. L. Axelrod and G. Costa, Contribution of fat loss weight loss in cancer, *Nutr Cancer.* 2:81 (1980).

71. M. Thompson and J. Koons, Modified lipoprotein lipase activities, rates of lipogenesis and lipolysis as factors leading to lipid depletion in C57BL mice bearing preputial gland tumor ESR 586, *Cancer Res.* 41:3228 (1981).

72. S.M. Shafie, Estrogen and the growth of breast cancer: New evidence suggests indirect action, *Science.* 209:701 (1980).

73. W.L. McGuire, D.L. Garza, and G.C. Chamness, Evaluation of estrogen receptor assays in human breast cancer tissue, *Cancer Res.* 37:637 (1977).

74. C.K. Osborne, E.B. Coronado, and J.P. Robinson, Human breast cancer in the athymic nude mouse: Cytostatic effect of long-term anti-estrogen therapy, *Eur J Cancer Clin Oncol.* 23:1189 (1987).

75. C.K. Osborne, K. Hobbs, and G.M. Clark, Effect of estrogen and anti-estrogens on growth of human breast cancer cells: role of the estrogen receptor, *Cancer Res.* 45:584 (1985).

76. C.K. Osborne, K. Hobbs, and J.M. Trent, Biological differences among MCF-7 human breast cancer cell lines from different laboratories, *Breast Cancer Res Treatmt.* 9:111 (1987).

77. L. Ozzello and M. Sordat, Behavior of tumors produced by transplantation of human mammary cell lines in athymic nude mice, *Eur J Cancer.* 16:553 (1980).

78. E.F. Adams, B. Rafferty, and M.C. White, Interleukin 6 is secreted by breast fibroblasts and stimulates 17β-oestradiol oxidoreductase activity of MCF-7 cells: possible paracrine regulation of breast 17β-oestradiol levels, *Int J Cancer.* 49:118 (1991).

79. K.M. Keating, B.G. Barisas, and D.A. Roess, Glucocorticoid effects on lipid lateral diffusion and membrane composition in lipopolysaccharide activated B-cell leukemia cells, *Cancer Res.* 48:59 (1988).

80. K.M. Keating, D.A. Roess, J.S. Peacock, and B.G. Barisas, Glucocorticoid effects on membrane lipid mobility during differentiation of murine B lymphocytes, *Biochim Biophys Acta.* 846:305 (1985).

81. J.A. Boullier, G. Melnykovych, and B.G. Barisas, A photobleaching recovery study of glucocorticoid effects on lateral mobilities of a lipid analog in S3G HeLa cell membranes, *Biochim Biophys Acta.* 596:320 (1980).

82. M. Chambon, H. Rochefort, H.J. Vial, and D. Chalbos, Progestins and androgens stimulate lipid accumulation in T47D breast cancer cells via their own receptors, *J Steroid Biochem.* 33:915 (1989).

83. S. Brandon, F. Vignon, D. Cjalbos, and H. Rochefort, RU486, a progestin and glucocorticoid antagonist inhibits the growth of breast cancer cells via the progesterone receptor, *J Clin Endocrinol Metab.* 60:692 (1985).

84. J. Malejczyk, M. Malejczyk, A. Urbanski, A. Kock, S. Jablonska, G. Orth, and T. Luger, Constitutive release of IL6 by human papillomavirus type 16 (HPV16)-harboring keratinocytes: A mechanism augmenting the NK-cell-mediated lysis of HPV-bearing neoplastic cells, *Cell Immun.* 136:155 (1991).

85. S.A. Miles, A.R. Rezai, J.F. Salazar-Gonzalez, M.V. Meyden, R.H. Stevens, D.M. Logan, R.T. Mitsuyasu, T. Taga, T. Hirano, T. Kishimoto, and O. Martinez-Maza, AIDS-Kaposi's-sarcoma-derived cells produce and respond to interleukin 6, *Proc Natl Acad Sci.* 40:4068 (1990).

86. M. Blick, S.A. Sherwin, M. Rosenblum, and J. Gutterman, Phase I study of recombinant tumor necrosis factor in cancer patients, *Cancer Res.* 47:2986 (1987).

87. M.T. Jennings, R.J. Maciunas, R. Carver, C.C. Bascom, P. Juneau, K. Misulis, and H.L. Moses, TGFβ₁ and TGFβ₂ are potential growth regulators for low-grade and malignant gliomas in vitro: Evidence in support of an autocrine hypothesis, *Int J Cancer.* 49:129 (1991).

88. M.R.I. Young, M.E. Young, Y. Lozano, M. Coogan M, and J.M. Bagash, Regulation of protein kinase A activation and prostaglandin E₂-stimulated migration of lewis lung carcinoma clones, *Int J Cancer.* 49:150 (1991).

89. Y. Nishizuka, The role of protein kinase C in cell surface signal transduction and tumor promotion, *Nature.* 308:693 (1984).

90. B.I. Weinstein, The origins of human cancer: Molecular mechanisms of carcinogenesis and their implications for cancer prevention and treatment, *Cancer Res.* 48:4135 (1988).

91. T. Pawson, Growth factors, oncogenes and breast cancer, *in:* "Fundamental Problems in Breast Cancer," A.H.G. Patterson and A.W. Lees, eds., Martinus Nijhoff Publishing, Boston (1987).

92. O. Farsano, D. Birnbaum, L. Edlund, J. Fogh, and M. Wigler, New human transforming genes by tumorigenicity assay, *Mol Cell Biol.* 4:1695 (1990).

93. C. Theillet, R. Lidereau, C. Escot, P. Hutzell, M. Brunet, J. Gest, J. Schlom, and R. Callahan, Loss of a C-H-ras-1 allele and aggressive human primary breast carcinomas, *Cancer Res.* 46:4776.

94. R. Lidereau, M.C. Escot, C. Theillet, M. Champene, M. Brunet, J. Gest, and R. Callahan, High frequency of rare alleles of the human C-Ha-ras-1 proto-oncogene in breast cancer patients, *J Natl Cancer Inst.* 77:699 (1986).

95. J. Downward, Y. Yarden, E. Mayes, G. Scrace, N. Totly, P. Stockwell, A. Ullrich, J. Schlessinger, and M. D. Waterfield, Close similarity of epidermal growth factor receptor and v-erb B oncogene protein sequences, *Nature.* 307:521 (1984).

96. C.L. Bargmann, M.C. Hung, and R.A. Weinberg, The new oncogene encodes an epidermal growth factor receptor-related protein, *Nature.* 319:226 (1986).

97. N.T. Telang, R.S. Bockman, M.J. Modak, and M.P. Osborne, The role of fatty acids in murine and human mammary carcinogenesis: An *in vitro* approach, *in:* "Carcinogenesis and Dietary Fat," S. Abraham, ed., Kluwer Academic Publishers, Boston (1989).

98. H. Sakai and K. Ogawa, Mutational activation of c-Ha-*ras* genes in intraductal proliferation induced by N-nitroso-N-methylurea in rat mammary glands, *Int J Cancer.* 49:140 (1991).

99. H. Zarbl, S. Sukumar, A.V. Arthur, D. Martin-Zanca, and M. Barbacid, Direct mutagenesis of Ha-*ras*-1 oncogenes by N-nitroso-N-methylurea during initiation of mammary carcinogenesis in rats, *Nature.* (Lond.) 315:382 (1985).

100. F. Rilke, M.I. Colnaghi, N. Cascinelli, S. Andreola, M.T. Baldini, R. Bufalino, G.D. Porta, S. Menard, M.A. Pierotti, and A. Testori, Prognostic significance of her-2/*NEU* expression in breast cancer and its relationship to other prognostic factors, *Int J Cancer.* 49:44 (1991).

101. S. Ramachandra, L. Machin, S. Ashley, P. Monaghan, and G. Gusterson, Immunohistochemical distribution of c-*erb* B-2 in *in situ* breast carcinoma, a detailed morphological analysis, *J Pathol.* 161:7 (1990).

102. C.R. De Potter, J. Quaracker, G. Maertens, S. Van Daele, C. Pauwels, C. Verhofstede, W. Eechaute, and H. Roels, The subcellular localization of the *neu* protein in human normal and neoplastic cells, *Int J Cancer.* 44:969 (1989).

103. R.F. Chen, R.A. Good, R.W. Engelman, N. Hamada, A. Tanaka, M. Nonoyama M, and N.K. Dey, Suppression of mouse mammary tumor proviral DNA and protooncogene expression: Association with nutritional regulation of mammary tumor development, *Proc Natl Acad Sci (USA).* 87:2385 (1990).

104. R. Weindruch and R.L. Walford, eds., The Retardation of Aging and Disease by Dietary Restriction, Charles C. Thomas, Springfield, USA (1988).

105. G. Fernandes, Nutritional factors: Modulating effects on immune function and aging, *Pharmacol Rev.* 36:123S (1984).

106. H.J. Chell and R.J. Wurtman, Short-term variations in diet composition change the patterns of spontaneous motor activity in rats, *Science.* 213:676 (1981).

107. G. Fernandes, Influence of nutrition on autoimmune disease, *in:* "Aging and the Immune Response," E. Goidl, ed., vol. 31, Marcel Dekker, Inc., New York, (1987).

108. R.A. Good and A.J. Gajjar, Diet, immunity, and longevity, *in:* "Nutrition and Aging," M.L. Hutchinson and H.N. Munro, eds., Academic Press, New York (1986).

109. P. Rous, The influence of diet on transplanted and spontaneous tumors, *J Exp Med.* 20:433 (1914).

110. A. Tannenbaum, The genesis and growth of tumors. Effects of caloric restriction per se, *Cancer Res.* 2:749 (1943).

111. D. Kritchevsky, M.M. Weber, and D.M. Klurfeld, Dietary fat versus caloric content in initiation and promotion of 7,12-dimethylbenzanthracene-induced mammary tumorigenesis in rats, *Cancer Res.* 44:3174 (1984).

112. H.P. Rusch and B.E. Kline, The effect of exercise on the growth of a mouse tumor, *Cancer Res.* 4:116 (1944).

113. R.A. Good and G. Fernandes, Enhancement of immunologic function and resistance to tumor growth in Balb/c mice by exercise, *Fed Proc.* 40:1040 (1981).

114. G. Fernandes, G. Jeng, and D. Baker, Effect of exercise during age on immune function in mice maintained on a normal and/or restricted caloric intake, *Fed Proc.* 44:2080 (1985).

115. G. Fernandes, M. Rozek, and D. Troyer, Reduction of blood pressure and restoration of T-cell immune function in SHR rats by food restriction and/or by treadmill exercise, *J Hyperten.* 4:S469 (1986).

116. D. Kritchevsky, Influence of caloric restriction and exercise on tumorigenesis in rats, *Proc Soc Exp Biol Med.* 193:35 (1990).

117. G. Fernandes, J.T. Venkatraman, E. Flescher, S. Laganiere, H. Iwai and P. Gray, Prevention in the decline of membrane-associated functions in immune cells during aging by food restriction, *in:* "Biological Effects of Dietary Restriction," L. Fishbein, ed., Life Science Institute ILSI series, Washington, D.C. (1991).

118. S. Laganiere and G. Fernandes, Study on the lipid composition of aging-Fischer-344 rat lymphoid cells: Effect of long-term calorie restriction, *Lipids.* 26:6:472 (1991).

119. J.T. Venkatraman and G. Fernandes, Modulation of age-related alterations in membrane composition and receptor associated immune functions by food restriction, *Mech & Aging Dev.* 63:27 (1992).

120. C.S. Enwemeka, L.C. Maxwell, and G. Fernandes, The effects of exercise and food restriction on rat skeletal muscles, *FASEB J.* 4:749A (1990).

121. A. Fernandes, J.T. Venkatraman, V. Tomar, and G. Fernandes, Effect of treadmill exercise and food restriction on immunity and endocrine hormone levels in rats, *FASEB J.* 4:751a (1990).

122. W.J. Evans and C.N. Meredith, Exercise and nutrition in the elderly, *in:* "Nutrition, Aging and the Elderly," H.N. Munro and D.E. Danford, eds., Plenum Publishing Corporation, New York (1989).

123. D.A. Mark, D.H. Bovbjerg, and M.E. Weksler, Voluntary Exercise, Life Span and Immunity, *in:* "Physical Activity, Aging and Sports," R. Harris and S. Harris, eds., Center for the Study of Aging, Albany, NY (1989).

Chapter 16

Dietary Fat, Calories, and Mammary Gland Tumorigenesis

CLIFFORD W. WELSCH

I. Introduction

In experimental animals (mice and rats), altering the levels and/or types of dietary fat markedly influences the development of mammary tumors. This phenomenon has now been demonstrated in an impressive array of carcinogen-induced,[1-106] transplantable,[107-121] "spontaneous"[122-139] and metastatic[140-150] experimental rodent mammary tumor systems. The purpose of this communication is to review and critique the relationships between dietary fat and mammary gland tumorigenesis in rodents. In particular, five issues are examined and critiqued, i.e., 1) amount of fat and rodent mammary tumorigenesis, 2) type of fat and rodent mammary tumorigenesis, 3) fat and rodent mammary tumor cell metastasis, 4) the fat-calorie-rodent mammary tumorigenesis relationship, and 5) influence of fat on development of human breast carcinoma transplants in immune-deficient mice. Although the amount and/or type of dietary fat have been reported to influence the development and/or growth of the normal and/or pre-neoplastic rodent mammary gland,[84,107,138,151-156] these relationships, albeit important, will not be discussed in this chapter. Specific mechanisms by which dietary fat influences mammary gland tumorigenesis in rodents have been discussed in previous reviews[157-162] and will not be a major focus of this communication. All amounts of dietary fat cited in this review are expressed as percent by weight. The terms "mammary tumor development" or "mammary tumorigenesis" denote mammary tumor growth, incidence, number, and/or multiplicity.

II. Amount of Dietary Fat and the Development of Mammary Tumors in Experimental Animals

It is clear that the amount of dietary fat has a profound effect on the development of mammary tumors in mice and rats. Increased amounts of ingested fat have been reported to increase the development of mammary tumors in an array of experimental animal models, e.g., "spontaneous" mammary tumors in mice[124,127,129-132,134-136] and rats,[122,125,128] induced (by

---

Clifford W. Welsch • Department of Pharmacology and Toxicology, Michigan State University, East Lansing, Michigan

Exercise, Calories, Fat, and Cancer, Edited by M.M. Jacobs
Plenum Press, New York, 1992

chemical carcinogens, irradiation, or hormones) mammary tumors in mice[12,46,77] and rats,[4-7,] [9-11,13-26,28-36,38,40,42,44,45,47-63,65,66,68,71-75,81,83-86,90,91,93,97,99,101,102,104-106] transplantable mammary tumors in mice[113-115,120,121,143,144] and rats,[116-119,147] and metastatic mammary tumors in mice and rats.[143-147,150] Most of the studies which have reported accelerated mammary tumorigenesis by increasing the quantity of ingested fat have utilized unsaturated fats derived from vegetable products, e.g., corn oil, sunflower-seed oil, safflower-seed oil, etc.[5-7,10,11,13,14,16,20,30-] [36,38,44,45,49,50,55,56,60,63,65,71,73,77,83,90,91,97,99,101,105] However, it should be pointed out that a large number of studies have reported enhanced mammary tumorigenesis upon feeding increased quantities of saturated fats such as lard and beef tallow.[4,9,24,28,29,47,48,84,85,98] Thus, it is quite clear that increased mammary tumorigenesis in rodents is observed upon hyperalimentation of fat, irrespective as to whether or not the fat is of vegetable or animal origin.

The determination of the time period (initiation stage, promotion stage, pre-natal, pre-puberty, post-puberty, young, old, etc.) during this tumorigenic process when hyperalimentation of fat is effective has been the focus of a number of laboratories. With regard to the initiation and promotion stages, the carcinogen-induced rat mammary tumor model has been most useful.[163] In this model, the initiation stage is defined as the transformation of a normal mammary ductal cell into a tumor cell by the administration of a carcinogen; test diets are fed commencing several weeks prior to carcinogen treatment and continuously until $\cong$ 1-5 days after carcinogen treatment. The promotion stage is defined as that time period commencing shortly after carcinogen administration and depicts growth processes of tumorous mammary cells. Increasing the quantity of ingested fats during the initiation stage does not appear to have a significant effect on this tumorigenic process,[14,36,50,60,85,98,104] although there are reports to the contrary.[25,75,84] Thus, a profound and consistent effect of increased quantities of dietary fat during the initiation stage of mammary gland tumorigenesis has not been demonstrated. In contrast, when increased quantities of fat are fed during the promotion stage of mammary gland tumorigenesis, a consistent increase in the development of mammary tumors was observed. This increased development of mammary tumors was observed upon feeding unsaturated fats of vegetable origin[5-7,10,11,13,14,16,20,30-36,38,44,45,49,50,54-] [56,60,63,65,71,73,77,83,90,91,97,99,101,104,105] or saturated fats of animal origin.[4,9,24,28,29,47,84,85] That increased quantities of dietary fat can enhance the development of a number of transplantable mammary tumors in rodents[107,117,142,143,146] is further support for the concept that fat can act at the promotional stage of this tumorigenic process. The enhancing effect of increased amounts of dietary fat on the promotion stage is most often observed when the fat is fed commencing early in this stage (usually in young animals). It should be pointed out, however, that increased quantities of fat can also enhance mammary tumorigenesis when fed commencing at late timepoints during the promotion stage (in older animals).[29,36,38,50,56,65,99] Thus, hyperalimentation of fat, commencing at either early or late timepoints during the promotion stage, significantly enhances the development of mammary tumors in rats treated with carcinogens. It should also be stressed that the duration in which high levels of fat are fed during the promotion stage is an important factor in this tumorigenic process. It is apparent that the longer the timespan of feeding high levels of fat, the greater the development of mammary tumors.[6,36] Upon the use of rodent models that develop mammary tumors "spontaneously," it also appears that the longer the timespan in which high-fat diets are fed, the greater the risk of developing mammary tumors[132]; the pre-puberty (weaning to puberty) or post-puberty periods do not appear to differ in their sensitivity to this dietary constituent.[132] That the amount[138] and type[124] of fat can increase the development of mammary tumors when fed solely during the perinatal period[138] and perinatal-neonatal period,[124] respectively, have been reported.

It has been suggested in a number of reports that once a critical level of fat is reached in a diet, a further increase in fat does not result in a parallel increase in mammary tumor development. For example, doubling the fat content of the diet from 10% to 20% did not result in a significant increase in the development of mammary tumors in carcinogen-treated rats.[4,11,15,30] This concept has been extended to the quantity of linoleic acid in the diet, i.e., a linear increase in mammary tumor development was observed upon increasing dietary lineoleic acid from 0.5 to 4.4%; further increasing the level of lineolic acid in the diet did not result in a further increase in the development of mammary tumors.[55] These results would suggest that a threshold level for dietary fat (e.g., 10%) and linoleic acid (e.g., 4.4%) does indeed exist, further increases in the levels of these nutrients does not result in a parallel increase in mammary tumor development. However, if the level of linoleic acid is maintained at a constant level (4.8%) in a series of diets with wide-ranging fat levels, a proportionate enhancement in mammary tumor development is observed with increasing levels of dietary fat (8% to 20%).[54] Thus, at least within this range of dietary fat levels and constant levels of linoleic acid, a threshold level of dietary fat may not exist, i.e., any increase in fat consumption may result in a parallel increase in mammary tumorigenesis. An absence of a threshold level of dietary fat in the range of 5 to 20% and mammary tumorigenesis also has been suggested by other studies.[11,13,30,71]

How increased quantities of dietary fat enhance this tumorigenic process is not known; such has been the subject of a number of relatively recent reviews.[159,160] Two points, however, may be germane to this issue. Firstly, since virtually all studies that report a significant enhancing effect of dietary fat on experimental mammary gland tumorigenesis compared very low levels of fat with high levels, i.e., 0.5-5.0% fat vs. 20-30% fat, it is conceivable that the animals consuming the low levels of fat were not receiving adequate quantities of an essential lipid nutrient (e.g., linoleic acid) required for optimal tumor growth processes. Mammary tumors, in a state of intense proliferation, may need increased quantities of such a nutrient, compared with normal tissues. Secondly, the animals consuming the high-fat diets may be consuming more usable energy than those fed the low-fat diets despite the use of isocalorie diets. Relevant to this issue is the evidence that the stimulatory effect of a high-fat diet in rodent mammary gland tumorigenesis is dependent upon an *ad libitum* type of feeding protocol,[30,99,105] i.e., this phenomenon may only occur in an environment of calorie (energy) excess; both of these issues are discussed in a subsequent section of this chapter.

III. Type of Dietary Fat and the Development of Mammary Tumors in Experimental Animals

A number of laboratories have addressed the relationship between the type of dietary fat and the development of mammary tumors in experimental animals. The animal model that has been utilized most often in these studies has been the carinogen-induced rat mammary tumor model.[1-4,11,13,15,19,23,27,33,34,37,39,41-43,45,47-49,67,68,75,81,86,90,93,94,98,103,106] Studies have been reported, however, using the carcinogen-induced mouse mammary tumor model[12,48] as well as an array of "spontaneous,"[122-129,131,132,136,137] transplantable,[107-117,119-121] and metastatic[141,142,145,148,149] rodent mammary tumor models.

Utilizing the carcinogen-induced rat mammary tumor model, only a few laboratories have examined whether or not the type of fat can affect the initiation stage of this tumorigenic process. Reports from these laboratories provide evidence that high dietary levels of saturated fats (e.g., lard, beef tallow), compared to high dietary levels of unsaturated fats (e.g., corn oil), when fed during the initiation stage, can stimulate the development of mammary tumors.[48,84,98] Such observations, however, have not always been confirmed by others.[85] Considering the paucity and inconsistencies of these studies, it is not possible to derive a definitive conclusion as to whether or not the type of fat can effect the initiation stage of rat mammary gland tumorigenesis.

In constrast, a multitude of studies provide evidence that the type of dietary fat can affect the promotional stage of this tumorigenic process. In general, high dietary levels of saturated fats of either animal (i.e., lard and beef tallow) or plant (i.e., coconut oil and palm oil) origin suppress the development of mammary tumors in carcinogen-treated rats when compared to high dietary levels of unsaturated fats of vegetable origin (i.e., corn oil, soybean oil, safflower-seed oil, and sunflower-seed oil).[11,33,34,37,41,45,47,48,55,86,94,106] It has been reported that supplementation of the saturated fats with a small amount of unsaturated fats (many saturated fats are deficient in the essential fatty acid linoleic acid, e.g., beef tallow and coconut oil), the mammary tumor development suppressing activities of a high saturated fat diet is abolished.[45,47] Thus, mammary tumor development is as high in rats fed a 20% sunflower-seed oil diet as it is in rats fed a 17% beef tallow-3% sunflower-seed oil diet[45] or a 17% coconut oil-3% ethyl linoleate diet.[47] When these studies were repeated, however, supplementating the saturated fat diet with a similar amount of unsaturated fat only partially reversed the mammary tumor suppressing activities of the saturated fat diet.[11] A relatively recent report provides evidence that the level of linoleic acid in a high saturated (coconut oil), low unsaturated (corn oil) fat diet blend is the major determinant in influencing the development of mammary tumors. When the level of linoleic acid reached 4.4%, a further increase in the ratio of saturated fats to unsaturated fats did not result in a parallel reduction in mammary tumor development.[55] Thus, high dietary levels of saturated fats, compared to unsaturated fats, can clearly inhibit the development of carcinogen-induced rat mammary tumors (promotion stage). However, and importantly, this inhibition by the saturated fat diet can often be reversed by modest dietary supplementation of a linoleic acid-rich oil (e.g., corn oil) or by linoleic acid itself. Parenthetically, it should be pointed out that all the studies cited above[11,33,34,37,41,45,47,48,55,86,94,106] specifically examined the promotion stage of rat mammary gland tumorigenesis. Many other studies have also demonstrated an inhibitory effect of high dietary levels of saturated fats, compared to unsaturated fats, on chemical carcinogenesis of the rat mammary gland.[15,23,27,42,43,59,67,68,81,93] In these studies, the test diets were fed continuously during both the initiation and promotion stages of this tumorigenic process and therefore are difficult to interpret. Results from studies examining other rodent mammary tumor models also provide evidence that high dietary levels of saturated fats, when compared to diets rich in unsaturated fats, suppress the development of mammary tumors. This has been demonstrated in "spontaneously" derived[122,128,129,136,137] and transplantable[107-111,113-115,120,121] mammary tumors in mice and rats. Again, supplementing the saturated fat diets with small amounts of unsaturated fats negates the mammary tumor suppressing activities of the saturated fat diets.[110,136] In accord, high-fat diets that are formulated to suppress cardiovascular disease in humans, i.e., a fatty acid composition of saturated, monounsaturated, and polyunsaturated fatty acids of 34%, 33%, and 33%, respectively, stimulate mammary tumor development in rats to a degree comparable to high-fat diets that mimic that consumed by Western world populations, i.e., a fatty acid composition of saturated, monounsaturated, and polyunsaturated fatty acids of 46%, 38%, and 16%, respectively.[8]

The influence of diets rich in monoenoic fatty acids, e.g., oleic acid as found in olive oil and palm oil, on the development of mammary tumors in rodents has in recent years received increased attention.[4,15,34,39,94,125,128,136,142,145] The results of these studies have been inconsistent. Using the carcinogen-induced rat mammary tumor model, the feeding of high dietary levels of olive oil ($\cong$79% oleic acid and 7% linoleic acid) has been reported to have no effect[15] or an inhibitory effect[34,78] on the development of mammary tumors. The latter studies examined the promotion stage of this tumorigenic process; the former study utilized a continuous initiation-promotion stage experimental protocol. Rats fed high dietary levels of an oleic acid rich mutant safflower-seed oil (77% oleic acid) during the promotion stage, developed virtually the same number[39] or even increased numbers[78] of carcinogen-induced mammary tumors as rats fed high levels of standard relatively low oleic acid containing safflower-seed oil (12% oleic acid). A positive association between oleic acid consumption and the enhancement of rat mammary gland carcinogenesis also has been reported.[23] In contrast, rats fed high levels of palm oil (≅43% oleic acid and 11% linoleic acid) during the promotion stage of rat mammary gland tumorigenesis had fewer mammary tumors than did rats fed corn oil (37% oleic acid) or soybean oil (21% oleic acid).[94] The ingestion of high levels of olive oil by C3H mice has been reported to inhibit[128] or to have no effect[136] on the development of "spontaneous" mammary tumors. The development of transplantable mouse[142] and rat[145] mammary tumors has been reported not to be influenced by the consumption of diets rich in olive oil. Thus, it is quite apparent from these studies that a consistent inhibitory activity of diets rich in monoenoic fatty acids on the development of mammary tumors in rodents has not been demonstrated. It is conceivable that diets rich in olive oil or palm oil may not contain levels of linoleic acid sufficient for optimal mammary tumor growth processes. Supplementation of olive oil diets with linoleic acid has been reported to block the inhibitory activities of an olive oil diet in rats treated with a chemical carcinogen.[78] Thus, the reported suppression of mammary tumorigenesis by these oils may not be a function of monoenoic fatty acid levels but merely due to inadequate levels of linoleic acid. Further studies, however, are warranted in an effort to more clearly define the role of monoenoic fatty acids in mammary tumor development processes.

Primrose oil, a seed extract of the evening primrose plant, like corn oil, is rich in a linoleic acid (≅75%). In addition, this oil contains relatively high levels (≅9%) of γ-linolenic acid, a fatty acid that is rapidly elongated to dihomo-γ-linolenic acid, a precursor of certain monoenoic fatty acids. Feeding diets containing primrose oil has been reported to inhibit the development of carcinogen-induced rat mammary tumors (promotion stage),[1,2] carcinogen-induced mouse mammary tumors,[12] and transplantable rat mammary tumors.[112,117] Inhibition of mammary tumor development by primrose oil does not appear to be dose dependent.[112,117] Although there is a paucity of reports on the effectiveness of this oil in the chemoprevention of mammary tumorigenesis, such reports are interesting and justify further studies.

In recent years there has been appreciable interest in the chemoprevention of mammary tumorigenesis by using diets rich in fish oils. Such oils, when obtained from cold-water fish, are often rich in a number of omega-3 fatty acids, the most abundant being eicosapentaenoic acid (EPA) and docosahexaenoic acid (DHA). When fed to mice or rats at relatively high dietary levels, a consistent inhibition of mammary tumorigenesis is observed. This has been observed using the carcinogen-induced rat mammary tumor model during the promotion stage[2,3,11,13] or when using the continuous initiation-promotion stage protocol.[64] In addition, inhibition of mammary tumorigenesis by dietary fish oil has been observed when using the carcinogen-induced mouse mammary tumor model,[12] transplantable mammary tumors in both mice[109] and rats,[116,119,149] and in a "spontaneous" mammary tumor mouse model.[128] Fish oils, as those used in the studies cited above, are most often deficient or marginal in linoleic acid; unfortunately, in a number of these studies, the fish oil diets were not supplemented with this essential fatty acid.[2,11-13,64,116,128] Supplementation of the fish oil diets with modest amounts of corn oil (e.g., 75% fish oil and 25% corn oil) has been reported to block,[110] or partially block,[3] the inhibition of mammary tumor development by a fish oil diet. High-fat diets rich in fish oil and supplemented with vegetable oils (79% fish oil and 21% corn oil, olive oil, or linseed oil), failed to influence the development of a transplantable rat mammary tumor when the diet was fed commencing the day of tumor cell inoculation.[149] In addition, a dose response to fish oil diets was indicated in one study,[64] but not in several other studies.[11,13,110,116] Thus, it is clear that diets rich in fish oil inhibit the development of an array of rodent mammary tumors; supplementation of the fish oil diets with modest amounts of linoleic acid-rich vegetable oils, however, often negates or partially negates, the tumor development inhibitory activities of a fish oil diet.

Other types of dietary fat also have been examined for their effect on mammary tumor developmental processes in rodents. Evidence has been provided that *trans* fats (partially hydrogenated soybean oil and cottonseed oil, 50:50, approximately 38% *trans* fatty acids) modified carcinogen-induced rat mammary gland tumorigenesis (promotion stage) no differently than *cis* fats (olive oil, cocoa butter, and coconut oil, 50:48:2); mammary tumorigenesis was reduced to a comparable degree when compared with rats fed a corn oil diet.[49,90] It is germane to point out that the diets used in these studies were adjusted so that the fatty acid composition in the *trans* and *cis* fats were similar. Thus, *trans* fats appear to behave like saturated fats in the modification of rat mammary gland tumorigenesis. Medium-chain triglycerides have also been examined in the carcinogen-induced rat mammary tumor model. Feeding high levels of medium-chain triglycerides (hydrolysis of coconut oil, > 70% of the fatty acids are 12 carbons or less in length) to carcinogen-treated rats during the promotion stage reduced mammary tumor development compared with rats fed a high level of corn oil.[32,35] Compelling evidence for an important role of cholesterol in rodent mammary gland tumorigenesis has not been reported.[28,41,164]

IV. Dietary Fat and the Metastasis of Mammary Tumor Cells in Experimental Animals

Relatively few laboratories have focused on the relationship between dietary fat and mammary tumor cell metastasis. A number of reports provide evidence that the amount and/or type of dietary fat can effect mammary tumor metastasis in rodents[142-147,150]; others report to the contrary.[119,140,141,148,149] Using the transplantable mouse mammary tumor model, it has been reported that increasing the linoleic acid content of the diet increases the rate of spontaneous mammary tumor cell metastasis.[143,144] The metastasis (experimental, cells injected via tail vein) of a transplantable mouse mammary tumor has been reported to be increased by a diet rich in beef tallow compared to a diet containing low amounts of this animal fat; a different rate of metastasis between low- and high-fat diets of vegetable origin (corn oil) was not observed.[150] In rats bearing a transplantable mammary tumor, the rate of metastasis increased as the fat (corn oil) content of the diet increased[145-147]; a phenomenon dependent upon the age of the animals[147] and the duration of high-fat diet feeding.[146]

The type of dietary fat may also regulate the metastasis of rodent mammary tumor cells. Mice fed a diet rich in *trans* fatty acids (soybean oil and cottonseed oil, 50:50, hydrogenated) had fewer mammary tumor cell metastases (experimental metastasis) than mice fed a diet rich in *cis* fatty acids (olive oil, cocoa butter, and coconut oil, 58:40:2). The fatty acid concentrations were similar in both diets.[142] In rats, the metastasis (spontaneous) of a transplantable mammary tumor has been shown to be increased in animals fed high dietary levels of corn oil compared with animals fed large amounts of olive oil or beef tallow.[145] In contrast, in other studies, dietary comparisons of corn oil vs. beef tallow,[150] safflower-seed oil vs. coconut oil,[141] or corn oil vs. fish oil[148,149] showed no differences in the degree of metastases of mouse[141,150] or rat[148,149] mammary tumor cells. It appears, therefore, that a definitive and consistent influence of dietary fat on mammary tumor cell metastasis in rodents has not been established, further studies are required to more specifically define this potentially important relationship.

V. Dietary Fat and Calories in Mammary Tumor Development in Experimental Animals

The relationship between dietary fat and calories in mammary tumorigenic processes in rodents has been examined and discussed in a number of recent reviews.[157-159,161,162] Clearly, caloric restriction has a profound and consistent inhibitory activity on the development of rodent mammary tumors.[8,10,30,69-71,75,76,80,92,96,99,105,135,165-179] A critical question is whether or not the enhancement of mammary tumorigenesis by hyperalimentation with fat results from the metabolic activity of the fat *per se* or is due to an excessive energy intake. It has been reported that a low-fat, high-calorie diet increased carcinogen-induced rat mammary gland tumorigenesis more than a high-fat, low-calorie diet.[75] Indeed, a direct linear relationship between the degree of energy restriction (10-40%) and the inhibition of carcinogen-induced rat mammary gland tumorigenesis (promotion stage) was observed. The diets were adjusted so that animals in the energy-restricted groups consumed comparable amounts of fat.[70] It was concluded from these studies that dietary energy may be a greater determinant than dietary fat in enhancing mammary tumorigenesis.

Evidence supporting the concept that enhancement of mammary tumorigenesis by a high-fat diet is a function of fat *per se* (independent of calories) is as follows. In animals fed isocaloric low- and high-fat diets (ingesting virtually identical amounts of calculated kcal per day), the development of mammary tumors has been reported to be greater in animals fed the higher level of fat. This has been reported using the carcinogen-induced rat mammary tumor model[24,35,40,42,45,91,105] and the "spontaneous" mouse mammary tumor model.[127,133,134] Furthermore, the striking differences in mammary tumor development in mice and rats fed diets containing indentical levels of fat but differing in fat composition (e.g., corn oil vs. beef tallow, primrose oil, palm oil, or fish oil) has been additional support for the concept of a direct, non-caloric activity of fat because such diets are virtually equicaloric. In those reports comparing isocaloric low- and high-fat diets, caloric consumption was computed using the customary Atwater values for metabolizable energy of 4, 4, and 9 kcal/g for carbohydrate, protein, and fat, respectively. Recently, it was reported that the Atwater value of 9 kcal/g of dietary fat may not be appropriate for rodents consuming large quantities of fat and that a value of 11.1 kcal/g or ≅124% of the expected value is a more appropriate estimate of metabolizable fat energy in such animals (since 9 kcal/g is the maximum energy yield of fat via calorimeter analysis, the relative energy yield from protein or carbohydrate would be less than the customary values of 4 kcal/g).[180] This suggestion is not novel, for a number of years ago it was proposed that as the fat content of the diet is increased, the amount of recovered energy is also increased.[181] Shortly thereafter, this concept was applied to tumorigenic (skin) processes.[182] In essence, more energy may be recovered or retained within the animal from a calorie of fat then from a calorie of carbohydrate or protein, in animals consuming increased amounts of fat. If this concept is correct, the assessment of the available energy from low- and high-fat diets, as calculated in virtually all of the studies cited in this communication, is erroneous. Such diets may not be isocaloric. In support of this contention, it was reported recently that when low- and high-fat isocaloric diets (corn oil) were fed to female rats (rats were individually housed and fed, and caloric consumption, calculated by using Atwater values, was virtually identical in the two groups of rats), a significant increase in body weight gain (≅13%) was observed in the rats fed the higher level of fat.[105] Thus, it is questionable (doubtful) that past dietary fat-mammary tumorigenesis rodent studies used isocaloric low- and high-fat diets. Clearly, whether or not the enhancement of mammary tumorigenesis by hyperalimentation with fat results from a specific metabolic activity of fat *per se* or is due to excess calories from the fat is a critical question that to date remains unresolved. That different types of fat of similar caloric value and fed at identical levels (e.g., corn oil vs. beef tallow, fish oil, primrose oil, or palm oil) can differentially influence mammary tumorigenesis in rodents would appear to support a calorie-independent activity of fat. However, recent studies have provided evidence that animals consuming fats such as fish oils have reduced carcass energy accumulation compared with animals fed equal amounts of corn oil.[183-185] Thus, different types of fat fed at the same level may not yield comparable amounts of usable energy.

One of the most impressive observations emerging from the studies of calories and fat and rodent mammary gland tumorigenesis has been the impact of caloric restriction on this tumorigenic process. In general, the longer the duration of caloric restriction, the greater the inhibition of mammary tumor development.[76] Furthermore, inhibition of mammary tumorigenesis by caloric restriction can occur even when calories are restricted late in the tumorigenic process.[54,76,171] In a recent study, energy consumption restricted by 10, 20, and 30% during the promotion stage of rat mammary gland tumorigenesis resulted in a ≅23, 33, and 68% inhibition, respectively, of this tumorigenic process.[70] Utilizing the same experimental animal model and a similar experimental design, it was observed that a reduction of caloric consumption by 25% resulted in a reduction in mammary tumor development of ≅75%; reduction of fat consumption by 25% resulted in only a ≅23% reduction in mammary tumor development.[54] In another more recent study, a mere 12% reduction in diet (energy) consumption during the promotion stage of rat mammary gland tumorigenesis inhibited mammary tumorigenesis by ≅42%; a 75% reduction in fat consumption was required to reduce mammary tumorigenesis to a quantitatively similar level.[105] Thus, a very small reduction in energy consumption will substantially reduce mammary tumorigenesis in rodents; extremely large reductions in fat consumption are required to produce a quantitatively equivalent inhibition of this tumorigenic process.

In view of the numerous reports demonstrating a direct positive relationship between caloric consumption and rodent mammary gland tumorigenesis,[25,26,70,105] recent studies have focused on whether or not modification of energy expenditure could influence this tumorigenic process. Exercise is a potential means for achieving this goal.[30,82,100,101] In a recent study, using the carcinogen-induced rat mammary tumor model (promotion stage), it was reported that voluntary exercise (free access to an activity wheel) of rats fed a high-fat diet (corn oil) resulted in a reduction in mammary tumor development to a degree comparable to that observed in control sedentary rats fed a low-fat diet.[30] Paradoxically, those rats that exercised the most had the smallest reduction in mammary tumor development. In contrast, in a study using virtually the same experimental animal model, involuntary exercise (motorized treadmill) of rats fed a high-fat diet (corn oil) resulted in a stimulation of mammary tumorigenesis,[101] an enhancing effect that was directly related to the intensity of exercise.[100] Although these reports appear contradictory, an increase in mammary tumorigenesis was observed when the intensity of exercise or stressful activity increased. Stress, including exercise-induced stress, can readily increase secretion of pituitary prolactin,[186,187] a known hormonal stimulant in the development of rodent mammary gland tumors.[163,188] Extremely severe stress can have the opposite effect.[163] Thus, using exercise to modify energy expenditure in the clarification of the relationship between energy, fat, and mammary tumorigenesis can be extremely useful but, in addition, can also be beset by an array of known and no doubt many unknown confounding variables.

The restriction of caloric consumption not only suppresses the development of mammary tumors in experimental animals but, in addition, appears to block the difference in mammary tumorigenesis between rats fed low- and high-fat diets.[30,99,105] Thus, in carcinogen-treated rats, reducing energy consumption by 25%[30] or as little as 12%[105] of that consumed by *ad libitum*-fed controls negates the significant mammary tumor development stimulation of a high-fat diet. Furthermore, groups of carcinogen-treated rats fed low- and high-fat diets and restricted in food consumption to a level equivalent to that consumed by the animals that consumed the least amount of food showed no differences in mammary tumor development.[99] Thus, it appears that the enhancement of mammary tumorigenesis in rodents by a high-fat diet is a phenomenon dependent upon an *ad libitum* type of feeding protocol. Virtually all of the studies cited here that clearly document an enhancing effect of a high-fat diet on mammary tumorigenesis in mice and rats followed an *ad libitum* type of feeding protocol. Why high-fat diets enhance mammary tumorigenesis in rodents only in an environment of caloric excess is unknown. It is also unknown how caloric restriction suppresses the development of mammary tumors (and possibly all tumors) in experimental animals. Caloric restriction may create an energy deficiency at the level of the mammary tumor cells or at the level of the tumor, resulting in a relative decrease in tumor cell proliferation. Alternatively, caloric restriction, even mild caloric restriction, may induce a decrease in the synthesis of and/or impede the responsiveness to hormones and/or growth factors required for optimal mammary tumor cell proliferative processes; such studies are currently being pursued[87-89] and should be encouraged. The combination of an energy deficiency and diminished prerequisite hormone and/or growth factor activities may explain the lack of mammary tumorigenic stimulation by high-fat diets in calorie-restricted animals.

VI. Dietary Fat and the Growth of Human Breast Carcinomas Maintained in Immune-Deficient Mice

Very recently, studies designed to evaluate the influence of dietary fat on growth of human breast carcinomas maintained in immune-deficient mice (athymic nude mice) have been reported.[189-193] All human breast carcinomas used in these studies were derived from well-characterized cell lines. High-fat diets (20% corn oil), have been reported to stimulate the development of MDA-MB231 human breast carcinomas when compared with development of tumors in mice fed a low-fat diet (5% corn oil).[192] The development of MCF-7 and MDA-MB231 human breast carcinomas in mice has been reported to be greatest in mice fed high levels of a vegetable oil (20% corn oil), intermediate in mice fed high levels of an animal fat (19% beef tallow and 1% corn oil), and lowest in mice fed high levels of a fish oil diet (19% Menhaden oil and 1% corn oil).[192] Inhibition of development of MCF-7 human breast carcinomas in mice fed evening primrose oil or fish oil compared with an olive oil control, also has been reported.[193] Diets rich in fish oil (Max EPA) suppressed the development of MX-1 human breast carcinomas in mice compared with diets rich in corn oil.[189-191] It is apparent from these studies, albeit few in number, that the influence of dietary fat, quantitatively and qualitatively, on development of human breast carcinomas in immune-deficient mice parallels that occurring in rodent mammary gland tumors.

Two potentially important aspects of the above studies should be noted. In three studies, diet modifications were imposed to evaluate their influence on chemotherapy[190] and immunotherapy.[189,191] Such studies should be encouraged. Secondly, in one of the above studies,[192] inhibition of development of human breast carcinomas induced by dietary fish oil was blocked by supplementation of the diet with potent anti-oxidants. Although most laboratories postulate that the modulation of mammary gland tumorigenesis by dietary fish oil is exerted via alterations in eicosanoic metabolism,[159,160] the possibility that this activity may be, at least in part, a function of the generation of cytostatic and/or cytolytic lipid peroxides cannot be ruled out.

Whether or not the amount and/or type of dietary fat can affect the risk of breast carcinoma development in human populations is at present not clear. This relationship has been the subject of a number of epidemiologic studies. Some studies support a positive association between fat consumption and breast cancer risk[194-201] and others report no association between the consumption of fat and the risk of developing this disease.[202-206] That dietary fat and/or calories profoundly influences the development of mammary tumors in rodents provides a compelling biologic basis for a potentially important relationship between dietary fat, calorie consumption, and breast carcinoma development in human populations.

VII. Summary

In this communication, a vast array of studies designed to examine the relationship between dietary fat and experimental mammary gland tumorigenesis was reviewed and critiqued. It is clear, as reported by many laboratories, that as the fat content of the diet is increased from a low or standard level to a high level, a consistent and substantial increase in the development of rodent mammary gland tumors is observed. The longer the duration the high-fat diet is fed, the greater the enhancing effect on tumorigenesis. Furthermore, the stimulatory effect of a high-fat diet is observed even when fed commencing late in an animal's life. A multitude of studies also have provided evidence that the type of fat can markedly influence the development of rodent mammary gland tumors. In general, high dietary levels of unsaturated fats (e.g., corn oil, sunflower-seed oil) stimulate this tumorigenic process more than high levels of saturated fats (e.g., beef tallow, coconut oil); diets rich in certain fish oils (e.g., Menhaden oil, Max EPA) are often the most inhibitory to this tumorigenic process. Importantly, however, supplementation of saturated fat or fish oil diets with modest amounts of unsaturated fats, e.g., corn oil, often negates the mammary tumor inhibitory activities of these fats. Thus, rather extreme differences in the types of fat are required for a differential in mammary gland tumorigenesis; common proportionate blends of different fats of animal, plant, and/or fish origin are often unable to differentially influence this tumorigenic process. Diets rich in monoenoic fatty acids, e.g., those containing high levels of olive oil, have been examined in a number of studies; results from these studies have been inconsistent.

A number of reports suggest that the increase in development of mammary tumors in rodents fed a high-fat diet, compared with those fed a low-fat diet, is due to specific metabolic activities of the fat *per se*, activities independent of a caloric mechanism. Careful analysis of these reports suggest that such a conclusion may not be totally warranted. Indeed, persuasive evidence is accumulating indicating that the major mammary tumor development enhancing activities of a high-fat diet may be via a caloric (energy) mechanism. Caloric restriction, even in animals fed a high-fat diet, significantly suppresses mammary tumor development. Even mild caloric restriction (e.g., 12%) can significantly suppress development of mammary tumors in rodents. Deprivation of mammary tumor cells of requisite levels of energy may explain this phenomenon. In addition, caloric restriction, even mild caloric restriction, may decrease synthesis of and/or impede the responsiveness to hormones and/or growth factors required for optimal mammary tumor development. Diets high in fat and rich in energy may provide the optimal environment for these cellular and/or physiologic processes. Diets low in fat (e.g., 0.5 to 5.0% corn oil), compared with diets high in fat (e.g., 20% corn oil), although allegedly isocaloric, may suppress mammary gland tumorigenesis in rodents by providing relatively less energy and/or insufficient amounts of an essential lipid component such as linoleic acid. Mammary tumor cells, in a state of intense proliferation, may have an energy and/or nutrient requirement that exceeds that required by normal cells. Fat may also have a mammary tumorigenesis modulating activity, however, that is independent of calories. The differential in mammary gland tumorigenesis in rodents fed high dietary levels of corn oil and those fed high levels of beef tallow or fish oil is often but not always completely abolished by the addition to the beef tallow or fish oil diets of adequate levels of essential nutrients such as linoleic acid. Differences in mammary tumorigenesis in rodents fed high levels of corn oil versus those fed high levels of palm oil or evening primrose oil have been reported; the latter fat, in particular, would appear to be clearly sufficient in essential fatty acids. That dietary fat and/or calorie intake can significantly influence the development of mammary tumors in rodents is unequivocal. Such studies provide a compelling biologic basis for a potentially important relationship between dietary fat and/or calorie consumption and breast carcinoma development in human populations.

Acknowledgment

Supported by NIH research grant CA-42876 and AICR research grant 90BW05. Address correspondence to C.W. Welsch, Dept. of Pharmacology and Toxicology, Michigan State University, East Lansing, MI 48824.

References

1. S.H. Abou-El-Ela, K.W. Prasse, R. Carroll, and O.R. Bunce, Effects of dietary primrose oil on mammary tumorigenesis induced by 7,12-dimethylbenzanthracene, *Lipids*. 22:1041 (1987).

2. S.H. Abou-El-Ela, K.W. Prasse, R. Carroll, A.E. Wade, S. Dharwadkar, and O.R. Bunce, Eicosanoid synthesis in 7,12-dimethylbenzanthracene-induced mammary carcinomas in Sprague-Dawley rats fed primrose, menhaden or corn oil diets, *Lipids*. 23:948 (1988).

3. S.H. Abou-El-Ela, K.W. Prasse, B.L. Farrell, R.W. Carroll, A.E. Wade, and O.R. Bunce, Effects of D,L-2-difluoromethylornthine and indomethacin on mammary tumor promotion in rats fed high n-3 and/or n-6 fat diets, *Cancer Res*. 49:1434 (1989).

4. M. Askoy, M.R. Berger, and D. Schmahl, The influence of different levels of dietary fat on the incidence and growth of MNU-induced mammary carcinoma in rats, *Nutr Cancer*. 9:227 (1987).

5. C.F. Aylsworth, M.E. Cullum, M.H. Zile, and C.W. Welsch, Influence of dietary retinyl acetate on normal rat mammary gland development and on the enhancement of 7,12-dimethylbenzanthracene-induced rat mammary tumorigenesis by high levels of dietary fat, *J Natl Cancer Inst*. 76:339 (1986).

6. C.F. Aylsworth, C. Jone, J.E. Trosko, J. Meites, and C.W. Welsch, Promotion by 7,12-dimethylbenzanthracene-induced mammary tumorigenesis by high dietary fat in the rat: possible role of intercellular communication, *J Natl Cancer Inst*. 72:637 (1984).

7. C.F. Aylsworth, D.A. VanVugt, P.W. Sylvester, and J. Meites, Role of estrogens and prolactin in stimulation of carcinogen-induced mammary tumor development by a high-fat diet, *Cancer Res*. 44:2835 (1984).

8. M. Beth, M.R. Berger, M. Aksoy, and D. Schmahl, Comparison between the effects of dietary fat level and of calorie intake on methylnitrosourea-induced mammary carcinogenesis in female SD rats, *Int J Cancer*. 39:737 (1987).

9. M. Beth, M.R. Berger, M. Aksoy, and D. Schmahl, Effect of vitamin A and E supplementation to diets containing two different fat levels on methylnitrosourea-induced mammary carcinogenesis in female SD rats, *Br J Cancer*. 56:445 (1987).

10. G.A. Boissonneault, C.E. Elson, and M.W. Pariza, Net energy effects of dietary fat on chemically induced mammary carcinogenesis in F344 rats, *J Natl Cancer Inst*. 76:335 (1986).

11. L.M. Branden and K.K. Carroll, Dietary polyunsaturated fat in relation to mammary carcinogenesis in rats, *Lipids*. 21:285 (1986).

12. E. Cameron, J. Bland, and R. Marcuson, Divergent effects of omega-6 and omega-3 fatty acids on mammary tumor development in C3H/Heston mice treated with DMBA, *Nutr Res*. 9:383 (1989).

13. K.K. Carroll, and L.M. Braden, Dietary fat and mammary carcinogenesis, *Nutr Cancer*. 6:254 (1985).

14. K.K. Carroll, and H.T. Khor, Effects of dietary fat and dose level of 7,12-dimethylbenzanthracene on mammary tumor incidence in rats, *Cancer Res*. 30:2260 (1970).

15. K.K. Carroll, and H.T. Khor, Effects of level and type of dietary fat on incidence of mammary tumors induced in female Sprague-Dawley rats by 7,12-dimethylbenzanthracene, *Lipids*. 6:415 (1971).

16. C.A. Carter, R.J. Milholland, W. Shea, and M.M. Ip, Effect of the prostaglandin synthetase inhibitor indomethacin on 7,12-dimethylbenzanthracene-induced mammary tumorigenesis in rats fed different levels of fat, *Cancer Res*. 43:3559 (1983).

17. W.T. Cave, J.T. Dunn, and R.M. MacLeod, Effects of iodine deficiency and high-fat diet on N-nitrosomethylurea-induced mammary cancers in rats, *Cancer Res.* 39:729 (1979).

18. W.T. Cave, and M.J. Erickson-Lucas, Effects of dietary lipids on lactogenic hormone receptor binding in rat mammary tumors, *J Natl Cancer Inst.* 68:319 (1982).

19. W.T. Cave, and J.J. Jurkowski, Dietary lipid effects on the growth, membrane composition, and prolactin-binding capacity of rat mammary tumors, *J Natl Cancer Inst.* 73:185 (1984).

20. P.C. Chan, and L.A. Cohen, Effect of dietary fat, antiestrogen, and antiprolactin on the development of mammary tumors in rats, *J Natl Cancer Inst.* 52:25 (1974).

21. P.C. Chan, and T.L. Dao, Effects of dietary fat on age-dependent sensitivity to mammary carcinogenesis, *Cancer Letters.* 18:245 (1983).

22. P.C. Chan, and T.L. Dao, Enhancement of mammary carcinogenesis by a high-fat diet in Fischer, Long-Evans and Sprague-Dawley rats, *Cancer Res.* 41:164 (1981).

23. P.C. Chan, K.A. Ferguson, and T.L. Dao, Effects of different dietary fats on mammary carcinogenesis, *Cancer Res.* 43:1079 (1983).

24. P.C. Chan, J.F. Head, L.A. Cohen, and E.L. Wynder, Influence of dietary fat on the induction of mammary tumors by N-nitrosomethylurea: associated hormone changes and differences between Sprague-Dawley and F344 rats, *J Natl Cancer Inst.* 59:1279 (1977).

25. S.K. Clinton, J.M. Alster, P.B. Imrey, S. Nandkumar, C.R. Truex, and W.J. Visek, Effects of dietary protein, fat and energy intake during an intitiation phase study of 7,12-dimethylbenzanthracene-induced breast cancer in rats, *J Nutr.* 116:2290 (1986).

26. S.K. Clinton, P.B. Imrey, J.M. Alster, J. Simon, C.R. Truex, and W.J. Visek, The combined effects of dietary protein and fat on 7,12-dimethylbenzanthracene-induced breast cancer in rats, *J Nutr.* 114:1213 (1984).

27. S.K. Clinton, A.L. Mulloy, and W.J. Visek, Effects of dietary lipid saturation on prolactin secretion, carcinogen metabolism and mammary carcinogenesis in rats, *J Nutr.* 114:1630 (1984).

28. L.A. Cohen, and P.C. Chan, Dietary cholesterol and experimental mammary cancer development, *Nutr Cancer.* 4:99 (1982).

29. L.A. Cohen, P.C. Chan, and E.L. Wynder, The role of a high-fat diet in enhancing the development of mammary tumors in ovariectomized rats, *Cancer.* 47:66 (1981).

30. L.A. Cohen, K. Choi, and C.X. Wang, Influence of dietary fat, caloric restriction and voluntary exercise on N-nitrosomethylurea-induced mammary tumorigenesis in rats, *Cancer Res.* 48:4276 (1988).

31. L.A. Cohen, K. Choi, J.H. Weisburger, and D.P. Rose, Effect of varying proportions of dietary fat on the development of N-nitrosomethylurea-induced rat mammary tumors, *Anticancer Res.* 6:215 (1986).

32. L.A. Cohen and D.O. Thompson, The influence of dietary medium chain triglycerides on rat mammary tumor development, *Lipids.* 22:455 (1987).

33. L.A. Cohen, D.O. Thompson, K. Choi, R.A. Karmali, and D.P. Rose, Dietary fat and mammary cancer. II. Modulation of serum and tumor lipid composition and tumor prostaglandins by different dietary fats: association with tumor incidence patterns, *J Natl Cancer Inst.* 77:43 (1986).

34. L.A. Cohen, D.O. Thompson, Y. Maeura, K. Choi, M.E. Blank, and D.P. Rose, Dietary fat and mammary cancer. I. Promoting effects of different dietary fats on N-nitrosomethylurea-induced rat mammary tumorigenesis, *J Natl Cancer Inst.* 77:33 (1986).

35. L.A. Cohen, D.O. Thompson, Y. Maeura, and J.H. Weisburger, Influence of dietary medium-chain triglycerides on the development of N-methylnitrosourea-induced rat mammary tumors, *Cancer Res.* 44:5023 (1984).

36. T.L. Dao and P.C. Chan, Effect of duration of high fat intake on enhancement of mammary carcinogenesis in rats, *J Natl Cancer Inst.* 71:201 (1983).

37. T.L. Dao and P.C. Chan, Hormones and dietary fat as promoters in mammary carcinogenesis, *Environ Health Perspect.* 50:219 (1983).

38. M.B. Davidson and K.K. Carroll, Inhibitory effect of a fat-free diet on mammary carcinogenesis in rats, *Nutr Cancer.* 3:207 (1982).

39. S. Dayton, S. Hashimoto, and J. Wollman, Effect of high-oleic and high-linoleic safflower oils on mammary tumors induced in rats by 7,12-dimethylbenzanthracene, *J Nutr.* 107:1353 (1977).

40. W.F. Dunning, M.R. Curtis, and M.E. Maun, The effect of dietary fat and carbohydrate on diethylstilbestrol-induced mammary cancer in rats, *Cancer Res.* 9:354 (1949).

41. H.F. Gabriel, M.F. Melhem, and K.N. Rao, Enhancement of DMBA-induced mammary cancer in Wister rats by unsaturated fat and cholestyramine, *In Vivo*, 1:303 (1987).

42. E.B. Gammal, K.K. Carroll, and E.R. Plunkett, Effects of dietary fat on mammary carcinogenesis by 7,12-dimethylbenzanthracene, *Cancer Res.* 27:1734 (1967).

43. N.A. Habib, C.B. Wood, K. Apostolov, W. Barker, M.J. Hershman, M. Aslam, D. Heinemann, B. Fermor, R.C.N. Williamson, W.E. Jenkins, J.R.W. Masters, and M.J. Embleton, Stearic acid and carcinogenesis, *Br J Cancer.* 56:455 (1987).

44. P. Hill, P. Chan, L. Cohen, E. Wynder, and K. Kuno, Diet and endocrine-related cancer, *Cancer.* 39:1820 (1977).

45. G.J. Hopkins and K.K. Carroll, Relationship between amount and type of dietary fat in promotion of mammary carcinogenesis induced by 7,12-dimethylbenzanthracene, *J Natl Cancer Inst.* 62:1009 (1979).

46. J.G. Hopkins, G.C. Hard, and C.E. West, Carcinogenesis induced by 7,12-dimethylbenzanthracene in C3H-A^{vy} fB mice: influence of different dietary fats. *J Natl Cancer Inst.* 60:849 (1978).

47. G.J. Hopkins, T.G. Kennedy, and K.K. Carroll, Polyunsaturated fatty acids as promoters of mammary carcinogenesis induced in Sprague-Dawley rats by 7,12-dimethylbenzanthracene, *J Natl Cancer Inst.* 66:517 (1981).

48. G.J. Hopkins, C.E. West, and G.C. Hard, Effect of dietary fats on the incidence of 7,12-dimethylbenzanthracene-induced tumors in rats, *Lipids.* 11:328 (1976).

49. J.E. Hunter, C. Ip, and E.J. Hollenbach, Isomeric fatty acids and tumorigenesis: a commentary on recent work, *Nutr Cancer.* 7:199 (1985).

50. C. Ip, Ability of dietary fat to overcome the resistance of mature rats to 7,12-dimethylbenzanthracene-induced mammary tumorigenesis, *Cancer Res.* 40:2785 (1980).

51. C. Ip, Dietary vitamin E intake and mammary carcinogenesis in rats, *Carcinogenesis.* 3:1453 (1982).

52. C. Ip, Factors influencing the anticarcinogenic efficacy of selenium in dimethylbenzanthracene-induced mammary tumorigenesis in rats, *Cancer Res.* 41:2683 (1981).

53. C. Ip, Modification of mammary carcinogenesis and tissue peroxidation by selenium deficiency and dietary fat, *Nutr Cancer.* 2:136 (1981).

54. C. Ip, Quantitative assessment of fat and calories as risk factors in mammary carcinogenesis in an experimental model, *Prog Clin Biol Res.* 346:107 (1990).

55. C. Ip, C.A. Carter, and M.M. Ip, Requirement of essential fatty acid for mammary tumorigenesis in the rat, *Cancer Res.* 45:1997 (1985).

56. C. Ip and M.M. Ip, Inhibition of mammary tumorigenesis by a reduction of fat intake after carcinogen treatment in young versus adult rats, *Cancer Letters.* 11:35 (1980).

57. C. Ip and M.M. Ip, Serum estrogens and estrogen responsiveness in 7,12-dimethylbenzanthracene as influenced by dietary fat, *J Natl Cancer Inst.* 66:291 (1981).

58. C. Ip and D. Sinha, Anticarcinogenic effect of selenium in rats treated with dimethylbenzanthracene and fed different levels and type of fat, *Carcinogenesis.* 2:435 (1981).

59. C. Ip and D. Sinha, Enhancement of mammary tumorigenesis by dietary selenium deficiency in rats with a high polyunsaturated fat intake, *Cancer Res.* 41:31 (1981).

60. C. Ip and D. Sinha, Neoplastic growth of carcinogen-treated mammary transplants as influenced by fat intake of donor and host, *Cancer Letters.* 11:277 (1981).

61. C. Ip and G. White, BCG-modulated mammary carcinogenesis is dependent on the schedule of immunization but is not affected by dietary fat, *Cancer Letters.* 31:87 (1986).

62. C. Ip, P. Yip, and L.L. Bernardis, Role of prolactin in the promotion of dimethylbenzanthracene-induced mammary tumors by dietary fat, *Cancer Res.* 40:374 (1980).

63. E.A. Jacobson, K.A. James, J.V. Frei, and K.K. Carroll, Effects of dietary fat on long-term growth and mammary tumorigenesis in female Sprague-Dawley rats given a low dose of DMBA, *Nutr Cancer*. 11:221 (1988).

64. J.J. Jurkowski and W.T. Cave, Dietary effects of Menhaden oil on the growth and membrane lipid composition of rat mammary tumors, *J Natl Cancer Inst*. 74:1145 (1985).

65. R. Kalamegham and K.K. Carroll, Reversal of the promotional effect of high-fat diet on mammary tumorigenesis by subsequent lowering of dietary fat, *Nutr Cancer*. 6:22 (1984).

66. Y. Katsuda, Effect of semisynthetic diets containing various amounts of corn oil upon development of DMBA-induced mammary cancer, *J Kansai Med Univ*. 33:360 (1981).

67. M.M. King, D.M. Bailey, D.D. Gibson, J.V. Pitha, and P.B. McCay, Incidence and growth of mammary tumors induced by 7,12-dimethylbenzanthracene as related to the dietary content of fat and antioxidant, *Cancer Res*. 63:657 (1979).

68. M.M. King and P.B. McCay, Modulation of tumor incidence and possible mechanisms of inhibition of mammary carcinogenesis by dietary antioxidants, *Cancer Res*. 43:2485s (1983).

69. D.M. Klurfeld, M.M. Weber, and D. Kritchevsky, Inhibition of chemically induced mammary and colon tumor promotion by caloric restriction in rats fed increased dietary fat, *Cancer Res*, 47:2759 (1987).

70. D.M. Klurfeld, C.B. Welch, M.J. Davis, and D. Kritchevsky, Determination of degree of energy restriction necessary to reduce DMBA-induced mammary tumorigenesius in rats during the promotion phase, *J Nutr*. 119:286 (1989).

71. D.M. Klurfeld, C.B. Welch, L.M. Lloyd, and D. Kritchevsky, Inhibition of DMBA-induced mammary tumorigenesis by caloric restriction in rats fed high-fat diets, *Int J Cancer*. 43:922 (1989).

72. G.M. Kollmorgen, M.M. King, A.A. Lehman, G. Fischer, R.E. Longley, B.J. Daggs, and W.A. Sansing, The methanol extraction residue of Bacillus Calmette-Guerin protects against 7,12-dimethylbenzanthracene-induced rat mammary carcinoma, *Proc Soc Exp Biol Med*. 162:410 (1979).

73. G.M. Kollmorgen, M.M. King, J.F. Roszel, B.J. Daggs, and R.E. Longley, The influence of dietary fat and non-specific immunotherapy on carcinogen-induced rat mammary adenocarcinoma, *Vet Pathol*. 18:82 (1981).

74. G.M. Kollmorgen, W.A. Sansing, A.A. Lehman, G. Fischer, R.E. Longley, S.S. Alexander, M.M. King, and P.B. McKay, Inhibition of lymphocyte function in rats fed high-fat diets, *Cancer Res*. 39:3458 (1979).

75. D. Kritchevsky, M.M. Weber, and D.M. Klurfeld, Dietary fat versus caloric content in initiation and promotion of 7,12-dimethylbenzanthracene-induced mammary tumorigenesis in rats, *Cancer Res*. 44:3174 (1984).

76. D. Kritchevsky, C.B. Welch, and D.M. Klurfeld, Response of mammary tumors to caloric restriction for different time periods during the promotion phase, *Nutr Cancer*. 12:259 (1989).

77. H.W. Lane, J.S. Butel, C. Howard, F. Shepherd, R. Halligan, and D. Medina, The role of high levels of dietary fat in 7,12-dimethylbenzanthracene-induced mouse mammary tumorigenesis: lack of an effect on lipid peroxidation, *Carcinogenesis*. 6:403 (1985).

78. J.B. Lasekan, M.K. Clayton, A. Gendron-Fitzpatrick, and D.M. Ney, Dietary olive oil and safflower oils in promotion of DMBA-induced mammary tumorigenesis in rats, *Nutr Cancer*. 13:153 (1990).

79. S.Y. Lee and A.E. Rogers, Dimethylbenzanthracene mammary tumorigenesis in Sprague-Dawley rats fed diets differing in content of beef tallow or rapeseed oil, *Nutr Res*. 3:361 (1983).

80. F.C. Leung, C.F. Aylsworth, and J. Meites, Counteraction of underfeeding-induced inhibition of mammary tumor growth in rats by prolactin and estrogen administration, *Proc Soc Exp Biol Med*. 173:159 (1983).

81. P.B. McCay, M.M. King, and J.V. Pitha, Evidence that the effectiveness of antioxidants as inhibitors of 7,12-dimethylbenzanthracene-induced mammary tumors is a function of dietary fat composition, *Cancer Res*. 41:3745 (1981).

82. C. Moore and P.W. Tittle, Muscle activity, body fat, and induced rat mammary tumors, *Surgery.* 73:329 (1973).

83. N. Oyaizu, S. Morii, K. Saito, Y. Katsuda, and J. Matsumoto, Mechanism of growth enhancement of 7,12-dimethylbenzanthracene-induced mammary tumors in rats given high polyunsaturated fat diet, *Jpn J Cancer Res.* 76:676 (1985).

84. A.E. Rogers, Influence of dietary content of lipids and lipotropic nutrients on chemical carcinogenesis in rats, *Cancer Res.* 43:2477s (1983).

85. A.E. Rogers, B. Conner, C. Boulanger, and S. Lee, Mammary tumorigenesis in rats fed diets high in lard, *Lipids.* 21:275 (1986).

86. A.E. Rogers and W.C. Wetsel, Mammary carcinogenesis in rats fed different amounts and types of fat, *Cancer Res.* 41:3735 (1981).

87. B.A. Ruggeri, D.M. Klurfeld, and D. Kritchevsky, Biochemical alterations in 7,12-dimethylbenzanthracene-induced mammary tumors from rats subjected to caloric restriction, *Biochimica et Biophysica Acta.* 929:239 (1987).

88. B.A. Ruggeri, D.M. Klurfeld, D. Kritchevsky, and R.W. Furlanetto, Caloric restruction and 7,12-dimethylbenzanthracene-induced mammary tumor growth in rats: alterations in circulating insulin, insulin-like growth factors I and II and epidermal growth factor, *Cancer Res.* 49:4130 (1989).

89. B.A. Ruggeri, D.M. Klurfeld, D. Kritchevsky, ansd R.W. Furlanetto, Growth factor binding to 7,12-dimethylbenzanthracene-induced mammary tumors from rats subject to chronic caloric restriction, *Cancer Res.* 49:4135 (1989).

90. S.L. Selenskas, M.M. Ip, and C. Ip, Similarity between trans fat and saturated fat in the modification of rat mammary carcinogenesis, *Cancer Res.* 44:1321 (1984).

91. J. Silverman, C.J. Shellabarger, S. Holtzman, J.P. Stone, and J.H. Weisburger, Effect of dietary fat on x-ray-induced mammary cancer in Sprague-Dawley rats, *J Natl Cancer Inst.* 64:631 (1980).

92. D.K. Sinha, R.L.Gebhard, and J.E. Pazik, Inhibition of mammary carcinogenesis in rats by dietary restriction, *Cancer Letters.* 40:133 (1988).

93. H. Sugihara, Suppression of growth of DMBA-induced mammary cancers in female rats fed on coconut oil diets, *J Kansai Med Univ.* 26:72 (1974).

94. K. Sundram, H.T. Khor, A.S.H. Ong, and R. Pathmanathan, Effect of dietary palm oils on mammary carcinogenesis in female rats induced by 7,12-dimethylbenzanthracene, *Cancer Res.* 49:1447 (1989).

95. P.W. Sylvester, C.F. Aylsworth, and J. Meites, Relationship of hormones to inhibition of mammary tumor development by underfeeding during the "critical period" after carcinogen administration, *Cancer Res.* 41:1384 (1981).

96. P.W. Sylvester, C.F. Aylsworth, D.A. VanVugt, and J. Meites, Influence of underfeeding during the "critical period" or thereafter on carcinogen-induced mammary tumors in rats, *Cancer Res.* 42:4943 (1982).

97. P.W. Sylvester, C. Ip, and M.M. Ip, Effects of high dietary fat on the growth and development of ovarian-independent carcinogen-induced mammary tumors in rats, *Cancer Res.* 46:763 (1986).

98. P.W. Sylvester, M. Russell, M.M. Ip, and C. Ip, Comparative effects of different animal and vegetable fats fed before and during carcinogen administration on mammary tumorigenesis, sexual maturation and endocrine functions in rats, *Cancer Res.* 46:757 (1986).

99. H.J. Thompson, D. Meeker, A.R. Tagliaferro, and J.S. Roberts, Effect of energy intake on the promotion of mammary carcinogenesis by dietary fat, *Nutr Cancer.* 7:37 (1985).

100. H.J. Thompson, A.M. Ronan, K.A. Ritacco, and A.R. Tagliaferro, Effect of type and amount of dietary fat on the enhancement of rat mammary tumorigenesis by exercise, *Cancer Res.* 49:1904 (1989)

101. H.J. Thompson, A.M. Ronan, K.A. Ritacco, A.R. Tagliaferro, and L.D. Meeker, Effect of exercise on the induction of mammary carcinogenesis, *Cancer Res.* 48:2720 (1988).

102. D.A. Wagner, P.H. Naylor, U. Kim, W. Shea, C. Ip, and M.M. Ip, Ineraction of dietary fat and the thymus in the induction of mammary tumors by 7,12-dimethylbenzanthracene, *Cancer Res.* 2:1266 (1982).

103. M. Watanabe and M. Sugano, Effects of dietary *cis-* and *trans-*monoene fats on 7,12-dimethylbenzanthracene-induced rat mammary tumors, *Nutr Rept Internatl.* 33:163 (1986).

104. C.W. Welsch and J.V. DeHoog, Influence of caffeine consumption on 7,12-dimethylbenzanthracene-induced mammary gland tumorigenesis in female rats fed a chemically defined diet containing standard and high levels of unsaturated fat, *Cancer Res.* 48:2074 (1988).

105. C.W. Welsch, J.L. House, B.L. Herr, S.J. Eliasberg, and M.A. Welsch, Enhancement of mammary carcinogenesis by high levels of dietary fat: a phenomenon dependent on *ad libitum* feeding, *J Natl Cancer Inst.* 82:1615 (1990).

106. W.C. Wetsel, A.E. Rogers, and P.M. Newberne, Dietary fat and DMBA mammary carcinogenesis in rats, *Cancer Det and Prevent.* 4:535 (1981).

107. S. Abraham, L.J. Faulkin, L.A. Hillyard, and D.J. Mitchell, Effect of dietary fat on tumorigenesis in the mouse mammary gland, *J Natl Cancer Inst.* 72:1421 (1984).

108. S. Abraham and L.A. Hillyard, Effect of dietary 18-carbon fatty acids on growth of transplantable mammary adenocarcinomas in mice, *J Natl Cancer Inst.* 71:601 (1983).

109. K.L. Erickson and I.K. Thomas, The role of dietary fat in mammary tumorigenesis, *Food Technol.* 39:69 (1985).

110. H. Gabor and S. Abraham, Effect of dietary Menhaden oil on tumor cell loss and the accumulation of mass of a transplantable mammary adenocarcinoma in Balb/c mice, *J Natl Cancer Inst.* 76:1223 (1986).

111. H. Gabor, L.A. Hillyard, and S. Abraham, Effect of dietary fat on growth kinetics of transplantable mammary adenocarcinoma in Balb/c mice, *J Natl Cancer Inst.* 74:1299 (1985).

112. T. Ghayur and D.F. Horrobin, Effects of essential fatty acids in the form of evening primrose oil on the growth of the rat R3230AC transplantable mammary tumour, *IRCS Med Sci.* 9:582 (1981).

113. M. Giovarelli, E. Padula, G. Ugazio, G. Forni, and G. Cavallo, Strain- and sex-linked effects of dietary polyunsaturated fatty acids on tumor growth and immune functions in mice, *Cancer Res.* 40:3745 (1980).

114. L.A. Hillyard and S. Abraham, Effect of dietary polyunsaturated fatty acids on growth of mammary adenocarcinomas in mice and rats, *Cancer Res.* 39:4430 (1979).

115. G.J. Hopkins and C.E. West, Effect of dietary polyunsaturated fat on the growth of a transplantable adenocarcinoma in C3HA^{vy} fB mice, *J Natl Cancer Inst.* 58:753 (1977).

116. R.A. Karmali, J. Marsh, and C. Fuchs, Effect of omega-3 fatty acids on growth of a rat mammary tumor, *J Natl Cancer Inst.* 73:457 (1984).

117. R.A. Karmali, J. Marsh, and C. Fuchs, Effects of dietary enrichment with gamma-linolenic acid upon growth of the R3230AC mammary adenocarcinoma, *J Nutr Growth and Cancer.* 2:41 (1985).

118. G.M. Kollmorgen, M.M. King, S.D. Kosanke, and C. Do, Influence of dietary fat and indomethacin on the growth of transplantable mammary tumors in rats, *Cancer Res.* 43:4714 (1983).

119. W.J. Kort, I.M. Weijma, A.M. Bijma, W.P. van Schalkwijk, A.J. Vergroesen, and D.L. Westbroek, Omega-3 fatty acids inhibiting the growth of a transplantable rat mammary adenocarcinoma, *J Natl Cancer Inst.* 79:593 (1987).

120. G.A. Rao and S. Abraham, Enhanced growth rate of transplanted mammary adenocarcinoma induced in C3H mice by dietary linoleate, *J Natl Cancer Inst.* 56:431 (1976).

121. G.A. Rao and S. Abraham, Reduced growth rate of transplantable mammary adenocarcinoma in C3H mice fed eicosa-5,8,11,14-tetraenoic acid, *J Natl Cancer Inst.* 58:445 (1977).

122. A.S. Bennett, Effect of dietary stearic acid on the genesis of spontaneous mammary adenocarcinomas in strain A/ST mice, *Int J Cancer.* 34:529 (1984).

123. J. Benson, M. Lev, and C.G. Grand, Enhancement of mammary fibroadenomas in the female rat by a high fat diet, *Cancer Res.* 16:135 (1956).

124. B. Boeryd and B. Hallgren, The incidence of spontaneous mammary carcinoma in C3H mice is influenced by dietary fat given from weaning and given to mothers during gestation and lactation, *Acta Path Microbiol Immunol Scand Sect A.* 94:237 (1986).

125. R.R. Brown, Effects of dietary fat on incidence of spontaneous and induced cancer in mice, *Cancer Res.* 41:3741 (1981).

126. R.K. Davis, G.T. Stevenson, and K.A. Busch, Tumor incidence in normal Sprague-Dawley female rats, *Cancer Res.* 16:194 (1956).

127. D.S. Gridley, J.D. Kettering, J.M. Slater, and R.L. Nutter, Modification of spontaneous mammary tumors in mice fed different sources of protein, fat and carbohydrate, *Cancer Letters.* 19:133 (1983).

128. D. Harman, Free radical theory of aging: effect of the amount and degree of unsaturation of dietary fat on mortality rate, *J. Gerontol.* 26:451 (1971).

129. W.J. Kort, P.E. Zondervan, L.O.M. Hulsman, I.M. Weijma, W.C. Hulsmann, and D.L. Westbroek, Spontaneous tumor incidence of female Brown Norway rats after lifelong diets high and low in linoleic acid, *J Natl Cancer Inst.* 74:529 (1985).

130. L.M. Olson, S.K. Clinton, J.I. Everitt, P.V. Johnston, and W.J. Visek, Lymphocyte activation, cell-mediated cytotoxicity and their relationship to dietary fat-enhanced mammary tumorigenesis in C3H/OUJ mice, *J Nutr.* 117:955 (1987).

131. P. Pennycuik, A. Fogerty, M. Wilcox, M. Ferris, R. Baxter, and A. Johnson, Tumour incidence, growth reproduction and longevity in female C3H mice fed polyunsaturated ruminant-derived foodstuffs, *Aust J Biol Sci.* 32:309 (1979).

132. J. Silverman, J. Powers, P. Stromberg, J.A. Pultz, and S. Kent, Effects on C3H mouse mammary cancer of changing from a high fat to a low fat diet before, at, or after puberty, *Cancer Res.* 49:3857 (1989).

133. H. Silverstone and A. Tannenbaum, The effect of the proportion of dietary fat on the rate of formation of mammary carcinoma in mice, *Cancer Res.* 10:488 (1950).

134. A. Tannenbaum, The genesis and growth of tumors. III. Effects of a high fiber diet, *Cancer Res.* 2:468 (1942).

135. A. Tannenbaum, The dependence of tumor formation on the composition of the calorie-restricted diet as well as on the degree of restriction, *Cancer Res.* 5:616 (1945).

136. I.J. Tinsley, J.A. Schmitz, and D.A. Pierce, Influence of dietary fatty acids on the incidence of mammary tumors in the C3H mounse, *Cancer Res.* 41:1460 (1981).

137. I.J. Tinsley, G. Wilson, and R.R. Lowry, Tissue fatty acid changes and tumor incidence in C3H mice ingesting cottonseed oil, *Lipids.* 17:115 (1982).

138. B.E. Walker, Tumors in female offspring of control and diethylstilbestrol-exposed mice fed high-fat diets, *J Natl Cancer Inst.* 82:50 (1990).

139. S.H. Waxler, G. Brecher, and S.L. Beal, The effect of fat-enriched diet on the incidence of spontaneous mammary tumors in obese mice, *Proc Soc Exp Biol Med.* 162:365 (1979).

140. E.S. Boylan and L.A. Cohen, The influence of dietary fat on mammary tumor metastasis in the rat, *Nutr Cancer.* 8:193 (1986).

141. C.C. Carrington and H.L. Hosick, Effects of dietary fats on the growth of normal, preneoplastic and neoplastic mammary epithelial cells *in vivo* and *in vitro, J Cell Sci.* 75:269 (1975).

142. K.L. Erickson, D.S. Schlanger, D.A. Adams, D.R. Fregeau, and J.S. Stern, Influence of dietary fatty acid concentration and geometric configuration on murine mammary tumorigenesis and experimental metastases, *J Nutr.* 114:1834 (1984).

143. N.E. Hubbard, R.S. Chapkin, and K.L. Erickson, Inhibition of growth and linoleate-enhanced metastasis of a transplantable mouse mammary tumor by indomethacin, *Cancer Letters.* 43:111 (1988).

144. N.E. Hubbard and K.L. Erickson, Enhancement of metastasis from a transplantable mouse mammary tumor by dietary linoleic acid, *Cancer Res.* 47:6171 (1987).

145. E.B. Katz and E.S. Boylan, Effect of the quality of dietary fat on tumor growth and metastasis from a rat mammary adenocarcinoma, *Nutr Cancer,* 12:343 (1989).

146. E.B. Katz and E.S. Boylan, Effects of reciprocal changes of diets differing in fat content on pulmonary metastasis from the 13762 rat mammary tumor, *Cancer Res.* 49:2477 (1989).

147. E.B. Katz and E.S. Boylan, Stimulatory effect of high polyunsaturated fat diet on lung metastasis from the 13762 mammary adenocarcinoma in female retired breeder rats, *J Natl Cancer Inst.* 79:351 (1987).

148. W.J. Kort, I.M. Weijma, T.E.M. Stehmann, A.J. Vergroesen, and D.L. Westbroek, Diets rich in fish oil cannot contract tumor cell metastasis, *Ann Nutr Metab.* 31:342 (1987).

149. W.J. Kort, I.M. Weijma, A.J. Vergroesen, and D.L. Westbroek, Conversion of diets at tumor induction shows the pattern of tumor growth and metastasis of the first given diet, *Carcinogenesis*. 8:611 (1987).

150. E.M. Scholar, L.A.D. Violi, J. Newland, E. Bresnick, and D.F. Birt, The effect of dietary fat on metastasis of the Lewis lung carcinoma and the Balb/c mammary carcinoma, *Nutr Cancer*. 12:109 (1989).

151. L.J. Faulkin, S. Abraham, D.J. Mitchell, and L.A. Hillyard, Effects of dietary fat on mammary development relative to age and hormones in BALB/c mice, *Proc Soc Exp Biol Med*. 181:575 (1986).

152. R.A. Knazek, S.C. Liu, J.S. Bodwin, and B.K. Vonderhaar, Requirement of essential fatty acids in the diet for development of the mouse mammary gland, *J Natl Cancer Inst*. 64:377 (1980).

153. M.J. Miyamoto-Tiaven, L.A. Hillyard, and S. Abraham, Influence of dietary fat on the growth of mammary ducts in Balb/c mice, *J Natl Cancer Inst*. 67:179 (1981).

154. C.W. Welsch, J.V. DeHoog, D.H. O'Connor, and L.G. Sheffield, Influence of dietary fat levels on development and hormone responsiveness of the mouse mammay gland, *Cancer Res*. 45:6147 (1985).

155. C.W. Welsch and D.H. O'Connor, Influence of the type of dietary fat on developmental growth of the mammary gland in immature and mature female Balb/c mice, *Cancer Res*. 49:5999 (1989).

156. L. Zhang, R.P. Bird, and W.R. Bruce, Proliferative activity of murine mammary epithelium as affected by dietary fat and calcium, *Cancer Res*. 47:4905 (1987).

157. D. Albanes, Total calories, body weight, and tumor incidence in mice, *Cancer Res*. 47:1987 (1987).

158. L.S. Freedman, C. Clifford, and M. Messina, Analysis of dietary fat, calories, body weight and the development of mammary tumors in rats and mice: a review, *Cancer Res*. 50:5710 (1990).

159. C.W. Welsch, Enhancement of mammary tumorigenesis by dietary fat: review of potential mechanisms, *Am J Clin Nutr*. 45:192 (1987).

160. C.W. Welsch and C.F. Aylsworth, Enhancement of murine mammary tumorigenesis by feeding high levels of dietary fat: a hormonal mechanism?, *J Natl Cancer Inst*. 70:215 (1983).

161. M.W. Pariza, Calorie restriction, *ad libitum* feeding, and cancer, *Proc Soc Exp Biol Med*. 183:293 (1986).

162. D. Kritchevsky and D.M. Klurfeld, Caloric effects in experimental mammary tumorigenesis, *Am J Clin Nutr*. 45:236 (1987).

163. C.W. Welsch, Host factors affecting the growth of carcinogen-induced rat mammary carcinomas: a review and tribute to Charles Brenton Huggins, *Cancer Res*. 45:3415 (1985).

164. D.M. Klurfeld and D. Kritchevsky, Serum cholesterol and 7,12-dimethylbenzanthracene-induced mammary carcinogenesis, *Cancer Letters*. 14:273 (1981).

165. G. Fernandes, E.J. Yunis, and R.A. Good, Suppression of adenocarcinoma by the immunological consequences of caloric restriction, *Nature (London)*. 263:504 (1976).

166. R.A. Huesby, Z.B. Ball, and M.B. Visscher, Further observations on the influence of simple caloric restriction on mammary cancer incidence and related phenomenon in C3H mice, *Cancer Res*. 5:40 (1945).

167. N.H. Sarkar, G. Fernandes, N.T. Telang, I.A. Kourides, and R.A. Good, Low-calorie diet prevents the development of mammary tumors in C3H mice and reduces circulating prolactin levels, murine mammary tumor virus expression, and proliferation of mammary alveolar cells, *Proc Natl Acad Sci (USA)*. 79:7758 (1982).

168. R. Shao, T.L. Dao, N.K. Day, and R.A. Good, Dietary manipulation of mammmary tumor development in adult C3H/Bi mice, *Proc Soc Exp Biol Med*, 193:313 (1990).

169. A. Tannenbaum, Relationship of body weight to cancer incidence, *Arch Path*. 30:509 (1940).

170. A. Tannenbaum, The initiation and growth of tumors: introduction: I. Effects of underfeeding, *Am J Cancer*. 38:335 (1940).

171. A. Tannenbaum, The genesis and growth of tumors. II. Effects of caloric restriction *per se*, *Cancer Res.*, 2:460 (1942).

172. A. Tannenbaum, The dependence of tumor formation on degree of caloric restriction, *Cancer Res.* 5:609 (1945).

173. A. Tannenbaum and H. Silverstone, Failure to inhibit the formation of mammary carcinoma in mice by intermittent fasting, *Cancer Res.* 10:577 (1950).

174. M.J. Tucker, The effect of long-term food restriction on tumours in rodents, *Intl J Cancer.* 23:803 (1979).

175. M.G. Visscher, Z.B. Ball, R.H. Barnes, and I. Silversten, The influence of caloric restriction upon the incidence of spontaneous mammary carcinoma in mice, *Surgery (St. Louis).* 11:48 (1942).

176. S.H. Waxler, The effect of weight reduction on the occurrence of spontaneous mammary tumors in mice, *J Natl Cancer Inst.* 14:1253 (1954).

177. S.H. Waxler, P. Tabar, and L.R. Melcher, Obesity and the time of appearance of spontaneous mammary carcinoma in C3H mice, *Cancer Res.* 13:276 (1953).

178. F.R. White, The relationship between underfeeding and tumor formation, transplantation, and growth in rats and mice, *Cancer Res.* 21:281 (1961).

179. F.R. White, J. White, G.B. Midler, M.G. Kelly, W.E. Heston, and P.W. David, Effect of caloric restriction in mammary-tumor formation in strain C3H mice and on the response of strain DBA to painting with methylcholanthrene, *J Natl Cancer Inst.* 5:43 (1944).

180. K. Donato and D.M. Hegsted, Efficiency of utilization of various sources of energy for growth, *Proc Natl Acad Sci (USA).* 82:4866 (1985).

181. E.B. Forbes, R.W. Swift, R.F. Elliot, and W.H. James, Relation of fat to economy of food utilization. I. By the mature albino rat, *J Nutr.* 31:213 (1946).

182. R.K. Boutwell, M.K. Brush, and H.P. Rusch, The stimulating effect of dietary fat on carcinogenesis, *Cancer Res.* 9:741 (1949).

183. P.J.H. Jones, Effect of fatty acid composition of dietary fat on energy balance and expenditures in hamsters, *Can J Physiol Pharmacol.* 67:994 (1989).

184. C.C. Parrish, D.A. Pathy, and A. Angel, Dietary fish oils limit adipose tissue hypertrophy in rats, *Metabolism.* 39:217 (1990).

185. R.J. Jandacek, E.J. Hollenbach, B.N. Holcombe, C.M. Kuehlthau, J.C. Peters, and J.D. Taulbee, Reduced storage of dietary eicosapentaenoic and docosahexaenoic acids in the weaning rat, *J. Nutr Biochem.* 2:142 (1991).

186. J. Meites, J.F. Bruni, D.A. vanVugt, and A.F. Smith, Relation of endogenous opioid peptides and morphine to neuroendocrine functions, *Life Sci.* 24:1325 (1979).

187. P.W. Sylvester, S. Forczek, M.M. Ip, and C. Ip, Exercise training and the differential prolactin response in male and female rats, *J Appl Physiol.* 67:804 (1989).

188. C.W. Welsch and H. Nagasawa, Prolactin and murine mammary tumorigenesis: a review. *Cancer Res.* 37:951 (1977).

189. E.W. Blank and R.L. Ceriani, Fish oil enhancement of ^{131}I-conjugated-anti-human milk fat globule monoclonal antibody experimental radio-immunotherapy of breast cancer, *J Steroid Biochem.* 34:149 (1989).

190. C.E. Borgeson, L. Pardini, R.S. Pardini, and C. Reitz, Effects of dietary fish oil on human mammary carcinoma and on lipid-metabolizing enzymes, *Lipids.* 24:290 (1989).

191. H. Gabor, E.W. Blank, and R.L. Ceriani, Effect of dietary fat and monocolonal antibody therapy on the growth of human mammary adeno-carcinoma MX-1 grafted in athymic mice, *Cancer Letters.* 52:173 (1990).

192. M.J. Gonzalez, R.A. Schemmel, J.I. Gray, L. Dugan, L.G. Sheffield, and C.W. Welsch, Effect of dietary fat on growth of MCF-7 and MDA-MB231 human breast carcinomas in athymic nude mice: relationship between carcinoma growth and lipid peroxidation product levels, *Carcinogenesis.* 12:1231 (1991).

193. G.A. Pritchard, D.L. Jones, and R.E. Mansel, Lipids in breast cancer, *Brit J Surg.* 76:1069 (1989).

194. B.K. Armstrong and R. Doll, Environmental factors and cancer incidence and mortality in different countries, with special reference to dietary practices, *Int J Cancer*. 15:617 (1975).

195. G.E. Gray, M.C. Pike, and B.W. Henderson, Breast cancer incidence and mortality rates in different countries in relation to known risk factors and dietary practices, *Br J Cancer*. 39:1 (1979).

196. L. Kaiser, N.F. Boyd, V. Kriukov, and D. Tritchler, Fish consumption and breast cancer risk: an ecological study, *Nutr Cancer*. 12:61 (1989).

197. A.B. Miller, A. Kelly, N.W. Choi, V. Matthews, R.W. Morgan, L. Munan, J.D. Burch, J. Feather, G.R. Howe, and M. Jain, A study of diet and breast cancer, *Am J Epidemiol*. 107:499 (1978).

198. R.L. Prentice, M. Pepe, and S.G. Self, Dietary fat and breast cancer: a quantitative assessment of the epidemiological literature and a discussion of methodological issues, *Cancer Res*. 49:3147 (1989).

199. A. Schatzkin, P. Greenwald, D.P. Byar, and C.K. Clifford, The dietary fat-breast cancer hypothesis is alive, *J Amer Med Assoc*. 261:3284 (1989).

200. P. Toniolo, E. Riboli, F. Protta, M. Charrel, and A.P.M. Coppa, Calorie-providing nutrients and risk of breast cancer, *J Natl Cancer Inst*. 81:278 (1989).

201. E.L. Wynder, Identification of women at high risk of breast cancer, *Cancer*. 24:1235 (1969).

202. P.J. Goodwin and N.F. Boyd, Critical appraisal of the evidence that dietary fat intake is related to breast cancer risk in humans, *J Natl Cancer Inst*. 79:473 (1987).

203. S. Graham, J. Marshall, C. Mettlin, T. Rzepka, T. Nemoto, and T. Byers, Diet in the epidemiology of breast cancer, *Am J Epidemiol*. 116:68 (1982).

204. D.Y. Jones, A. Schatzkin, S.B. Green, G. Block, L.A. Brinton, R.G. Ziegler, R. Hoover, and P.R. Taylor, Dietary fat and breast cancer in the National Health and Nutrition Examination Survey I Epidemiologic Follow-up Study, *J Natl Cancer Inst*. 79:465 (1987).

205. S.C. Newman, A.B. Miller, and G.R. Howe, A study of the effect of weight and dietary fat on breast cancer survival time, *Am J Epidemiol*. 123:767 (1986).

206. W.C. Willett, M.J. Stampfer, G.A. Colditz, B.A. Rosner, C.H. Hennekens, and F.E. Speizer, Dietary fat and the risk of breast cancer, *N Engl J Med*. 316:22 (1987).

Chapter 17

Dietary Fat and Breast Cancer: A Search for Mechanisms

THOMAS L. DAO and RUSSELL HILF

I. Introduction

In considering nutrition as an interventional approach to alter cancer incidence and mortality, most attention has focused on dietary lipids, a result of considerable experimental animal studies and the observations from numerous epidemiologic investigations internationally and nationally on the relationship between fat intake and breast cancer rates. Taken together, it has been suggested that high dietary fat intake is an important factor in breast cancer development and reduction of dietary fat is recommended. Although indisputable evidence for a beneficial outcome remains to be obtained and the controversy among epidemiologists pertaining to the association between dietary fat intake and breast cancer risk is disconcerting, it appears plausible to examine two important postulates regarding mechanisms by which dietary fat enhances breast cancer incidence or mortality. These can be stated simply as 1) dietary fat has a direct effect on initiation and/or promotion on mammary carcinogenesis and 2) dietary fat has indirect effects on initiation and/or promotion *via* alterations in the host's hormonal milieu. It is noted that these do not have to be mutually exclusive, since the level and content of fat could affect cell membrane composition and fluidity and signal transduction *via* membrane receptors may be altered. This chapter will examine current literature pertinent to the aforementioned postulates and to consider further research needed to support the validity of these hypotheses.

II. Overview: Dietary Fat and Breast Cancer in Rodents

The first observations suggesting an association between dietary fat and breast cancer were reported by Tannenbaum in 1942.[1] His experiments demonstrated that dietary fat enhanced both chemically induced and spontaneously developing mammary tumors in mice. The author provided evidence that fat, rather than calories, was responsible for the promoting

---

Thomas L. Dao ● Professor of Surgery Emeritus, Roswell Park Memorial Institute, 666 Elm Street, Buffalo, New York; Russell Hilf ● Biochemistry Department, University of Rochester, School of Medicine and Dentistry, Box 607, 601 Elmwood Avenue, Rochester, New York

Exercise, Calories, Fat, and Cancer, Edited by M.M. Jacobs
Plenum Press, New York, 1992

effect in mammary tumorigenesis, since the mice were fed isocaloric high- or low-fat diets. Decades later, a renewed interest in dietary factors and cancer ensued. Using a chemical carcinogen 7,12-dimethybenz(a)anthracene (7,12-DMBA)-induced mammary cancer model in the rat, Carroll and Khor[2,3] demonstrated that high dietary fat, particularly the polyunsaturated fat, enhanced mammary tumor development. Similar observations have since been reported by numerous investigators using the DMBA-induced model as well as N-nitrosomethylurea (NMU)-induced mammary tumors in the rat.[4-7]

The relationship between amount and type of dietary fat in promotion of mammary carcinogenesis was investigated by several researchers. Hopkins and Carroll[8] reported that the mammary tumor incidence in rats fed a high-fat diet of different types was similar if these diets contained 3% linoleate. This finding led these investigators to conclude that concentration, rather than type, of dietary fat was the important factor in the increased incidence of mammary tumors. In contrast, King et al.[9] observed that rats fed a diet containing 18% stripped, hydrogenated coconut oil plus 2% linoleic acid had a lower mammary tumor yield than did those rats fed a diet containing 20% stripped corn oil. Rogers and Wetsel[10] reported that rats fed a diet containing 30% beef tallow supplemented with 2% vegetable oil had a lower mammary tumor yield than did rats fed a diet containing 15% vegetable oil. These observations disagreed with those from Hopkins and Carroll's experiments. Chan, Ferguson and Dao[11] examined 4 different dietary fats on mammary carcinogenesis in female Fischer rats. The rats were given low corn oil, high corn oil, high lard, high beef tallow, and high coconut oil diets. Mammary tumor incidence at 28 weeks after NMU treatment was 33, 85, 64, 50, and 43% respectively. The data show that an increase in fat intake enhanced mammary tumorigenesis, but the magnitude of the increase was dependent on the type of fat. Further analyses showed that the total oleic and linoleic acid intake in the five groups of rats correlated positively (r=0.95) with mammary tumor incidence. The data suggest that the total oleic and linoleic acid intake in the high-fat diet is the major factor influencing the incidence of mammary tumors. Altogether, the data led to the conclusion that the type of fat, rather than the concentration, is the important factor in the increased incidence of mammary tumors induced by a chemical carcinogen.

The effect of dietary fat on enhancement of mammary carcinogenesis in different strains of rats, including susceptible and resistant strains of rats to carcinogen-induced mammary carcinogenesis, was examined by Chan and Dao[12] in Fischer, Long-Evans, and Sprague-Dawley rats. The data show that the susceptibility to NMU-induced mammary carcinogenesis in the three strains of rats was in the order of Sprague-Dawley>Fischer>Long-Evans. The mammary tumor incidence was highest in rats fed a high-fat diet, intermediate in rats fed a low-fat diet and lowest in those fed a NP (nonpurified) Teklad mouse/rat diet. These experiments demonstrated a that high-fat diet can promote mammary tumor development in the genetically resistant Long-Evans rat.

Although the majority of investigators seem to agree with the conclusion that high dietary fat exerts its enhancing effect during the promotion phase, few experiments have been carried out to examine the effect of dietary fat during the initiation phase. The design of earlier experiments precluded an answer to the question whether dietary fat exerts its effect during initiation. Dao and Chan[13] presented convincing evidence that the enhancing effect of a high-fat diet on mammary carcinogenesis was directly related to the duration of high-fat diet intake and that an increment of approximately 1.53% tumor incidence requires about a week duration of high-fat diet ingestion. These authors' data clearly showed that a 4-week period of feeding of a high-fat diet either prior to or after carcinogen treatment had little or no effect on tumor incidence. This finding suggests that the failure to significantly increase mammary tumor incidence when a high-fat diet is fed to rats prior to carcinogen treatment (initiation phase) is due to insufficient intake of the high-fat diet. The authors concluded that dietary fat is not just a promoter but is in fact co-carcinogenic in mammary tumor induction by chemical carcinogens.

III. Dietary Fat and Breast Cancer in Humans

The possible association of dietary fat and breast cancer in women was proposed by the observation of a positive correlation between national estimates of per capita dietary fat intake and corresponding breast cancer rates as reported by Carroll and colleagues in 1968.[14] Numerous studies have since been carried out in an attempt to establish this relationship. Although positive correlations were observed internationally between per capita intake of fat, particularly from animal sources, and rates of breast cancer, concerns were raised regarding the quality of the mortality data and accuracy of the dietary intake estimates.[15-17] The consistent increase in the incidence of breast cancer among later generations of Japanese immigrants compared to that in the native Japanese women is suggestive of a link to a Western life-style, implying increased urbanization and high dietary fat consumption. Hirayama[18] in a study of 12 districts in Japan, reported a highly positive correlation (r=0.84) between dietary fat intake and breast cancer mortality (age-adjusted). The author pointed out that the breast cancer mortality rates were higher in large cities and among women from higher socioeconomic groups. In a recent paper comparing cancer epidemiology between the U.S. and Japan, Wynder et al.[19] examined vital statistics from 1955 through 1985 for Japanese natives and U.S. whites as one approach to elucidate changes in cancer mortality and related antecedent patterns of life-style in these two populations. The results show that as the Japanese life-style and diet continue to become more "westernized," the rates of breast, ovary, corpus uteri, prostate, pancreas, and colon cancers also continue to rise. In contrast, the breast cancer mortality among U.S. women has remained relatively constant over the last half century. Further, it is noted that the percentage of fat calories in the Japanese diet has increased from about 10% in 1950 to nearly 25% in 1987, concurrent with the two-fold increase in breast cancer mortality. The percentage of fat calories in the U.S. diet for the same period of time has consistently been about 40%.

Several case-control studies were carried out in North America using a dietary history questionnaire. Miller et al.[20] reported that in pre-menopausal breast cancer patients, the consumption of total and saturated fat was higher than in control women. In a U.S. case-control study Graham et al.,[21] using a food-frequency questionnaire to estimate animal fat consumption, reported no association between dietary fat and breast cancer in 2024 breast cancer cases and 1463 control patients without malignant diseases. The choice of the food-frequency method was based on the authors' experience in ascertaining the most reliable approach for both interviewer and interviewee. In a recent prospective study Willett et al.[22] observed little or no association between per capita intake of fat, particularly fat from animal sources, and rates of breast cancer in more detailed studies of individual women.

IV. Mechanisms of Action

Although the association between dietary fat and mammary cancer development has been conclusively demonstrated in animal experiments, the presence of this association in humans continues to be debated. Questions can be raised on the rationale for large-scale clinical trials to test a weak dietary fat-breast cancer hypothesis. Questions can also be raised about the existence of plausible biologic mechanisms of dietary fat on mammary carcinogenesis. We will review experiments from many laboratories that we believe are relevant to the eulicidation of mechanisms of an association between dietary lipids and breast cancer.

A. A Direct Effect of Fat on Mammary Cells and Carcinogenesis

1. The Ability of Dietary Fat to Overcome the Refractoriness of the Mammary Gland to Chemical Carcinogenesis

The effect of age on mammary carcinogenesis induced by DMBA in rats was first described by Huggins et al. in 1961[23] and later confirmed by Dao.[24] In female Sprague-Dawley rats, the mammary tumor incidence reached a maximum when the carcinogen was administered at 50-60 days of age and then declined as the age of rats increased. Only rarely can mammary tumors be induced in rats over 100 days of age. The basis of this susceptibility of the mammary gland to DMBA carcinogenesis in relation to age was investigated. It was conclusively shown by Sinha et al.[25] that the DNA synthesis pattern played a major role during carcinogenesis. These experiments disclosed that the progression of mammary gland development was accompanied by high thymidine labeling index in the end bud and alveolar bud cells (ranging from 14.7 and 19.8%) between the ages of 10 to 55 days. Thereafter, the labeling indexes declined and the cell proliferative activities were practically nil when the rats were 90 to 150 days old and, in these older rats, the carcinogen did not induce any tumors. Together, these results strongly suggest that an optimal level of DNA synthesis required for tumor induction was absent in aging rats. Lin et al. also observed that increased waves of DNA synthesis made the mouse mammary gland more susceptible to carcinogenesis.[26]

The evidence that dietary lipids exert a direct effect on mammary carcinogenesis has come from experiments that demonstrated the ability of dietary fat to overcome the resistance of the mammary glands in aging rats to carcinogenesis. To investigate any interdependence of fat intake and age as modifiers of mammary carcinogenesis, Ip[27] reported that a differential effect of high-fat and low-fat diets on mammary tumorigenesis can be demonstrated regardless of the age at which the carcinogen DMBA is given. In a more detailed study by Chan and Dao,[28] eight groups of rats, four receiving high-fat (20% corn oil) and four receiving low-fat (0.5%) diet throughout the experiments from weaning, a single dose of the carcinogen NMU was given to rats at 35, 50, 90, and 130 days of age from each diet group. The results showed that although the mammary tumor incidence declined in rats as their ages increased, irrespective of whether they were fed high- or low-fat diet, the tumor incidence was significantly higher in rats fed the high-fat diet than in those fed a low-fat diet. These experimental results using NMU as the carcinogen agree with the results obtained using DMBA as the carcinogen.[27] However, since NMU is a direct carcinogen these experiments removed the possibility of a relationship between the possible effects of age or dietary fat on the metabolism of the carcinogen. The fact that high dietary fat can produce a significant increase in tumor incidence in 130- and 150-day-old rats that are considered to be resistant to chemical carcinogens is highly suggestive of a direct action on mammary carcinogenesis. These in vivo experiments are supported by results in vitro, described in the following section.

2. Effects of Free Fatty Acids on Growth of Normal and Neoplastic Mammary Epithelial Cells in Vitro

Using a primary culture system adapted from Janss et al.,[29] Wicha et al.[30] cultured normal mammary epithelial cells and DMBA-induced mammary tumor cells to study the effects of free fatty acids on their growth. The epithelial nature of the mammary cell cultures was confirmed by light and electron microscopy, by association of cells with basement membrane, and by production of α-lactalbumin. The results show that in the presence of insulin, hydrocortisone, progesterone, estrogen, prolactin, and delipidized fetal calf serum, both the normal mammary and tumor cells were stimulated in their growth by addition of unsaturated fatty acids to the growth medium. For normal cells, linoleic or linolenic acid at 1.0 and 0.1 µg/ml, respectively, and for DMBA-induced mammary tumor cells, oleic and linoleic acid at 0.5 and 1.0 µg/ml, respectively, produced greater than a doubling of the growth rate compared to cultures with no added free fatty acids. It should be noted, however, that cultures of normal cells showed no appreciable growth in the absence of hormones when linoleic acid was added. With hormones only, the cells had a doubling time of 58 hours whereas with hormones plus linoleic acid, the doubling time was 34 hours, suggesting that maximal stimulation requires both hormones and linoleic acid. These results from the experiments *in vitro* relate well to the experiments *in vivo* on the unsaturated fatty acid enhancement of mammary carcinogenesis.

Recent studies of the effect of linoleic acid on the growth of human breast cancer cells were reported by Rose and Connolly.[31] Two human breast cancer cell lines, the hormone dependent MCF-7 and hormone-independent MDA-MB-231 were used. The results showed that MDA-MB-231 cells cultured in IMDM (Iscove's modified Dulbecco's medium), with or without 1% fetal bovine serum, plus delipidized BSA, and LA-BSA (linoleic acid) complex additions over the range of 1 to 150 µg/ml (5 to 750 ng/ml of linoleic acid) resulted in a stimulation of cell growth, which was positively correlated over the entire range of linoleic acid levels. In MCF-7 cell cultures in IMDM in the presence of 1% FBS, SA, insulin, and estradiol, linoleic acid stimulated cell growth (mitogenesis) with an increase in cell number that was maximal (at a linoleic acid concentration of 500 ng/ml) after 6 days of incubation. Under serum-free conditions, but in the presence of insulin and estradiol, linoleic acid had no effect on MCF-7 cell growth. These authors suggested that growth factors and other nutrients present in the fetal bovine serum might be necessary in addition to unsaturated fatty acid, to stimulate the cell growth.

Although more experiments appear necessary to confirm those earlier studies using human cell lines, the data imply that linoleic acid stimulates directly the growth of some human cell lines *in vitro*.

3. Dietary Lipids and Inhibition of Prostaglandin Synthesis

Additional support for a direct effect of dietary lipids on mammary tumor growth comes from reports that inhibition of prostaglandin synthesis impairs mammary tumor development by chemical carcinogens, and the substitution of menhaden oil (i.e., dietary n-3 lipids) for n-6 lipids inhibits mammary tumorigenesis.[32] The mechanism common to both is reduction in arachidonate metabolism, either by inhibition of the biosynthesis enzymes or by competition with substrates that are not metabolized to prostaglandins.[33-35]

The mechanisms whereby direct effects of dietary lipids manifest a growth stimulation of mammary tumors, i.e., a promotional effect, are yet to be defined. The importance of fatty acid metabolism or, more specifically, the products formed from enzymatic conversion of polyunsaturated fatty acids by cyclooxygenases to prostaglandins or to those arising via lipoxygenases to leukotrienes, has been inferred from the observations that dietary interventions can alter mammary tumor production and/or growth. The production of a varying array of these eicosanoids (a generic term for the oxygenated metabolites of 20-carbon polyunsaturated fatty acids) may be the basis for the observation that substitution of menhaden oil, an n-3 lipid, for n-6 lipid, such as corn oil, resulted in a reduction in NMU-induced tumorigenesis. In one early report, Jurkowski and Cave[36] clearly demonstrated that as the percentage of menhaden oil in the diet was increased, the latent period of tumor appearance was lengthened and the incidence of tumors was reduced, as was the total tumor burden. The amount of eicosapentaenoic acid was significantly higher in tumor and liver cell membranes of the animals fed the elevated levels of menhaden oil. Metabolism of this fatty acid by cyclooxygenases yields prostaglandins of the three series and leukotrienes of the five series, compared to prostaglandins of the two series and leukotrienes of the four series resulting from the metabolism of arachidonic acid derived from the linoleic acid in corn oil.

Braden and Carroll,[37] using the DMBA-induced mammary tumor model in rodents, observed that increased tumor yield was correlatable with increasing dietary levels of corn oil but tumor yield was lower and latent periods were longer in animals fed higher levels of menhaden oil. Several studies followed to determine the effects of various dietary mixtures of polyunsaturated fatty acids, i.e., menhaden or fish oil and corn oil.[38-40] Analysis of cell membrane fatty acids demonstrated a good correlation between the proportion of membrane linoleic acid and the amount of corn oil in the diet, as did the proportion of membrane eicosapentaenoic acid and the level of dietary menhaden oil.[39] These studies, along with others[41,42] led to the suggestion that increased tumor growth and development resulted from increased eicosanoid synthesis, and that elevations in those arachidonic acid metabolites could be reduced by inhibition of the biosynthetic enzymes, e.g., cyclo-oxygenase, lipoxygenase, or by substrate competition for the same enzymes.[33,42] To address this important aspect of mechanism of action, Abou-El-Ela and co-workers[43] extended their studies of n-6 and n-3 fatty acid diets to include administration of the ornithine decarboxylase (ODC) inhibitor, DFMO, and the cyclooxygenase inhibitor, indomethacin. Their results showed that DFMO was capable of reducing the average number of DMBA-induced tumors and of extending the duration of the latent period. These events were apparently correlatable with significant reductions in the PGE and leukotriene B_4 levels in tumors and in ODC activity in the lesions. Although indomethacin reduced prostaglandin synthesis and ODC activity, leukotriene B_4 synthesis was increased and, importantly, no effect on tumor growth was seen. They suggest that leukotriene B_4 may be involved in mammary tumor production whereas the relationship of PGE and tumor growth was not apparent in the studies using indomethacin to inhibit PGE synthesis. Others had reported a lack of correlation between reduced PGE levels and tumor growth response to indomethacin treatment.[44,45] The recent proposal for a role of leukotrienes in tumorigenesis and/or tumor growth will need confirmation. Hopefully, such investigations will also answer whether the time course of changes precedes changes in tumor growth behavior, whether such altered metabolism occurs in the normal gland and, if so, whether such a milieu has an altered response to an administered carcinogen.

Even if all agree that production of arachidonic acid is critical, there remains the mechanistic question of how arachidonate or its metabolites are important stimulators of tumor growth. Arachidonic acid arises from metabolic pathways of fatty acid chain elongation and desaturation, as well as directly from dietary ingestion; the majority of it is esterified in phospholipids, and as such, is not utilizable for eicosanoid biosynthesis. There are however a number of ways that arachidonic acid can be liberated: by hydrolysis, from the 2-acyl position of membrane phospholipids; action by phospholipase A2, phospholipase C and mono- and diglyceride lipases; via phospholipase A, followed by phospholipase B; by phospholipase D followed by phosphatidate phosphohydrolase and glyceride lipases; by inhibition of those pathways involved in acylation of arachidonate into phospholipids. A recent review by Naor[46] postulates that arachidonic acid could play a second messenger role in signal transduction, particularly as an activator of one or more of the protein kinase C subspecies and/or a mobilizer or intracellular calcium. A relationship between arachidonic acid formation or inositol phosphates and diacylglycerol, activation of protein kinase C, and calcium mobilization is not unreasonable. Currently, research is being conducted to provide proof for such scenarios, although these will be difficult studies to conduct because of the transitory nature of the messenger. On the other hand, phopholipase C-α has been reported to be induced by estradiol. This enzyme catalyzes metabolism of membrane-bound phosphatidylinositol 4,5-bisphosphate (PIP_2), yielding inositol 1,4,5-triphosphate (IP_3) and diacylglycerol, which in turn can act as a precursor for synthesis of numerous arachidonic acid metabolites, including prostaglandins and leukotrienes, and as an activator of protein kinase C. It is obvious that a more detailed examination of the lipid-phospholipid protein-hormone interaction and the production of mediators that are secondary effectors is necessary before a direct role of dietary lipids can be defined.

B. An Indirect Effect of Dietary Lipids on Mammary Carcinogenesis

Indirect mechanisms have been explored in some depth in both the laboratory animals and in humans. The mechanisms usually considered are: 1) dietary fat can affect hormone secretion, metabolism, pharmacokinetics, thereby resulting in a hormonal milieu that favors tumor development and growth, or 2) that dietary fat can alter the sensitivity of responsive tissues by altering the physical environment of the cells.

1. Effect of Dietary Lipids on Hormone Metabolism

a. Studies in Laboratory Animals

The role of hormones in mammary carcinogenesis has been extensively investigated in rodents. Among the various anterior pituitary and steroidal hormones, estrogen and prolaction appear to be the most critical regulators of growth.[47] DMBA-induced mammary tumors are dependent on these two hormones and it has been demonstrated that prolactin stimulation of mammary tumor growth is dependent on the presence of ovarian hormones.[48] The possible modulation of endocrine functions by high dietary fat has been proposed by several investigators and data on the effect of a high-fat diet on the levels of several hormones, including prolactin and estrogen, have been reported.

High-Fat Diet and Serum Prolactin. It was proposed that a high-fat diet enhanced prolactin secretion. Chan et al.[48] reported earlier that afternoon serum prolactin levels were significantly higher in proestrous rats on a high-fat diet than in rats on a low-fat diet. These authors further demonstrated that enhancement of mammary tumorigenesis by high-fat diet can be blocked by the administration of an ergot drug (CB-154), a compound that inhibits prolactin secretion. Reduction of serum prolactin levels probably resulted from both a direct action on the pituitary and by increasing hypothalamic prolactin inhibitory factor.[49] These data provide indirect evidence for a relationship between a high-fat diet and prolactin secretion. Unfortunately, several investigators failed to confirm these earlier data.[50-52] It should be pointed out, however, that in most of the experiments reporting the negative results the data were often derived from a single sampling of blood during the entire estrous cycle. It appears that many of these experiments neglected to consider the importance of episodic fluctuations of prolactin levels and also the changes during the estrous cycles.

High-Fat Diet and Serum Estrogen. Estrogens and prolactin are the major mammotrophic hormones that are critically involved in the normal development and pathogenesis of cancer in the mammary gland. Since prolactin synthesis and secretion by the pituitary is regulated in part by estrogen, it seems logical to examine the effect of dietary fat on estrogen biosynthesis and secretion. Chan et al.[53] reported that tumor-bearing rats on a high-fat diet had a slightly higher estrogen level than those on a low-fat diet. Later, Ip and Ip[54] observed that serum estrogen level appeared to reflect the amount of fat in the diet. These data are not conclusive. Indirect evidence suggesting a possible relationship between a high-fat diet and ovarian function was reported by Frisch et al.[55] who observed early vaginal opening and estrous in rats on high-fat diets. This observation was confirmed by others[56] and led to the conclusion that a high-fat diet has an effect on the ovarian function. On the other hand, Wetsel et al.[57] found no effect of dietary corn oil on plasma prolactin, progesterone, or estrogen in rats during the entire estrous cycle.

Although the proposal that high dietary fat enhances secretion of mammotrophic hormones, which in turn promote the growth of mammary tumors appears plausible, the experimental evidence so far are contradictory and inconclusive. It should be noted that the role of prolactin, estrogens, and progesterone in mammary carcinogenesis is interrelated; simple measurement of serum levels of these hormones cannot elucidate the mechanism by which dietary fat affects mammary carcinogenesis. The effect of dietary fat on the biosynthesis of estrogens and progesterone remains to be examined in detail, recognizing the complexity of estrogen metabolism in mammary carcinogenesis. Equally important is the need to determine whether the effects of dietary fat in mammary carcinogenesis are mediated via neuroendrocrine mechanisms.

b. Studies in Humans

The pivotal role of ovarian and pituitary hormones in the pathogenesis of mammary cancer is well established in experimental carcinogenesis. This is less certain in humans, however. Metabolism of estrogens in women with breast cancer has been extensively investigated and reviewed.[58] Although there is overwhelming evidence that estrogens are involved in the pathogenesis of breast cancer, the exact role estrogens play in the etiology of breast cancer is not defined. Attempts to find consistent differences in plasma and/or urinary estrogens between breast cancer patients and normal women have failed. The report in 1981 by Suter et al.[59] that plasma non-protein-bound estradiol was elevated in breast cancer patients revived much interest in this approach; the logic that it is the free estradiol that is able to enter the cells and stimulate them was indisputable. Unfortunately, not all of the reports since Suter's have been confirmatory and in those studies where the free plasma estradiol was elevated in breast cancer patients, the increase was very small.[60]

The biologic activity of estradiol is governed, in part, by the extent to which it is bound to plasma sex hormone-binding globulin (SHBG); only the free estradiol is available for tissue uptake and binding to intracellular estrogen receptors. It is suggested that the amount of non-protein-bound estrogen is inversely proportional to the level of sex hormone- binding globulin in breast cancer patients. Several investigators have reported that patients with breast cancer have decreased levels of SHBG.[59,61,62]

Dietary Fat and Estrogens. Armstrong et al.[63] in their study of American vegetarians and omnivores of similar age, height, and body weight, found lower levels of urinary estrogen (entirely in the estriol fraction) and serum prolactin, along with high SHBG in the vegetarians. Schultz and Leklem[64] reported that, comparing pre-menopausal Seventh Day Adventists (SDA) and pre-menopausal omnivores, the SDA vegetarian women consumed significantly less fat, especially saturated fatty acids and their plasma levels of estrone and estradiol were lower than those of omnivores. Goldin et al.[65] measured urinary and plasma estrogens in premenopausal vegetarian and omnivorous women eating a high-fat, Western diet and found lower plasma estrogen levels in the vegetarians. It was also noted that there was an inverse correlation between plasma estrogen levels and fecal estrogen excretion. Rose et al.[66] reduced the fat intake (by dietary counseling) from 35 to 21% in 16 pre-menopausal women with cystic breast disease and observed a significant decrease of serum estrone and estradiol after 3 months on the low-fat diet. Goldin et al.[67] also conducted studies on recent Asian immigrants to Hawaii and showed that plasma estrone and estradiol were positively correlated with total and saturated fatty acid intake.

Obesity and Estrogens. De Waard et al.[68] suggested that breast cancer in post-menopausal women was due to altered estrogen production secondary to over-nutrition. The hypothesis came from a case-control study in which the author observed that obesity increased the breast cancer risk in post-menopausal women. Obesity or over-weight was assessed by the percent deviation from ideal weight-for-height in this study. In a later prospective study by De Waard and Baanders-Van Halewign[69] the effect of both body weight and height on breast cancer risk were included. Although several confirmatory reports were published[70-72] contrary results demonstrating a lack of an association between obesity and breast cancer were reported.[73-75] In a more recent paper by Schapira et al.,[76] the authors examined the effect of body fat distribution on breast cancer risk in newly diagnosed breast cancer patients and age-matched controls. The data showed a progressive rise in breast cancer risk with increasing upper body fat localization (android obesity). It was found that women in the highest quartile for upper body fat localization were at an approximately six-fold increased risk of developing breast cancer as compared to women in the lowest quartile (lower body fat localization). In a retrospective analysis of anthropometric data from the Framingham study, Ballard-Barbash et al.[77] reported that upper body fat localization was associated with breast cancer risk.

At menopause, ovarian function declines rapidly and continues progressively into the post-menopausal years. Circulating estrogens in post-menopausal women are derived primarily from the peripheral metabolic transformation of adrenal androstenedione to estrone and estradiol. The adipose tissue is the predominant site of this transformation. This conversion process increases with the increase of body fat.[78] However, measurement of plasma estrogens in post-menopausal women have yielded conflicting results. It should be noted however, that the more critical factors in the relationship between obesity and breast cancer may be the availability of the precursor hormone and the local tissue levels of estrogens.

Many investigators have examined the relationship between obesity and levels of SHBG in the plasma. DeMoor and Joossen[79] reported an inverse relation between body weight and the level of the SHBG in human plasma. Obese women have lower levels of SHBG than their leaner counterparts. Schapira et al.[80] recently investigated whether obesity and body-fat distribution affected the levels of SHBG, testosterone, and estrone in age-matched and weight-matched breast cancer patients and controls. Results disclosed that increasing obesity correlated with a progressive fall in SHBG level and an increase in testosterone level. Pre-menopausal breast cancer patients were found to have significantly lower levels of SHBG compared with age-matched and weight-matched controls. This difference in SHBG level was not observed in post-menopausal patients. The SHBG level decreased with increasing upper body fat localization in breast cancer patients and controls.

2. Effect of Dietary Lipids on Physical Characteristics of Responsive Tissues

When considering one possible indirect mechanism whereby dietary lipids influence tumorigenesis and/or tumor growth, attention invariably focuses on cell membranes as a critical site. Eukaryotic cell membranes are composed primarily of phospholipids, proteins, and cholesterol, the phospholipids providing the backbone of the bilayer due to their amphiphatic properties, i.e., a polar (hydrophilic) head group and hydrophobic fatty acids. The term membrane fluidity refers to the relative degree of order or lack of order (random-ness) that results from the packing and interactions of the long-chain fatty acids. Saturated fatty acids are rather straight and rigid, yielding a less fluid environment, whereas the unsaturated double bond produces a bend that results in a decrease in packing of the fatty acid chains, hence a more fluid environment. Because alteration in dietary lipids can significantly modify the fatty acid composition of membranes in a variety of cells, including mammary cancer (see Section A.3.), it has been suggested that such changes in membrane composition could result in an altered physical and chemical environment, i.e., fluidity, which in turn could affect the activity or responsiveness of protein molecules in the membrane. The most obvious membrane components that could be affected are receptors and transporters.

Experiments to evaluate the effects of dietary lipids on prolactin-binding were carried out by Cave and co-workers.[32,81] They found that there was an association between low dietary corn oil ingestion, reduced tumor growth and lowered prolactin binding capacity in NMU-induced rat mammary tumors. However, once the dietary threshold of polyunsaturated lipid was attained (about 3% corn oil), the increased tumor growth resulting from increased dietary corn oil was not accompanied by a concomitant increase in prolactin-binding capacity. They concluded that some minimal membrane desaturation is needed for optimal prolactin receptor number and/or function, but beyond this, other factors must play a role.

One such factor may be insulin, which has been suggested as playing a growth regulatory role in rodent mammary tumors.[82] There are several reports that dietary lipids could alter membrane fatty acid composition and influence insulin receptors. Ginsburg et al.[83] reported that an increased unsaturated fatty acid composition in Friend erythroleukemia cells led to increased insulin binding. Grunfeld et al.[84] found decreased insulin binding in 3T3-L1 cells maintained in a medium containing saturated fatty acids, and adipocytes and membranes from livers of rats fed high-fat diets displayed lower insulin binding.[85,86] Feldman and Hilf[87] studied insulin receptors in the R3230AC transplantable rat mammary adenocarcinoma and observed that insulin binding to tumor membranes from high fat (20% corn oil)-fed animals was greater than insulin binding to tumor membranes from low fat (0.5% corn oil)- or no fat-fed rats. Interestingly, these changes might be related inversely to serum insulin levels, although it was clear that ovarian status was an important determinant of insulin binding. It was most interesting that estrogen-induced inhibition of tumor growth and down-regulation of insulin binding was greatest in rats ingesting the low-fat diet, a result that could have important implications if a similar observation can be found for anti-estrogen treatment.

A number of important questions remain. With the recent interest and implications of growth factor involvement as paracrine and/or autocrine regulators of mammary tumor growth, it would be of considerable interest to assess whether altered lipid membrane composition can modify growth factor receptor characteristics and their functional activity. It would not be surprising that changes in receptors for IGF-1 and EGF might occur as a result of changes in dietary lipid intake. A second important question is whether response or regulation of these growth factor receptors by other hormonal factors is altered by dietary intervention. A third consideration should be given to the effects of dietary modification or production of growth factors by stromal elements and their ability to affect adjacent neoplastic cells. The difficulty with any of these approaches is to dissect out cause and effect and to conclusively demonstrate that altered membrane composition is responsible for altered tumor growth in the face of a multi-hormonal and multi-growth factor responsive disease such as breast cancer.

V. Conclusion

Experiments in laboratory animals have conclusively demonstrated an association between dietary fat and mammary carcinogenesis. Mechanistic investigations in rodent mammary tumor systems however, have failed to show an endocrine-mediated mechanism. Unfortunately, most of these studies were based on a rather simplistic approach by measuring the serum levels of mammotrophic hormones, e.g., estrogens and prolactin. It is not surprising that conflicting results have been reported. The complex metabolism of hormones in rodents had not been investigated in depth as it has been in humans. To study the effect of dietary fat on hormone metabolism by measuring hormone levels in a few serum samples is not likely to provide meaningful information to elucidate the mechanism of enhancement of mammary carcinogenesis by high dietary fat. Indeed it would be naive to suggest that there is a negative relationship. The *in vitro* experiments demonstrating a direct effect of linoleic and oleic acid to stimulate the growth of normal and neoplastic mammary cells in a medium containing mammotrophic hormones, is highly suggestive of an interaction between the fatty acids and hormones on mammary tumor growth. In the absence of hormones, the fatty acids were unable to stimulate growth of either the normal mammary cells or the neoplastic epithelial cells. Perhaps experiments should be designed to examine how the interaction of fatty acids and hormones may lead to the enhancement of mammary carcinogenesis. In this regard, one must consider the role of prostaglandin as a crucial determinant of susceptibility to carcinogenesis. Several tumor-promoting agents have been shown to increase tissue prostaglandin levels including phenobarbitol, tetradecanoyl phorbol acetate, and dietary linoleate.[88-90] Some prostaglandin synthesis inhibitors have been shown to inhibit tumorigenesis.[34] It is appropriate to suggest that more detailed and in-depth examination of the relationship between dietary fat and prostaglandin synthesis may lead to a better understanding of the mechanisms of action of dietary fat on mammary tumorigenesis.

Although epidemiologic investigations of a link between dietary fat and breast cancer incidence and mortality have yet to come to an agreement, there is nonetheless strong evidence to suggest the existence of such an association. Dietary fat or obesity has been shown to have an effect on hormone metabolism in the majority of investigations. Significantly, many authors have reported that dietary fat or obesity is associated with increased levels of free estradiol (non-protein-bound estradiol) and decreased levels of sex hormone-binding globulin. Further studies could be directed to examine the membrane receptors for hormone and growth factors, e.g., EGF, IGF-1, etc., in breast tumors from women consuming diets of different lipid content and composition. This may be another way to explore mechanisms of regulation of tumor growth. Finally, whether a linkage between dietary fat/obesity and hormone metabolism is indicative of a susceptibility to breast cancer, can only be proven by a carefully constructed prospective cohort study.

Acknowledgment

Address correspondence to Thomas L. Dao, 40 Sturbridge Lane, Williamsville, NY 14221.

References

1. A. Tannenbaum, Genesis and growth of tumors: effects of a high fat diet, *Cancer Res.* 2:168 (1942).
2. K.K. Carroll and G.J. Khor, Effects of dietary fat and dose level of 7,12-dimethyl-benz(a)anthracene on mammary tumor incidence in rats, *Cancer Res.* 30:2260 (1970).
3. K.K. Carroll and G.J. Khor, Effects of level and type of dietary fat on incidence of mammary tumors induced in Sprague-Dawley rats by DMBA, *Lipids.* 6:415 (1971).
4. P.C. Chan and L.A. Cohen, Dietary fat and growth promotion of rat mammary tumors, *Cancer Res.* 35:3384 (1975).
5. G.J. Hopkins and C.E. West, Possible roles of dietary fats in carcinogenesis, *Life Sci.* 19:1103 (1976).
6. S.H. Waxler, G. Brecher, and S.L. Bead, The effect of fat enriched diet on the incidence of spontaneous mammary tumors in obese mice, *Proc Soc Exp Biol and Med.* 62:365 (1979).
7. W.C. Westsel, A.E. Rogers, and P.M. Newberne, Dietary fat and DMBA mammary carcinogenesis in rats, *Cancer Detect Prev.* 4:535 (1981).
8. G.J. Hopkins and K.K. Carroll, Relationship between amount type of dietary fat in promotion of mammary carcinogenesis induced by DMBA, *J Natl Cancer Inst.* 62:1009 (1979).
9. M.M. King, D.M. Bailey, D.D. Gibson, J.V. Pitha, and P.B. McCay, Incidence and growth of mammary tumors induced by DMBA as related to the dietary content of fat and antioxidant, *J Natl Cancer Inst.* 63:657 (1979).

10. A.E. Rogers and W.C. Wetsel, Mammary carcinogenesis in rats fed different amounts and types of fats, *Cancer Res.* 41:3735 (1981).

11. P.C. Chan, K.A. Ferguson, and T.L. Dao, Effects of different dietary fats on mammary carcinogenesis, *Cancer Res.* 43:1079 (1983).

12. P.C. Chan and T.L. Dao, Enhancement of mammary carcinogenesis by a high fat diet in Fischer, Long-Evans and Sprague-Dawley rats, *Cancer Res.* 41:164 (1981).

13. T.L. Dao and P.C. Chan, Effect of duration of high fat intake on enhancement of mammary carcinogenesis in rats, *J Natl Cancer Inst.* 71:201 (1983).

14. K.K. Carroll, E.B. Gammal and E.R. Plumbett, *Canadian Medical Association Journal.* 98:590 (1968).

15. B. Armstrong and R. Doll, Environmental factors and cancer incidence and mortality in different countries with special reference to dietary practices, *Int J Cancer.* 15:617 (1975).

16. G. Hems, Contributions of diet and childbearing to breast cancer, *Br J Cancer.* 37:974 (1978).

17. G.E. Gray, M.C. Pike, and B.E. Henderson, Breast cancer incidence and mortality rates in different countries in relation to known risk factors and dietary practices, *Br J Cancer.* 39:1 (1979).

18. T. Hirayama, Epidemiology of breast cancer and special reference to the role of diet, *Prev Med.* 7:173 (1978).

19. E.L. Wynder, Y. Frijita, R.E. Harris, T. Hirayama and T. Hiyama, Comparative epidemiology of cancer between the United States and Japan, *Cancer.* 67:746 (1991).

20. A.B. Miller, A. Kelly, and N.W. Choi, A study of diet and breast cancer, *Amer J Epidemiology.* 107:499 (1978).

21. S. Graham, J. Marshall, and C. Mettlin, Diet in the epidemiology of breast cancer, *Amer J Epidemiology.* 116:68 (1982).

22. W.W. Willett, M.J. Stamfer, and G.A. Colditz, Dietary fat and the risk of breast cancer, *New Engl J Med.* 316:22 (1987).

23. C. Huggins, L.C. Grand, and E.P. Brillantes, Mammary cancer induced by a single feeding of polycyclic hydrocarbons and its suppression, *Nature.* 198:204 (1961).

24. T.L. Dao, Mammary cancer induction by 7,12-dimethylbenz(a)anthracene relation to age, *Science.* 165:810 (1969).

25. D.K. Sinha, J.E. Pazick, and T.L. Dao, Progression of rat mammary development with age and its relationship to carcinogenesis by a chemical carcinogen, *Int J Cancer.* 31:321 (1983).

26. F.K. Lin, M.R. Banerjee, and L.R. Crump, Cell cycle related hormone carcinogen interaction during chemical carcinogen induction of nodule-like mammary lesions in organ culture, *Cancer Res.* 36:1607 (1976).

27. C. Ip, Ability of dietary fat to overcome the resistance of mature female rats to 7,12-dimethylbenz(a)anthracene induced mammary tumorigenesis, *Cancer Res.* 40:2785 (1980).

28. P. Chan and T.L. Dao, Effect of dietary fat on age-dependent sensitivity to mammary carcinogenesis, *Cancer Letter.* 18:245 (1983).

29. D. Janss, E.H. Hillman, L.B. Malan-Shibley, and T.L. Ben, Method of culture for isolation and culture of normal human breast epithelial, *Methods in Cell Biology.* 21:107 (1980).

30. M.S. Wicha, L.A. Liotta, and W.R. Kidwell, Effects of free fatty acids on the growth of normal and neoplastic rat mammary epithelial cells, *Cancer Res.* 39:426 (1979).

31. D.P. Rose and J.M. Connolly, Stimulation of growth of human breast cancer cell lines in culture by linoleic acid, *Biochem and Bioph Research Communications.* 164:277 (1989).

32. W.T. Cave, Jr. and J.J. Jurkowski, Dietary lipid effects on the growth, membrane composition and prolactin-binding capacity of rat mammary tumors, *J Natl Cancer Inst.* 73:185 (1984).

33. L.A. Hillyard and S. Abraham, Effect of dietary polyunsaturated fatty acids on growth of mammary adenoarcinoma in mice and rats, *Cancer Res.* 39:4430 (1979).

34. C.A. Carter, R.J. Milholland, W. Shea and M.M. Ip, Effect of the prostaglandin synthetase inhibitor indomethacin on 7,12-dimethylbenz(a)anthracene induced mammary carcinogenesis in rats fed different levels of fat, *Cancer Res.* 43:3559 (1983).

35. B.R. Culp, B.G. Tilns, and W.M. Landes, Inhibiting of prostaglandin biosynthesis by eiscosapentaenoic acid, *Prostaglandins Med.* 3:263 (1979).

36. J.J. Jurkowski and W.T. Cave, Dietary effects of menhaden oil on the growth and membrane lipid composition of rat mammary tumors, *J Natl Cancer Inst.* 74:1145 (1985).

37. L.M. Braden and K.K. Carroll, Dietary polyunsaturated fat in relation to mammary carcinogenesis in rats, *Lipids.* 21:285 (1986).

38. C. Ip, M.M. Ip, and P. Sylvester, Relevance of trans fatty acids and fish oil in animal tumorigenesis studies, *in:* "Dietary Fat and Cancer," C. Ip, D.F. Birt, A.E. Rogers, and C. Mettlin, eds., *Prog Clin Biol Res Series*, Alan R. Liss, Inc., New York (1986).

39. W.T. Cave and J.J. Jurkowski, Comparative Effects of Omega-3 and Omega-6 Dietary Lipids on Rat Mammary Tumor Development, *in:* "Proceedings of the AOCS Short Course on Polyunsaturated Fatty Acids and Eicosanoids," W.E.M. Lands, ed., American Oil Chemists Society, Champaign, Illinois (1989).

40. R.A. Karmali, R.U. Doshi, L. Adams, and K. Choi, Effect of n-3 fatty acids on mammary tumorigenesis, *in:* "Advances in Prostaglandin, Thromboxane and Leukotriene Research," B. Samuelsen, R. Paoletti, and P.W. Ramwell, eds., Raven Press, New York (1989).

41. R.A. Karmali, Fatty acids: inhibition, *Am J Clin Nutr.* 45:225 (1987).

42. S.H. Abou-El-Ela, K.W. Prasse, R. Carrol, A.E. Wade, S. Dharwadkar, and O.R. Bunce, Eicosanoid synthesis in 7,12-dimethylbenz(a)anthracene induced mammary carcinomas in Sprague-Dawley rats fed primose, menhaden or corn oil diets, *Lipids.* 23:948 (1988).

43. S.H. Abou-El-Ela, K.W. Prasse, R.L. Farrell, R.W. Carroll, A.E. Wade, and O.R. Bunce, Effects of D,L-2-difluoromethylornithine and indomethacin on mammary tumor promotion in rats fed high n-3 and/or n-6 fat diets, *Cancer Res.* 49:1434 (1989).

44. D. Hofer, A.M. Dubitsky, P. Reilly, M.G. Santoro, and B.M. Jaffe, The interactions between indomethacin and cytotoxic drugs in mice bearing B-16 melanoma, *Prostaglandins.* 20:1033 (1980).

45. J.M. Feldman and R. Hilf, Failure of indomethacin to inhibit growth of the R3230AC mammary tumor in rats, *J Natl Cancer Inst.* 75:751 (1985).

46. Z. Naor, Is arachidonic acid a second messenger in signal transduction, *Mol Cell Endocrinol.* 80:C181 (1991).

47. D. Sinha, D. Cooper, and T.L. Dao, The nature of estrogen and effect on mammary tumorigenesis, *Cancer Res.* 33:411 (1973).

48. P.C. Chan, F. Didato, and L.A. Cohen, A high dietary fat, elevation of rat serum prolactin and mammary cancer, *Proc Soc Exp Biol & Med.* 149:133 (1975).

49. P.C. Chan and L.A. Cohen, Effect of dietary fat, antiestrogen and antiprolactin on development of mammary tumors in rats, *J Natl Cancer Inst.* 52:25 (1974).

50. G.J. Hopkins, T.G. Kennedy, and K.K. Carroll, Polyunsaturated fatty acids as promoters of mammary carcinogenesis induced in Sprague-Dawley rats by 7,12-dimethylbenz(a)anthracene, *J Natl Cancer Inst.* 66:517 (1981).

51. C.F. Aylsworth, D.A. Van Vergt, P.W. Sylvester and J. Meites, Failure of high dietary fat to influence serum prolactin levels during the estrous cycle in female Sprague-Dawley rats, *Proc Soc Exp Biol and Med.* 175:25 (1984).

52. W.T. Cave, J.T. Dunn and R.M. Macleod, Effect of iodine deficiency and high-fat diet on N-nitrosomethylurea-induced mammary cancer in rats, *Cancer Res.* 39:729 (1979).

53. P.C. Chan, J.F. Head, L.A. Cohen and E.L. Wynder, Influence of dietary fat on induction of mammary tumors by N-nitrosomethylurea associated hormone changes and differences between Sprague-Dawley and F344 rats, *J Natl Cancer Inst.* 59:1279 (1977).

54. C. Ip and M.M. Ip, Serum estrogen and estrogen responsiveness in 7,12-dimethybenz(a)anthracene-induced mammary tumors as influenced by dietary fat, *J Natl Cancer Inst.* 66:291 (1981).

55. R.E. Frisch, D.M. Hegsted, and K. Yoshinaga, Body weight and food intake as early status of rats on high fat diet, *Proc Natl Acad Sci.* 72:4172 (1975).

56. M.M. King, D.M. Bailey, D.D. Gibson, J.V. Pitha, and P.B. McCay, Incidence and growth of mammary tumors induced by 7,12-dimethylbenz(a)anthracene as related to the dietary content of fat and antioxidant, *J Natl Cancer Inst.* 63:657 (1979).

57. W.C. Wetsel, A.E. Rogers, A. Rutledge, and W.W. Leavitt, Absence of an effect of dietary corn oil content on plasma prolactin progesterone and 17 ß-estradiol in female Sprague-Dawley rats, *Cancer Res.* 44:1420 (1984).

58. T.L. Dao, Metabolism of estrogens in breast cancer, *Biochemica et Biophysica Acta.* 560:397 (1979).

59. P.K. Suter, G.L. Hammond, and J.A. Nicker, Increased availability of serum estrogens in breast cancer: a new hypothesis, *in*: "Banberry Report: Hormones and Breast Cancer," M.C. Pike, P.K. Siiteri, and C.W. Welsch, eds., Cold Spring Harbor Laboratories, New York (1981).

60. M.S. Langley, G. L. Hammond, A. Bardsley, R.A. Sellwood, and D.C. Anderson, Serum steroid binding protein and the bioavailability of estradiol in relation to heart diseases, *J Natl Cancer Inst.* 75:823 (1985).

61. P.F. Brining, J.M.G. Bonfrer, and A.A.M. Hart, Non-protein bond estradiol, sex hormone binding globulin, breast cancer and breast cancer risk, *Brit J Cancer.* 51:479 (1985).

62. J.W. Moore, G.M.G. Clark, and R.D. Bulbrook, Serum concentrations of total and non-protein bound estradiol in patients with breast cancer and in normal controls, *Int J Cancer.* 29:17 (1982).

63. B.K. Armstrong, J.B. Brown, and H.T. Clark, Diet and reproductive hormones: a study of vegetarian and nonvegetarian postmenopausal women, *J Natl Cancer Inst.* 67:761 (1981).

64. T.D. Schultz and J.E. Leklem, Nutrient intake and hormonal status of premenopausal vegetarian Seventh-Day Adventists and premenopausal non-vegetarians, *Nutr Cancer.* 4:247 (1983).

65. B.R. Goldin, H. Adlercreutz, and S.L. Gorbach, Estrogen excretion patterns and plasma levels in vegetarians and omnivorous women, *N Engl J Med.* 307:1524 (1982).

66. D.P. Rose, A.P. Boyon, C. Cohen, and L.E. Strong, Effect of a low-fat diet on hormone levels in women with cystic-heart disease, serum steroids and gonadotrophins, *J Natl Cancer Inst.* 78:623 (1987).

67. B.R. Goldin, H. Adlercruetz, S.L. Gorbach, *et al.*, The relationship between estrogen levels and diets of caucasian americans and oriental immigrant women, *Am J Clin Nutr.* 44:945 (1986).

68. F. De Waard, E.A. Baanders-Van Halewign, and J. Hiriginga, The biomodal age distribution of patients with mammary carcinoma, *Cancer.* 7:141 (1964).

69. F. De Waard and E.A. Baanders-Van Halewign, A prospective study in general practice on breast cancer risk in postmenopausal women, *Inst J Cancer.* 14:153 (1974).

70. F. De Waard, J. Portman, and B.J.A. Collette, Relationship of weight to the promotion of breast cancer after menopause, *Nutr Cancer.* 2:237 (1981).

71. A.P. Misra, P. Cole, and B. MacMahon, Breast cancer in an area of high parity: Sao Paulo, Brazil, *Cancer Res.* 31:77 (1971).

72. V.G. Valaoras, B. MacMahon, and B. Trichopaulos, Location and reproductive histories of breast cancer patients in greater Athens, *Int J Cancer.* 4:350 (1969).

73. M.O. Admi, A. Rimstein, and R. Stenquist, Influence of height, weight and obesity on risk of breast cancer in unselected Swedish population, *Brit J Cancer.* 36:787 (1977).

74. E.L. Wynder, F.A. MacCormak, and S.D. Stellman, The epidemiology of breast cancer in 785 United States caucasian women, *Cancer.* 41:2341 (1978).

75. K. Stavraky and S. Emmons, Breast cancer in premenopausal and postmenopausal women, *J Natl Cancer Inst.* 853:647 (1974).

76. D.V. Schapira, N.B. Kumar, G.H. Lyman, and C.E. Cox, Abdominal obesity and breast cancer risk, *Annals Int Med.* 114:182 (1990).

77. L. Ballard-Barbash, A. Schatzkin, and C.L. Carlos, Body fat distribution and breast cancer in the Framingham study, *J Natl Cancer Inst.* 82:286 (1990).

78. J.P. Deslypene, L. Verdonck, and A. Vermeulen, Fat tissue: a steroid reservoir and site of steroid metabolism, *J Clin Sadocrin Metab.* 61:564 (1985).

79. P. De Moor and J.V. Joossen, An inverse relationship between body weight and the activity of the steroid binding ß globulin in human plasma, *Steroidologia.* 1:129 (1970).

80. D.V. Schapira, R.D. Kumar, and G.H. Lyman, Obesity, body fat distribution and sex hormones in breast cancer patients, *Cancer*. 67:2215 (1991).

81. W.T. Cave, Jr. and M.J. Erickson-Lucas, Effects of dietary lipids on lactogenic hormone binding in rat mammary tumors, *J Natl Cancer Inst*. 68:319 (1982).

82. R. Hilf, The actions of insulin as a hormonal factor in breast cancer, *Banbury Rep*. 8:317 (1988).

83. B.H. Ginsburg, T.J. Brown, S. Ido and A.A. Spector, Effect of membrane lipid environment on the properties of insulin receptors, *Diabetes*. 30:773 (1981).

84. C. Grunfeld, K.L. Baird and C.R. Kahn, Maintenance of 3T3-L1 cells in culture media containing saturated fatty acids decreases insulin binding and insulin action, *Biochem Biophys Res Commun*. 103:219 (1981).

85. C. Ip, H.M. Tepperman, P. Holohan, and J. Tepperman, The effect of diet fat on rat adipocyte glucose transport, *Metabol Res*. 9:218 (1977).

86. J.V. Sun, H.M. Tepperman, and J. Tepperman, A comparison of insulin binding by liver plasma membranes of rats fed a high glucose diet or a high fat diet, *J Lipid Res*. 118:533 (1977).

87. J.M. Feldman and R. Hilf, A role of estrogens and insulin binding in the dietary lipid alteration of R3233OAC mammary carcinoma growth in rats, *Cancer Res*. 45:1964 (1985).

88. S. Hendrich, S.K. Krueger, H.W. Chen, and L. Cook, Phenobarbital increases rat hepatic prostaglandin $F_{2\alpha}$ glutathione S-transferase activity and oxidative stress, *Prostagl Leukotri Essen Fatty Acids*. 42:45 (1991).

89. G. Furstenburger, M. Gross and F. Marks, Eicosanoids and multistage carcinogenesis in NMRI mouse skin: role of prostaglandin E and F in conversion (first stage of tumor promotion) and promotion (second stage of tumor promotion), *Carcinogenesis*. 10:91 (1989).

90. J. Dupont, Essential fatty acids and prostaglandins, *Prev Med*. 16:485 (1987).

Chapter 18

Selected Recent Studies of Exercise, Energy Metabolism, Body Weight, and Blood Lipids Relevant to Interpretation and Design of Studies of Exercise and Cancer

ADRIANNE E. ROGERS

I. Introduction

The elucidation of the relationship between intake of calories, particularly from fat, and tumorigenesis in humans or animal models requires investigation of the other side of the energy equation, namely utilization of calories. The intake and utilization of dietary energy sources are governed by many exogenous and endogenous factors, any one or any grouping of which might influence cancer induction and development. Review of the chapters on metabolism of fats, carbohydrates, and energy and of the metabolic charts provided in a recent textbook[1] gives a well-balanced picture of the myriad aspects to be considered. Asking questions about the interactions between energy supply and utilization in exercise adds further complexity, as may be discerned from reading the literature on exercise and plasma lipids in humans. Moving from studies in human subjects to studies in animal models, which must be done to develop definitive data on many aspects of carcinogenesis, imposes a further layer of uncertainty and a clear need to standardize methods and to model as closely as possible human experience and responses.

It is clear from studies in laboratory rodents that tumorigenesis is reduced by restriction of caloric intake to levels at which the animals gain weight less rapidly than controls fed *ad libitum*. It is equally clear from studies in rodents that provision of plentiful calories as fat, particularly as triglycerides containing large amounts of N-6 polyunsaturated fatty acids, is a powerful stimulus to development of mammary gland tumors, and, under some experimental conditions, of tumor development at several other sites. In most studies, the excessive intake of fat yields a consistent, if small, increase in weight gain compared to controls (Welsch, this volume). In examination of either restricted or excessive intake, measurement

Adrianne E. Rogers ● Department of Pathology, Boston University School of Medicine and the Mallory Institute of Pathology, Boston City Hospital, 80 East Concord Street, Boston, Massachusetts

Exercise, Calories, Fat, and Cancer, Edited by M.M. Jacobs
Plenum Press, New York, 1992

or manipulation of caloric utilization has not been included in the experimental protocols. In recent studies in which increased caloric utilization through exercise has been investigated, the effects on tumorigenesis have not been consistent. This inconsistency is evident even when the studies have been performed in the tumor models that generally are the most responsive to both fat and caloric effects, such as chemically induced mammary tumors in rats (Thompson, Cohen *et al.* this volume). The development of better methods to manipulate and measure caloric utilization and to model the intensity, duration and physiologic effects of human physical activity is important in the pursuit of such studies. Hypotheses may be generated and methods may be gathered from experience in research into other multifactorial, nutrition-related diseases, including obesity and atherosclerotic cardiovascular disease. A small sample of recent studies in areas related to the two subjects is discussed.

II. Factors that Influence Intake and Utilization of Calories

A. Diet Composition

Laboratory rodents generally govern dietary intake to maintain caloric balance when provided nutritionally complete diets that vary in the macronutrient sources of calories, but they may over-consume calories when fed diets high in fat.[2-5] They respond to specific nutrient deficiency, however, by over- or under-consumption of diet with respect to calories, the response depending upon the nature and extent of nutrient deficiency encountered. Protein-deficient diets tend to be ingested in greater than expected amounts, but not well-utilized for growth, and vitamin- or mineral-deficient diets in less than expected amounts.

In post-pubertal (9- to 10-week-old) male Sprague-Dawley (S-D)[6] or Fischer 344[7] rats fed isoenergetic diets containing 2-25%[6] or 4-20%[7] high-quality protein (by weight) for 6-10 weeks, body weight gain increased with increasing protein in the diet up to a point between 8 and 15%, but feed consumption per 100 g body weight was increased at the lowest levels of dietary protein; feed efficiency, therefore, was decreased compared to rats fed higher levels of protein. Body morphometrics and composition[6] and liver weight[7] indicated little effect of protein levels of 4% or greater on lean body mass, but indicated that the increase in body weight with higher protein intakes was the result of greater body-fat deposition. Indices of thermogenesis were increased by low-protein diets,[7] as expected from earlier, more detailed studies of diet-induced thermogenesis in weanling male S-D rats fed low-protein diets.[7,8] Diet-induced thermogenesis (DIT) is the increase over resting metabolic rate (RMR) that follows food intake and is the result of the energy cost of absorbing, digesting and metabolizing the food[1]; it increases in rats that increase diet (caloric) intake in response to low dietary protein, regardless of whether the major source of calories in the diet is fat or carbohydrate (CHO).[8] DIT is lower for fat than for CHO, evidence of the efficient utilization of fat calories.[1]

Harris and Jones[2] have published recently a nutritional study relevant to designing studies of and hypothesizing about relationships between dietary calories, fat, caloric balance and mammary cancer in rats. They studied 250-g female S-D rats fed diets that varied widely in fat type and amount; in some diets a textured protein was substituted for some of the fat. They found that ingestion of the highest fat diet containing 10% corn oil and 30% Crisco® was not well controlled and that rats fed it ate and gained more than rats fed a control, 10% corn oil diet. The increased weight gain was accounted for by increased body fat and associated with development of hyperinsulinemia and increased hepatic fatty acid metabolism. Substitution of textured protein for half of the Crisco® (by weight) did not correct the over-consumption of calories or the weight gain but did reduce serum insulin and return hepatic fatty acid metabolism to the normal range. The fat-substituted diet did not differ appreciably from the control diet in caloric density and nutrient/calorie ratios and offers a potential new model for exploration of relationships between fat, calories, and mammary cancer if the diet designs can be further modified to be consistent in nutrient supply and fat type.

The contribution or significance of the source of excess calories to weight gain in adult animals and humans is a subject of great interest and controversy and is highly relevant to consideration of fat calories, exercise, and cancer. In adult (4- to 9-month-old) female CD-1 mice fed, in a cross-over experiment, nutritionally and calorically balanced diets that provided either 13 or 45% of energy as mixed fats, weight gain was increased by the higher fat diet and was composed approximately 60% of fat and 40% of lean body mass.[3] The mice had access to running wheels, and their energy balance and CHO and fat oxidation were monitored over 160 days. The results showed that oxidation of fat was governed by the energy gap between total energy expenditure and energy available from CHO and protein, regardless of the fat content of the diet. CHO oxidation was governed primarily by CHO intake, again independently of the fat in the diet. Because of the relatively tighter balance on CHO than on fat oxidation the author concluded, and reviewed work of others who have concluded, that energy balance is more readily maintained by both humans and laboratory rodents if the diet is relatively low in fat. He concluded also from his and others' earlier studies that sustained exercise that increases fat oxidation should help limit or reverse development of obesity independently of diet composition.[9]

B. Physical Activity

Physical activity, of course, influences calorie utilization and is a major determinant of fat oxidation. There are broad variations in energy utilization in response to physical activity that contribute to variability of the data in studies of energy balance and exercise. Poehlman et al.[10] reviewed many recent studies of effects of exercise, with or without diet restriction, on RMR in people ranging from athletes in training to over-weight subjects. They were interested in the questions of whether exercise influences RMR or general energy expenditure outside exercise time. The question of a prolonged effect of exercise on metabolic rate is a major one in evaluating the influence of exercise on weight control and has been extensively investigated. The results are relevant to hypotheses about exercise and caloric effects on cancer and to design of studies in humans or animals. Poehlman et al.[10] concluded that exercise intensity and duration, as well as post-exercise eating or fasting, determined the presence and magnitude of elevation of the post-exercise metabolic rate. The increase in energy utilization was very small (9-30 kcal) for any but the most intense and prolonged exercise. There appeared to be no difference in response between men and women in the studies they cited. In their own studies they found that the RMR was about 11% greater in highly aerobically trained men than in less highly trained men, but there was no consensus on this question in the literature, and subjects' responses were highly variable.

In an evaluation of the influence of exercise on energy expenditure in other physical activity, Poehlman et al.[10] found very few studies and proposed that more be done using doubly-labeled water to measure total daily energy expenditure. From studies reported in rats, they concluded that forced treadmill exercise resulted in lower spontaneous activity and over-all lower daily energy expenditure, observations that emphasize the need for measurement of all activity rather than just exercise activity. In contrast from two studies reported in humans, they concluded that nonexercise physical activity and energy expenditure may increase with increased exercise. In studies without diet restriction, participation in moderate to strenuous exercise had no effect on body weight or fat but raised the RMR slightly in some cases. In studies that included diet restriction, there was not a consistent pattern of difference in weight loss or RMR induced by exercise. In many studies the RMR decreased with weight loss, as is expected in nonexercising subjects, although in some, exercising appeared to prevent the decrease in RMR and to preserve fat-free weight. Weight loss was generally not increased by addition of exercise to a restricted diet regimen, but some investigators reported relatively greater loss of body fat with exercise.

Poehlman et al.[10] raised several interesting questions about the results that should be considered in design of studies of exercise physiology and are applicable to studies of exercise and cancer. They pointed out the heterogeneous metabolic responses of people to diet and exercise, the need for standardized exercise and diet programs, and the need to measure the actual energy deficit induced by the program. In addition they suggested that the energy deficit conditions might be different between dieters and dieters plus exercisers.

In recently published studies of relationships among physical activity, body composition and energy utilization, primarily in pre-menopausal women, it has been found that:

1. The sleeping metabolic index (sleeping metabolic rate/basal metabolic rate [BMR]) is positively and significantly ($P < 0.001$) correlated with the physical activity index (calculated from the average daily metabolic rate, measured using doubly-labeled water over a 7-14 day period, and the BMR). The result was not dependent upon body mass (Quetelet) index and extended over a range from under- to over-weight.[11] This is an example of the type of study suggested by Poehlman et al.[10] for application to studies of exercise effects.

2. Introduction of a moderate 12-week exercise program that gave a 5-14% increase in maximum aerobic capacity (VO_2 max) in subjects of normal weight who did not previously exercise regularly led to a statistically significant reduction in body fat, a modest, not significant, reduction in body weight, and a significant increase in diet intake.[12]

3. In moderately over-weight women assigned to an approximately 25% reduced-calorie diet that provided 30% of energy as fat and a regimen of moderate exercise, the body weight and body fat decreased to greater extent, but not significantly so, than in women assigned to the dietary change only. Calorie and fat intakes decreased to the same extent, in both groups. In contrast, men who were assigned to the exercise plus diet group and who showed no greater training effect on aerobic capacity than the exercising women, had significantly greater loss of body weight and body fat than their diet-only controls. Their caloric intake decreased somewhat, but not significantly, and fat intake decreased significantly more than in the diet-only controls.[13]

4. In moderately over-weight women given a moderate exercise program for 3 months with no required dietary change, caloric intake and body fat decreased significantly, and lean body mass increased significantly. In a second group, also somewhat over-weight but with lower weight and body fat than the first group, neither caloric intake, weight, nor body fat decreased significantly despite development of evidence of a similar training effect. Exercising men in the same program lost both weight and body fat with no change in caloric intake.[14]

5. In chronically trained and periodically highly trained women athletes studied by Snow et al.,[15] body weight and body fat decreased in the periods of heavy training and increased upon return to a lower level of training; information on changes in dietary intake was not given.

It is obvious from the results of these studies of exercise, diet, and body weight and from many earlier studies that caloric balance is not easily calculated, measured, or predicted. Standardized protocols are needed for study of interactions of diet, exercise, and body weight and composition and, certainly, for extension of such studies to look for relationships to cancer.

The suggestion of male-female differences is present in the results cited. There are many sex-specific and site-specific differences in adipose tissue metabolism and in its response to hormones and to changes in calorie supply as reviewed in Liebel *et al.*[16]

Genetics influences the physiologic effects of exercise as demonstrated by Fagard *et al.*[17] in studies of peak O_2 uptake and aerobic power in young men who were monozygotic or dizygotic twins. Anthropometric differences and differences in extent of current exercise practice also had significant influences on the exercise parameters measured.

III. Exercise and Blood Lipids

The literature on effects of exercise on blood lipids provides information on which it may be possible to develop hypotheses useful in investigating exercise-dietary fat-cancer interactions and evidence, again, of the need to standardize methods. Haskell[18] reviewed effects of exercise on blood lipids, noting that a number of factors interact to determine the levels and types of plasma lipoproteins. They include genetics, age, body composition, diet and alcohol, and tobacco use. From the studies reviewed, he concluded that total cholesterol content of plasma showed no consistent response to exercise across all studies, but a decrease was more likely to occur if the exercise program was vigorous and of extended duration. Total plasma triglycerides (TG) were more consistently reported to be reduced compared to sedentary controls in endurance athletes than in less vigorously exercising subjects and not to rise with age as is found in less active subjects. There was an acute decrease in plasma TG immediately following exercise, much more marked in hypertriglyceridemic than in normal men, in whom little or no decrease may occur, and unrelated to changes in weight or diet in subjects engaged in ongoing exercise programs.

Low-density lipoprotein cholesterol (LDL-C) tended to be somewhat reduced and high-density lipoprotein cholesterol (HDL_2-C) somewhat increased in both male and female long-distance runners compared to sedentary controls or less vigorously exercising subjects. HDL-C was increased by 20-35%. Reductions of 8-12% in LDL-C were reported as a result of training in previously sedentary men, particularly if they lost weight. There were generally no correlations between LDL-C and regular, habitual exercise, but HDL-C was generally increased in association with even moderate, regular physical activity in men and, less consistently, in women. In cases in which total cholesterol decreased with exercise or in which HDL-C was high before exercise, HDL-C decreased rather than increased with exercise.

Haskell summarized his review by saying that serum TG tended to respond, if at all, acutely to exercise and that plasma total cholesterol was more likely to respond to a prolonged period of increased activity, particularly to endurance exercise than to lower levels of exercise, a conclusion similar to the conclusions discussed above of the need for vigorous exercise to demonstrate any effect on RMR.[18]

Recently published studies of exercise effects on blood lipids in males include the following. Wallace *et al.*[19] studied the acute response of blood lipids in healthy young men performing resistance exercise, a form of exercise studied less extensively and, when studied, found to have little consistent influence on blood lipids in studies reviewed by Haskell.[18] Wallace *et al.*[19] found a significant increase in plasma HDL_3-C but not HDL_2-C and a significant decrease in plasma TG 24 hours after high-volume but not after low-volume resistance exercise performed in a fasting state. The high-volume exercise was equivalent in energy expenditure to endurance exercise known to alter plasma lipoproteins. The authors presented a useful discussion of factors that should be measured or controlled since they can influence the results of such studies. The factors include the exercise-induced decrease in plasma volume, the total energy expenditure in the exercise period, diet, fed or fasting state, use of alcohol, tobacco, or steroid hormones, composition of plasma lipids prior to exercise, the exercise protocols, and the subjects' state of fitness.

Mendoza *et al.*[20] studied the effects of exercise therapy in men aged 27-44 at periods of 2-10 months after they had suffered a myocardial infarction. They reported that plasma HDL-C increased an average of 23% and mean apo-A_2 increased 19%. Mean LDL-C decreased an average of 13%, and, interestingly, serum estradiol decreased nearly 50% after 3 months. Since plasma content of hepatic lipoprotein lipase decreased significantly, they postulated that the increased HDL-C might be, in part, the result of reduced breakdown rather than increased formation. Their subjects, who were Venezuelan and living and exercising at an altitude of 5400 feet, showed a significant training effect and did not lose weight. They had, in fact, been instructed not to lose weight and were given no dietary therapy.

A group of healthy Japanese, male, 40- to 61-year-old, factory employees were studied for a relationship between habitual exercise and blood lipids. The results were similar to results in Western males, in that habitual, vigorous, endurance exercise was associated with increased HDL-C; however, the results were confounded by the lower incidence of smoking in the vigorous exercisers compared to men with lower levels of exercise and sedentary men. Alcohol intake was positively correlated with HDL-C in all activity groups.[21]

IV. Endocrine Responses to Exercise

Endocrine effects of exercise have been postulated to underlie relationships between exercise and cancer, in general with respect to immunologic influences on cancer and in particular in women with respect to breast cancer (Frisch, this volume and Reference 22). Endocrine responses to exercise include activation of the sympathetic-adrenal medullary system and of the hypothalamic-adrenal cortical system, as well as activation of glucagon, all of which have major effects upon energy metabolism. Responses to training, conditioned in part by decreased body fat, include also increased insulin sensitivity of tissues.[1,23] The magnitude of the endocrine changes appears to be governed by the relative exercise intensity (percent of maximal aerobic capacity) rather than by the absolute intensity and is, therefore, responsive to training.[23]

An acute reduction following exercise in immunologic responses of lymphocytes has been reported in many studies and is thought to be related to increased blood cortisol induced by exercise.[24] In a study of healthy young men of different levels of fitness, resting plasma cortisol was significantly increased in the least fit group compared to all others, but all groups showed an increase with endurance exercise.

V. Conclusion

Data from these and other studies of responses to exercise in normal and abnormal subjects are needed to begin to understand the role of caloric balance or, perhaps, caloric flux in carcinogenesis, to evaluate fully the contribution of dietary fat to carcinogenesis, and to design studies to determine whether exercise is a factor in carcinogenesis.

References

1. M.C. Linder, "Nutritional Biochemistry and Metabolism with Clinical Applications," Elsevier, N.Y. (1991).
2. R.B.S. Harris and W.K. Jones, Physiological response of mature rats to replacement of dietary fat with a fat substitute, *J Nutr.* 121:1109 (1991).
3. J.P. Flatt, Assessment of daily and cumulative carbohydrate and fat balances in mice, *J Nutr Biochem.* 2:193 (1991).

4. R.B.S. Harris, Growth measurements in Sprague-Dawley rats fed diets of very low fat concentration, *J Nutr.* 121:1075 (1991).

5. M.L. Fernandez and D.J. McNamara, Regulation of cholesterol and lipoprotein metabolism in guinea pigs mediated by dietary fat quality and quantity, *J Nutr.* 121:934 (1991).

6. P. Donald, G.C. Pitts, and S.L. Pohl, Body weight and composition in laboratory rats: effects of diets with high or low protein concentrations, *Science.* 211:185 (1981).

7. F. Horio, L.D. Youngman, R.C. Bell, and T.C. Campbell, Thermogenesis, low-protein diets, and decreased development of AFB_1-induced preneoplastic foci in rat liver, *Nutr Cancer.* 16:31 (1991).

8. N.J. Rothwell and M.J. Stock, Influence of carbohydrate and fat intake on diet-induced thermogenesis and brown fat activity in rats fed low protein diets, *J Nutr.* 117:1721 (1987).

9. J.P. Flatt, Opposite effects of variation in food intake on carbohydrate and fat oxidation in *ad libitum* fed mice, *J Nutr Biochem.* 2:186 (1991).

10. E.T. Poehlman, C.L. Melby, and M.I. Goran, The impact of exercise and diet restriction on daily energy expenditure, *Sports Medicine.* 11:78 (1991).

11. K.R. Westerterp, G.A.L. Meijer, W.H.M. Saris, P.B. Soeters, Y. Winants, and F. Ten Hoor, Physical activity and sleeping metabolic rate, *Med Sci Sports Exerc.* 23:166 (1991).

12. C.A. Jensen, C.M. Weaver, and D.A. Sedlock, Iron supplementation and iron status in exercising young women, *J. Nutr Biochem.* 2:368 (1991).

13. P.D. Wood, M.L. Stefanick, P.T. Williams, and W.L. Haskell, The effects on plasma lipoproteins of a prudent weight-reducing diet, with or without exercise, in overweight men and women, *N Engl J Med.* 325:461 (1991).

14. B. Andersson, X. Xuefan, M. Rebuffe-Scrive, K. Terning, M. Krotkiewski, and P. Bjorntorp, The effects of exercise training on body composition and metabolism in men and women, *International Journal of Obesity.* 15:75 (1990).

15. R.C. Snow, R.L. Barbieri, and R.E. Frisch, Estrogen 2-hydroxylase oxidation and menstrual function among elite oarswomen, *J Clin Endocrinol Metabl.* 69:369 (1989).

16. R.L. Leibel, N.K. Edens, and S.K. Fried, Physiologic basis for the control of body fat distribution in humans, *Annual Review of Nutrition.* 9:417 (1989).

17. R. Fagard, E. Bielen, and A. Amery, Heritability of aerobic power and anaerobic energy generation during exercise, *J Appl Physiol.* 70:357 (1991).

18. W.L. Haskell, The influence of exercise on the concentrations of triglyceride and cholesterol in human plasma, *Exerc Sport Sci Rev.* 12:205 (1984).

19. M.B. Wallace, R.J. Moffatt, E.M. Haymes, and N.R. Green, Acute effects of resistance exercise on parameters of lipoprotein metabolism, *Med Sci Sports Exerc.* 23:199 (1991).

20. S.G. Mendoza, H. Carrasco, A. Zerpa, F. Briceno, B.F. Rodriguez, J. Speirs, and C.J. Glueck, Effect of physical training on lipids, lipoproteins, apolipoproteins, lipases, and endogenous sex hormones in men with premature myocardial infarction, *Metabolism.* 40:368 (1991).

21. H. Koyama, M. Ogawa, and S. Suzuki, Relationship between total cholesterol and high-density lipoprotein cholesterol and the effects of physical exercise, alcohol consumption, cigarette smoking and body mass index, *J Nutr Sci Vitaminol.* 36:377 (1990).

22. R.E. Frisch, G. Wyshak, N.L. Albright, I. Schiff, K.P. Jones, J. Witschi, E. Shiang, E. Koff, and M. Marguglio, Lower prevalence of breast cancer and cancers of the reproductive system among former college athletes compared to non-athletes, *Br J Cancer.* 52:885 (1985).

23. P.A. Deuster, G.P. Chrousos, A. Luger, J.E. DeBolt, L.L. Bernier, U.H. Trostmann, S.B. Kyle, L.C. Montgomery, and D.L. Loriaux, Hormonal and metabolic responses of untrained, moderately trained, and highly trained men to three exercise intensitites, *Metabolism.* 38:141 (1989).

24. B. MacNeil, L. Hoffman-Goetz, A. Kendall, M. Houston, and Y. Arumugam, Lymphocyte proliferation responses after exercise in men: fitness, intensity, and duration effects *J Appl Physiol.* 70:179 (1991).

Poster Abstracts

Modulation of Nitrosamine Mutagenicity and DNA Alkylation by High-Fat Diets

T. LAWSON

Eppley Institute for Research in Cancer,
University of Nebraska Medical Center, Omaha, NE

Dietary fat is implicated in human cancer etiology and enhances the carcinogenicity of many chemicals including N-nitrosobis(2-oxopropyl)amine (BOP) in the hamster pancreas. High-fat diets (HFD) did not enhance BOP carcinogenicity when given with it, suggesting that HFD's role was on the development/promotion phase of carcinogenesis. This suggestion appears to be a facet of the carcinogens used rather than of HFD action. Hepatocytes from hamsters fed HFD were used to activate N-nitrosobis(2-hydroxypropyl)amine (BHP) and BOP in the V79 mutagenicity assay. BHP mutagenicity increased five-fold whereas that of BOP by less than two-fold. O^6 methylguanine in DNA from these cells trebled when BHP was the alkylating agent but also increased **four-fold** when BOP was the alkylating agent. The increase in BHP mutagenicity was due to an increase in cytochrome P-45OIVA2 activity, which stimulates the conversion of BHP to BOP. BOP is α-hydroxylated and breaks down to produce a methylating agent. Similar increases in BHP mutagenicity were seen when pancreas acinar and duct tissue homogenates from HFD-fed hamsters were used as the activating system. HFD stimulated this activity more in acinar cells than in duct tissue suggesting a role for them in the activation of nitrosamines containing a β-hydroxyl group, such as BHP. These data show that the initiation phase of carcinogenesis can be affected by feeding HFD and suggest that HFD's role in carcinogenesis has been underestimated.

Supported by the American Institute for Cancer Research grant 90A11, National Cancer Institute Core grant CA36727, and American Cancer Society grant SIG 16.

The Effects of Beta-Alanyl-Melphalan in Mouse Liver Cells and Mouse Ehrlich Ascites Tumor Cells

B-L. TSAY and L. WOLFINBARGER, JR.

Center for Biotechnology, Department of Biological Sciences, Old Dominion University, Norfolk, VA

The targeting of proven anti-cancer drugs specially to cancer cells would provide a unique opportunity to restrict neoplasms without damaging the cancer patient. The present research utilizes the phenomenon of illicit transport, i.e., the coupling of normally impermeant metabolites to permeant metabolites, in targeting the drug melphalan to mouse Ehrlich ascites tumor cells. The dipeptide beta-alanyl-melphalan was synthesized and tested *in vitro* for potential toxicity toward mouse Ehrlich ascites tumor cells, mouse liver cells, and mouse 3T3 embryonic cells. Toxicity of this dipeptide towards these cell lines was compared to toxicity of melphalan. Melphalan was shown to be toxic to all three cell systems studied, whereas beta-alanyl-melphalan was toxic only towards the mouse Ehrlich ascites tumor cells and mouse 3T3 embryonic cells. *In vivo* chemotherapy assays, using mouse Ehrlich ascites tumor cells injected into the abdominal cavity of mice, revealed that melphalan, at concentrations of 5 and 10 mg/kg, was an effective anti-cancer drug providing for T/C ratios of 179 and 193, respectively. The dipeptide, beta-alanyl-melphalan, was also an effective anti-cancer drug, exhibiting reduced toxicity towards the tumor-bearing animal when compared to the parent drug melphalan, providing for T/C ratios of 152 at a drug concentration of 40mg/kg.

Differential Effects of Dietary Fat on Skin and Mammary Carcinogenesis

M. LOCNISKAR,[1] R.E. MALDVE,[2] D.H. BECHTEL[3] and S.M. FISCHER[2]

[1]University of Texas at Austin, Division of Nutrition, Austin, TX;
[2]University of Texas, M.D. Anderson Cancer Center, Science Park,
Smithville, TX; and [3]Best Foods, Inc., Union, NJ

Evidence has demonstrated that high levels of dietary corn oil, rich in the polyunsaturated fatty acid linoleic acid (LA), are associated with a greater tumor incidence in the chemically induced rat mammary and pancreas models. We hypothesized that an increase in consumption of linoleic acid would also result in an enhancement in skin tumor development when fed during the tumor promotion stage of the mouse skin initiation-promotion model. The effects of seven different levels of dietary LA, supplied as corn oil in a 15% fat diet, on the incidence and rate of skin papilloma and carcinoma development were determined. Female SENCAR mice were placed on one of the experimental diets, containing 0.8%, 2.2%, 3.5%, 4.5%, 5.6%, 7.0%, or 8.4% LA, 1 week after initiation with 7,12-dimethylbenz[a]anthracene (DMBA) and 3 weeks prior to beginning twice weekly promotion with 12-O-tetradecanoylphorbol-13-acetate (TPA). At 15 weeks of TPA treatment there were significant differences in papilloma number among the diet groups such that an inverse correlation (r=0.92) was observed between tumor number and level of LA. The 0.8% LA diet group had an average of 11.7 tumors/mouse while the 8.4% LA group had 5.4 tumors/ mouse. However, there was no significant difference in papilloma incidence among the diet groups. In addition, the 8.4% LA diet group had the lowest carcinoma incidence supporting a relationship between diet and carcinoma incidence. To determine whether the unexpected inverse correlation between dietary LA and tumor yield in the skin model was due to species differences or organ model differences, a mammary carcinogenesis experiment was performed in the SENCAR mouse. Female SENCAR mice were maintained on one of three diets: 0.8%, 4.5%, and 8.4% LA, and the carcinogen DMBA was administered by intragastric gavage at 1 mg/week for 6 weeks. Mammary tumor data were calculated as percentage of mice bearing a histologically verified adenocarcinoma. A dose-dependent relationship between dietary LA and adenocarcinoma incidence was observed during tumor development such that the highest incidence was associated with the 8.4% LA diet. In conclusion, high levels of dietary LA inhibited skin tumor development, but enhanced mammary tumorigenesis in the SENCAR mouse. The observations from these studies suggest that the effect of dietary LA on tumor development is organ specific rather than species specific.

Supported by National Institutes of Health grant CA 46886, Best Foods, Inc., and the American Institute for Cancer Research grant 91A56.

Anti-Neoplastic Function of Dietary InsP$_6$

I. VUCENIK and A. M. SHAMSUDDIN

School of Medicine, University of Maryland at Baltimore,
Department of Medical and Research Technology,
Baltimore, MD

It has been recognized that dietary fiber or other substances may have a cancer protective effect. One of these active substances could be inositol hexaphosphate (InsP$_6$), a naturally occuring carbohydrate, contained in substantial amount in cereal and legume products. Lower phosphorylated forms of inositol (Ins) are believed to play important roles in cellular signal transduction, regulating the cell growth and differentiation. Recent *in vivo* and *in vitro* studies in our laboratory have demonstrated novel anti-neoplastic properties of InsP$_6$. Its chemopreventive properties were demonstrated in experimental models of colon cancer in both rats and mice. It has been shown to exert an anti-tumor effect on murine transplantable and metastatic fibrosarcoma models. On a human cancer cell line it exibited growth inhibition and increased differentiation. It has also been observed that Ins potentiates the action of InsP$_6$. After long-term administration of InsP$_6$, we did not find any significant difference in body weight, and in serum Mg^{2+}, Zn^{2+}, Ca^{2+}, Fe^{2+} levels of animals between InsP$_6$ treatment and tap water control. Since InsP$_6$ and Ins are virtually nontoxic and are natural compounds, we believe that InsP$_6$+Ins may have great potential as chemopreventive and adjuvant chemotherapeutic agent.

Supported by the American Institute for Cancer Research grant 87B46 (A.M.S.) and 915G04 (I.V.).

Role of Lipotrope-Modified Diets in Mammary Gene Expression

C.B. CHOI, W. KELLER and C.S. PARK

North Dakota State University, Fargo, ND

Evidence indicates that lipotrope-deficient diets induce and enhance hepatocellular carcinogenesis. However, in lipotrope-deficient rats, the supplementation of lipotropes decreases the incidence of hepatocarcinomas. Although the majority of reports on lipotrope-modified diets focus on liver abnormalities, lipotrope deficiency affects almost every organ in the body, particularly when animals are in a state of high metabolic activity and growth. This study was conducted to provide information on the potential use of lipotrope-modified (deficient or supplemented) diets on the prevention of breast cancer. The specific aim was to examine the changes in DNA methylation and the expression of cellular protooncogenes and ornithine decarboxylase (ODC) activity in mammary tissue of rats fed lipotrope-modified diets. Female Sprague-Dawley rats (8-weeks-old) were fed for 3 weeks on one of three diets: control-synthetic diet (CSD); methyl-deficient diet, lacking choline, methionine, folic acid, and vitamin B_{12} (MDD); or methyl-additive diet (MAD) supplemented with twice the amount of each lipotrope as in CSD. There was no significant difference in 5-methylcytosine (5mC) levels among treatments in mammary tissues. The MDD group had 21- and 18-fold greater *v-fos* transcription than the control group in liver and mammary, respectively. The expression of *v-Ha-ras* oncogene in liver and mammary of the MAD group was increased by six- and nine-fold when compared to control. ODC activity in liver and mammary was higher in the MDD group compared to either the CSD group or the MAD group. This study suggests that lipotrope-deficient diets are related to cell proliferation and carcinogenesis in mammary tissue as well as in liver.

Supported by American Institute for Cancer Research grant 90SG13.

Synergistic Effect of the Combination of Glutathione and 5-Fluorouracil on the Cytotoxicity in HT29 Human Adenocarcinoma Cell Line

M.F. CHEN, L.T. CHEN and H.W. BOYCE, JR.

Departments of Internal Medicine and Anatomy,
University of South Florida College of Medicine, Tampa, FL

The cytotoxicity of many chemotherapeutic drugs has been shown to be affected by the intra-cellular concentration of reduced glutathione (GSH). GSH is the major intra-cellular nonprotein sulfhydryl in mammalian cells and its concentration has been shown to be affected by diet. In the present study, we investigated whether an increase in the intra-cellular GSH concentration can potentiate the cytotoxicity of 5-flourouracil (5-FU) in a human colon adenocarcinoma cell line, HT29. HT29 cells, obtained from the American Type Culture Collection, were cultured in RPMI 1640 medium containing fetal calf serum (10%), sodium bicarbonate (1 g/l), and gentamycin sulfate (50 mg/l) at 37°C, 5% CO_2, and 100% relative humidity. The effects of added GSH to the culture medium (30 mM final concentration) on the intra-cellular GSH level in HT29 cells were examined. GSH was added during the exponential phase of cell growth. The percentage of increase in intra-cellular GSH levels at various time intervals following the addition of GSH to the medium is as follows:

Time	0 min.	3 min.	½ hour	1 hour	5 hour	8 hour	22 hour
% Increase	0	9	23	40	62	65	59

The effects of various GSH concentrations in the culture medium for 8 hours on the intra-cellular GSH levels in HT29 cells are shown below:

GSH concentration	1.9 mM	3.8 mM	7.5 mM	15 mM	30 mM
% Increase	23	28	36	33	49

Various concentrations of GSH (1 to 50 mM, final concentration) and 5FU (0.5 to 50μM, final concentration) were added to the culture medium to determine whether GSH potentiates the toxicity of 5FU in HT29 cells. Several combinations of GSH and 5FU were tested. GSH was added before or after the addition of 5FU. 5FU was added on day 4 to HT29 cells in 96-well culture plates; day 0 being the day that the cells were seeded in the plates. The MTT (Tretrazolium) assay was used for measuring cytotoxicity. A multiple drug-effect analysis program was used to compute whether the different combinations of GSH/5FU were synergistic or antagonistic. GSH, in certain combinations, was synergistic with 5FU. In the presence of higher cellular GSH concentration, lower 5FU dosage was needed to achieve a given effect as compared to 5FU alone. Compounds that are known to raise intra-cellular GSH levels, such as N-acetyl-1-cysteine and 2-oxo-4-thiazolidinecarboxylic acid, were also found to be synergistic with 5FU. Buthionine sulfoximine, a specific inhibitor of GSH biosynthesis, however, was antagonistic. The results suggest that the toxicity of 5 FU in HT29 cells can be potentiated by higher intra-cellular GSH concentration.

Supported by the American Institute for Cancer Research grant 90SG22.

Tumorigenesis Inhibition by Isocaloric Alteration of the Dietary Arginine-Methionine Balance

R.M. MILLIS and C.A. DIYA

*Department of Physiology and Biophysics, College of Medicine and
Department of Human Nutrition, School of Human Ecology,
Howard University, Washington, DC*

Previous studies have shown that urinary polyamines may be indicative of tumorigenesis. Since dietary arginine and methionine are precursors for urinary polyamines, we hypothesized that isocaloric alteration of dietary arginine and methionine may inhibit tumor growth and suggest nutritional strategies for cancer treatment without caloric restriction. In a prior report, we showed that alteration of the normal dietary arginine-methionine balance decreased the weights of subcutaneously transplanted Morris hepatoma tumors. However, the essential sulfur-containing amino acid L-methionine is expensive to use as a dietary supplement, and has been reported to produce unacceptable flavors. Therefore, we designed this study to determine whether dietary replacement of L-methionine with N-acetyl-L-methionine (NALM) produces greater food intake and growth in rats without compromising the beneficial effects of altering the dietary arginine-methionine balance on tumorigenesis. Groups of healthy adult male host ACI rats (n=5-8, 250-300 g) were subjected to subcutaneous transplantation of viable Morris hepatoma inoculum from donor rats. Control groups were fed mixtures of amino acids in replacement of protein (22%) with carbohydrate (61%) and fat (10%) and with normal levels of minerals, fiber, and vitamins. Choline was decreased (0.2%) to ensure that it would not be used as a supplementary vitamin for methylation in animals fed methionine-deficient diets. Compared to the control diet, experimental diets were made up of combinations of deficiencies in arginine (-65%) or NALM (-50%) and excesses of arginine (+20%) or NALM (+24%). Animals were fed the diets and water *ad libitum*. Daily food intake and body weight were measured for 28 days, after which time tumors were excised and weighed. Statistical significance ($P<0.05$) of differences between controls and experimentals was analyzed using Duncan's multiple range test (SPSS). Results showed that (mean $\pm$SEM) daily food intake (6.23 ± 0.36 g to 7.70 ± 0.53 g) was unaffected by the experimental diets. The control group gained body weight (19.07 ± 1.93 g). Body weight increases of experimental groups were 18.36 ± 2.55 g to 26.67 ± 5.05 g. Tumor weight of controls was found to be $10.65 \pm 0.24\%$ of body weight. The experimental diets which produced significant decrements in tumor weight were: (1) the excess-arginine/NALM-deficient diet; and (2) the excess-arginine/NALM-normal diet. The group fed the deficient-arginine/NALM-deficient diet had significant increases in tumor weight. Compared to prior studies of the effects of altering the dietary arginine-methionine balance on tumor growth, food intakes, body weight gains and absolute tumor weights were significantly greater when NALM was substituted for L-methionine; however, the tumor weights expressed as percentages of body weights were similar. It is concluded that there is an association between inhibition of hepatoma growth and dietary alterations of both the arginine-methionine and the arginine-NALM balances. The increased body weight gains associated with dietary substitution of NALM for L-methionine suggests that NALM may be useful both as an inhibitor of tumorigenesis and as a body growth promoter in tumor-bearing animals. The results of these studies also suggest a usage for NALM as a replacement for L-methionine in hyperalimentation of cachexic cancer patients and that tumorigenesis may be inhibited by alteration of the dietary arginine-methionine balance without caloric restriction.

Effect of Fat Administration and the Perioxisome Proliferator Nafenopin on Lipid Peroxidation and Rat Liver Carcinogenesis

W. HUBER, B. KRAUPP-GRASL, C. GSCHWENTNER and
R. SCHULTE-HERMANN

*Institut für Tumorbiologie & Krebsforschung,
University of Vienna, Austria*

Peroxisome proliferators like nafenopin are nongenotoxic liver carcinogens in rodents. These compounds induce a pronounced increase in peroxisomal β-oxidation of fatty acids. It is discussed that the hydrogen peroxide thus generated might be the carcinogenic agent by causing lipid peroxidation. This hypothesis is investigated. First, we investigated possible correlations between tumor rate and several biochemical indicators of lipid peroxidation in two groups of male Wistar rats (old vs. young) that showed pronounced differences in susceptibility towards the carcinogenic effect of nafenopin. Although far more tumors were induced in the old animals there were no age differences in lipid peroxidation. Moreover, lipid peroxidation rather tended to be reduced than increased by nafenopin. Second, we investigated possible correlations between lipid peroxidation and nafenopin-induced fat metabolism by administration of high doses of substrate for peroxisomal β-oxidation (=corn oil). These corn oil doses, indeed, led to a significant increase of triacylglycerol in blood and liver which was clearly less pronounced under nafenopin. Nafenopin also reduced the triacylglycerol levels in animals fed *ad libitum* or rhythmically with standard chow, which were investigated in comparison. Lipid peroxidation, however, was essentially the same in all animals regardless of treatment. Only in the animals given corn oil were there some slightly higher values in the controls than after nafenopin treatment. In order to rule out any influence by the timepoint of sacrifice we sacrificed the animals in several groups over a period of 24 hours. In summary, neither was there any relevant correlation found between nafenopin-induced fat metabolism and lipid peroxidation nor between lipid peroxidation and carcinogenesis. From the present data it seems unlikely that nafenopin and high nutritional fat levels work synergistically towards liver carcinogenesis by the discussed mechanism.

The Effect of Lactobacillus Species Strain GG on DMH-Induced Rat Intestinal Tumor Formation

B.R. GOLDIN, L. GUALTIERI, R. MOORE[1] and S.L. GORBACH

Department of Community Health, Tufts University School of Medicine and [1]Tufts University School of Veterinary Medicine, Boston, MA

A rat dimethylhydrazine (DMH)-induced intestinal tumor model has been used to investigate the ability of a human bacterial isolate designated Lactobacillus species strain GG to inhibit tumor formation. Male F344 rats were given 20 mg/kg body weight of DMH weekly for 16 weeks and were sacrificed 8 weeks after the last injection. One group of animals was fed 10^8 Lactobacillus GG in each gram of food daily for 3 weeks prior to being injected with DMH and throughout the course of the experiment. This group had on average 1.6×10^6 Lactobacillus GG per gram of their feces. The GG strain was not found in the feces of animals not fed the organism. All animals were maintained on a 20% corn oil diet throughout the study.

A group of animals serving as a negative control receiving saline injections weekly had a mean weight gain of 157 g during the 16-week injection period. The animals administered DMH alone gained a mean of 96 g and the group fed Lactobacillus GG and injected with DMH gained on average 119 g over the 16-week period. The incidence of malignant colon tumors in the animals administered DMH alone was 100% and for the rats given Lactobacillus GG plus DMH the incidence was 71.4% this was significantly lower (P=0.012). The colon tumor load was 3.80 ± 0.49 tumors per tumor-bearing animal for rats receiving DMH alone and 1.66 ± 0.21 for the animals administered DMH and Lactobacillus GG; this was significantly lower (P < 0.01). The tumor's invasivness as judged by the Duke's classification or the degree of penetration through the wall of the colon was similiar for both groups. These data suggest that Lactobacillus species strain GG inhibits colonic tumor formation in rats fed a high-fat diet.

A second protocol has been completed and necropsies performed, however, the histologic analysis has not been completed, therefore the results described below have to be classified as preliminary. The second protocol differed from the protocol described above, with respect to when the Lactobacillus was introduced to the animals. The bacteria were introduced at the begining of week 10 of the 16-week DMH injection period. The preliminary results reveal that there was a 90.5% incidence of colonic tumors in the rats receiving DMH alone and a 71.4% for the animals given the Lactobacillus species strain GG plus DMH. The number of tumors per tumor-bearing animal was 3.26 and 3.00 for the rats receiving DMH alone and DMH plus Lactobacillus GG, respectively. These numbers if supported by histologic analysis, suggest a weaker protection by this organism when it was introduced in the later stages (promotional phase) of the tumorigenesis process.

Supported by the American Institute for Cancer Research grant 90A23.

Vitamin B$_6$ Deficiency and Cancer:
A Hypothesis

F.G.R. PRIOR

Eastern General Hospital, Edinburgh, Scotland

Factors involved in carcinogenesis all increase the requirement for DNA bases. Thymidine deficiency can result in DNA mutations (*Nature*, 255:764, 1970; *Mutat Res.* 105:433, 1982). Vitamin B$_6$ deficiency may result in thymidine deficiency. Thus a B$_6$ deficiency occuring at the same time as contact with carcinogens may be significant in the development of malignancies.

Cancer is a disease of cell multiplication. Two identical strands of DNA should be produced each time a cell multiplies. Errors in this process lead to DNA mutation. While small quantities of preformed DNA bases are absorbed from the GI tract, most of the requirement is synthesised from dietary components (JPEN, 14:18, 1990). DNA synthesis is halted when the synthesis of all four bases is blocked by an anti-metabolite. However, deficiency of a single base can lead to DNA base mutation, increase in replication errors (*Nature*, 255:764, 1970; *PNAS USA*, 77:1956, 1980), and induction of SOS repair functions (*PNAS, USA*, 75:1657, 1978). Of the many co-enzymes utilized in base synthesis, only one is involved in the production of just one base, namely vitamin B$_6$ in the synthesis of thymidine. A deficiency of thymidine is likely to be mutagenic (*Nature*. 255:764, 1970; *Mutat Res.* 105:433, 1982).

Contact with carcinogens causes either an increase in DNA mutation or an increase in cell multiplication rate. Contact with carcinogens in a subject who is also B$_6$ deficient, could result in insufficient thymidine biosynthesis for normal DNA repair or multiplication. Such profuse mutation could lead to cancer.

Estrogen lowers B$_6$ levels (*Am J Clin Nutr*, 27:326, 1974) and has been related to an increase in cervical (*Lancet*, 8356:930, 1983) and possibly breast (*Lancet*, 8356:926, 1983) cancer. Isoniazid also reduces B$_6$ levels and has been reported to be hepatocarcinogenic (*Br J Cancer*, 20:307, 1966). Dietary B$_6$ deficiency in baboons has been reported to cause hepatocarcinomas (*JNCI*, 53:1295, 1974). Incorporation of deoxycytosine in place of thymidine has been shown in the DNA of a range of cancers (*Free Radical Res, Res Comm*, 7:3, 1989.

The relationship between B$_6$ deficiency, thymidine misincorporation, and cancer warrants further investigation.

Nutrition and Cancer

E.K.M. BOSKAMP

Oldsum 72, Germany

Cancer, solid tumors as well as leukemia cells, are characterized as undifferentiated, remaining in a juvenile state. Potentially a lack of certain essential nutritional factors blocks completion of these cells. Considering the fact that only completed cells have the ability to emit signals to stop further cell production, the key factor behind the uncontrolled growth of cancer cells may be due to these cells having never reached their stage of completion.

It is supposed that certain nutritional deficiencies in the diet of cancer patients result from an insufficient intake of lipids with the complete series of sterols and other natural fats accompanying substances like the vitamins A, D, and E. A declining cholesterol, vitamin A and E level during the progression of illness and even before indicates this lack. The parabolic relationship between cancer progression and cholesterol is described elsewhere (*Lab Med* 10:26, 1986). Unfortunately, most of these nutritional factors are eliminated during the processing of oilseeds to oil and margarine and during the milling of wheat to meal or are avoided by nutritional habits. A dietetic anamnesis of cancer patients is proposed, followed by a dietetic therapy with the aim to increase the cholesterol level to stop further progression and the development of metastasis.

Response of Murine Natural Killer Cells to Moderate-Intensity Endurance Training: Relevance to Experimental Metastasis of B16-BL6 Melanoma

S.E. BLANK, C.A. ELSTAD, L. PFISTER,
K.L. WOODALL, R.M. GALLUCCI and G.G. MEADOWS

*Department of Physical Education, Sport and Leisure
Studies, College of Pharmacy, Pharmacology/Toxicology
Graduate Program, Washington State University, Pullman, WA*

Natural killer (NK) cells play an important role in combating hematogenous metastasis. Previously, we demonstrated that 10 weeks of moderate-intensity endurance training does not alter: (1) *in vitro* NK cell cytolytic activity of unmodified splenocytes and (2) the percent and total number of splenic NK cells from non-tumor-bearing female C57BL/6J mice, when assessed 48 or 72 hours after exercise. Following nylon wool passage, NK cell cytolytic activity was suppressed approximately 60% of controls in splenocytes from trained (TR) mice. The biologic significance of these findings is unknown. The purpose of this study was to assess the effects of moderate-intensity endurance training on NK cells and experimental metastasis of B16-BL6 melanoma. Mice (7-week-old female, C57BL/6) were single housed, matched by body weight, and assigned to the sedentary (SED, n=11) or TR (n=12) group. TR mice were progressively trained to run on a motorized treadmill at 12 m/min, 60 min/day, 5 days/week for 13 weeks without the use of electrical stimulation. At the end of 10 weeks, 4×10^4 viable tumor cells were inoculated into the lateral tail vein (48 hour post-exercise for TR mice). After 13 weeks (48 hours post-exercise for TR mice), the extent of pulmonary and extrapulmonary metastases were quantified. Splenic NK cell activity was determined by ^{51}Cr release assay and the numbers of NK1.1+ and the LGL-1+ subpopulation determined by flow cytometry.

Final body weight and daily food intake did not differ between groups. Spleen weight (91.4 ± 3.8 mg and 77.4 ± 3.8 mg, average values $\pm$ SEM for SED and TR groups, respectively), splenocyte number ($3.4 \pm 0.2 \times 10^7$ and $2.1 \pm 0.5 \times 10^7$), and splenocyte number per spleen weight ($3.6 \pm 0.5 \times 10^5$ and $2.8 \pm 0.2 \times 10^5$) were significantly ($p<0.05$) higher in SED versus TR mice. Lung weight (153.9 ± 13.0 mg and 175.2 ± 6.4 mg) and median number of pulmonary tumor colonies (15, range 0-66; and 18, range 1-64) were not significantly different between groups. In SED mice, NK cell cytolytic activity of unmodified splenocytes was 1.5 ± 0.2 lytic units per 10^6 effector cells. Training did not alter NK cell activity or the percentage of splenic NK1.1$^+$ cells ($6.9 \pm 0.5\%$), splenic LGL-1$^+$ cells ($3.4 \pm 0.3\%$), peripheral blood NK1.1$^+$ cells ($8.0 \pm 0.5\%$) and LGL-1$^+$ cells ($3.8 \pm 0.3\%$). Due to the lower number of splenocytes in TR mice, the total number of splenic NK$^+$1.1 and LGL-1$^+$ cells were significantly lower in TR versus SED mice.

It was concluded that experimental metastasis of B16-BL6 melanoma in mice was not altered with moderate-intensity endurance training. Under tumor-bearing conditions, training had no effect on splenic NK cell cytolytic activity or the percentage of splenic and peripheral blood NK1.1$^+$ and LGL-1$^+$ cells.

Supported by the American Institute for Cancer Research grant 85B79R88.

Alterations in Fat Metabolism Associated with Tumor Growth

T. FOLEY-NELSON, A. STALLION,
W.T. CHANCE and J.E. FISCHER

*Department of Surgery, University of Cincinnati
Medical Center, Cincinnati, OH*

Problems associated with cancer cachexia emphasize the need for understanding skeletal muscle substrate metabolism in tumor-bearing (TB) organisms. In catabolic conditions, protein conservation occurs via a shift from carbohydrate to lipid as a fuel. While lipid stores are mobilized in the TB organism, there is some question as to whether lipids are utilized as a fuel source. Hypertriglyceridemia is one indicator of inefficient lipid utilization. To investigate the effects of tumor burden on blood triglyceride (TRIG) levels, methylcholanthrene sarcomas were transplanted into 31 rats. Sixteen rats received sham inoculations. Groups of TB and sham rats were sacrificed 7, 14, 21, and 28 days post-tumor for analysis of plasma TRIG concentrations. TB rats exhibited significant increases in plasma TRIG levels by 14 days post-tumor (Table 1A). This effect peaked at 21 days and occurred prior to the onset of significant anorexia. Rats were, however, cachectic, as indicated by a significant decrease in gastrocnemius protein content by 7 days. Muscle protein loss in the TB rat can be decreased by the β_2-agonist, cimaterol. Experiment II (Table 1B) assessed the impact of cimaterol on plasma TRIG levels and determined the impact of tumor-induced alterations in food intake on plasma TRIG by including a pair-fed (PF) control group. Procedures were identical to Experiment I except testing occurred 21 days post-tumor and TB rats received injections of either cimaterol (0. 15 mg/kg, sc) (CIM) or saline (1 ml/kg, sc) (SAL) daily for one week prior to testing. Blood TRIG levels were significantly increased in TB-SAL rats relative to controls. This effect was associated with a significant decrease in muscle protein. Cimaterol, however, lowered plasma TRIG to control levels and resulted in significant muscle protein savings. Tumor-induced alterations in food intake did not contribute to hypertriglyceridemia or skeletal muscle protein loss.

	Table 1A					Table 1B			
Group (days past tumor)	Control (n = 16) (n = 4/week)	TB (n = 8) 7 days	TB (n = 7) 14 days	TB (n = 8) 21 days	TB (n = 8) 28 days	Control (n = 9) 21 days	TB-SAL (n = 7) 21 days	TB-CIM (n = 7) 21 days	PF-SAL (n = 7) 21 days
Food intake (g/100 g BW)	9.7 ± 0.4	10.1 ± 0.6	10.5 ± 0.4	7.4 ± 0.3[a]	5.2 ± 0.4[a]	7.9 ± 0.2	5.8 ± 0.8[b]	5.4 ± 0.5[b]	5.6 ± 1.0[b]
Gastrocnemius protein (mg/muscle)	251.9 ± 14.8	188.0 ± 7.8	184.0 ± 13.6[a]	182.3 ± 9.9[a]	132.7 ± 8.1[a]	256.1 ± 7.6	206.0 ± 15.0[a]	231.0 ± 15.0	252.0 ± 13
Tumor weight (g)	—	1.0 ± 1.0	10.0 ± 1.0	36.0 ± 2.0	70.0 ± 4.0	—	49.0 ± 6.0	51.0 ± 5.0	—
TRIG (mg/dl)	70.0 ± 7.0	46.0 ± 6.0	138.0 ± 38.0[a]	224.0 ± 31.0[a]	109.0 ± 35.0	129.0 ± 11.0	349.0 ± 51.0[a]	154.0 ± 23[c]	127.0 ± 11.0

[a] p<0.01
[b] p<0.05 vs. control
[c] p<0.01 TB-SAL vs. TB-CIM

Supported by the American Institute for Cancer Research grant 90A44.

Biochemical Effects of Transfer of Polychlorinated Biphenyl-Loaded Mice to High-Fat vs. Low-Fat Diet

Y.E. KIM, L.E. BEEBE, L. FORNWALD and L.M. ANDERSON

Laboratory of Comparative Carcinogenesis, National Cancer Institute, Frederick Cancer Research and Development Center, Frederick, MD

Polychlorinated biphenyls (PCBs), widespread environmental contaminants that accumulate in body fat, are tumorigenic and tumor-promotive in rodents; in mice even a limited dose of the PCB mixture Aroclor 1254 effectively promotes nitrosamine-initiated liver and lung tumors. PCBs are detectable in body fat of most humans, and mobilization of fat, as in dieting, may release PCBs to the circulation. The potential toxic impact, including tumor promotion, of stored PCBs and those released during fat breakdown can be studied with animal models. Tumor promotion by PCBs is closely associated with induction of specific cytochromes P450. While possible mechanistic associations between this induction and tumor promotion are still problematic, nevertheless increased enzyme levels are a reliable experimental marker for biologically effective doses of PCBs and elevated risk of tumor promotion.

In this study, adult Swiss male mice received a single 500 mg/kg dose of Aroclor 1254 or oil. After 1 week subgroups were switched to low-fat (0.4%) or high-fat (12%) diets and killed at intervals of 2 days, 1 week, and 4 weeks. Livers were assayed for total cytochrome P450 and benzyloxyresorufin-o-dealkylase (BenzRod), a specific marker enzyme for P450 IIB1, inducible by many PCB congeners. At all timepoints mice kept on normal diet (6% fat) after Aroclor exhibited a two-fold increase in P450 compared to controls, whereas those on high-fat diet showed a three-fold increase, and on low-fat, a three- to five-fold increase. Differences in BenzRod activities were even more striking, with a two- to four-fold induced increase in mice on normal diet, a five- to seven-fold increase on high-fat diet, and a 14-fold increase on low-fat diet. These changes correlated well with changes in body weights. These results imply enhancement of specific cellular pre-toxic effects in mice given a low-fat diet after PCB loading, presumably from release of adipose-stored congeners. The significance of this phenomenon for tumor promotion is under investigation.

Physical Activity and Breast Cancer Risk in the Framingham Study

J. DORGAN,[1] A SCHATZKIN,[1] C. BROWN,[1] B. KREGER,[2,3]
M. BARRETT,[1] D. ALBANES[1] and G. SPLANSKY[2,3]

[1]National Cancer Institute, Bethesda, MD; [2]Boston University
School of Medicine, Boston, MA; and [3]National Heart,
Lung, and Blood Institute, Bethesda, MD

We examined the relation between physical activity and breast cancer in a prospective cohort of women who participated in the Framingham Study. Self-reports of physical activity were obtained from 2304 women, 35 to 68 years old, at the fourth biennial examination in 1954. Women were followed for up to 29 years, during which time 119 breast cancers (six pre-menopausal, 112 post-menopausal, and one with unknown menopausal status) were diagnosed.

Physical activity was assessed by asking women how many hours a day they usually spent at work and during leisure time at basal, sedentary, slight, moderate, and heavy levels of activity. The number of hours at each level of activity, weighted by the relative oxygen consumption of that activity, were summed to create a physical activity index. The association of this index with development of breast cancer was assessed using Cox proportional hazards with age as the underlying time variable in the model. Adjustment was made for age at assessment of physical activity, education, parity, and menopausal status. Height and body mass index did not substantially affect results and were not included in the model.

Physical activity was not associated with reduced breast cancer risk in this relatively sedentary cohort. If anything, results suggested a direct relation between physical activity and subsequent breast cancer. Compared to women in the 1st (lowest) quartile of physical activity, those in the 2nd, 3rd, and 4th (highest) quartiles had odds (95% CI) of developing breast cancer of 1.14 (0.64-2.03), 1.33 (0.74-2.42), and 1.65 (0.92-2.96), respectively. The trend was marginally significant ($p = 0.07$).

Problems and Opportunities in Voluntary Exercise Methodology

T. C. GILES and B.D. ROEBUCK

Department of Pharmacology and Toxicology,
Dartmouth Medical School, Hanover, NH

Voluntary exercise has been demonstrated to inhibit carcinogenesis in several organ systems in laboratory rats. Investigation into the response of rats to voluntary running wheels reveals certain consistent behavior patterns while raising new issues that warrant further exploration. Observations from several experiments suggest that both weanling and adolescent rats exhibit a characteristic running pattern such that running increases immediately upon exposure to the wheel, reaches a maximum within 2-3 weeks, and usually declines gradually after several weeks of exercise. In two separate studies, the "area under the running curve" was greater for female than for male rats, since for the former both the height and length of the curve was greater. However, there is tremendous individual variation in both the pattern and the quantity of daily exercise within like groups of rats. Regardless of gender or age, rats restrict their running activity to the dark period of the light-dark cycle unless disturbed by human activity in the room; the majority of running occurs early in the dark period and is alternated with eating activity. Changes in food intake patterns in response to exercise may be sex dependent, as suggested by our observations that exercising female rats increase their food intake in comparison to sedentary rats, while male rats maintain or decrease their food consumption. Additionally, voluntary exercise appears to decrease "body fat stores" independent of changes in food intake levels, suggesting mechanistic possibilities for observed carcinogenesis outcomes. While these observations help to define the parameters of voluntary running that require measurement or control, they also raise concerns of whether observed variations in individual running behavior may affect experiment outcome.

Supported by the American Institute for Cancer Research grant 88A29.

Potentiation by High-Fat Diet and Effects of Cholecystokinin Receptor Blockade on Pancreatic Tumor Induction

M.K. HERRINGTON, J. PERMERT, K. KAZAKOFF, P.M. POUR and T.E. ADRIAN

Department of Biomedical Sciences, Creighton University School of Medicine, and the Eppley Cancer Institute, Omaha, NE

Considerable etiologic evidence links fat intake with pancreatic cancer. A possible mechanism for this is through the hormone cholecystokinin (CCK), which is released by dietary fat and causes pancreatic growth. Studies on the role of CCK in models of pancreatic cancer are controversial, either demonstrating enhanced tumor promotion with exogenous CCK or inhibition of tumor initiation when CCK is administered before the carcinogen.

Our aims were to investigate the potentiation by high-fat diet on pancreatic cancer in a model resembling the human disease, and to investigate the effect of CCK receptor blockade during tumor initiation on subsequent cancer incidence.

Four groups of 25 hamsters were studied at 9 weeks of age. Two groups of animals received continuous infusion of CCK receptor antagonist (MK329, 25 nmol/kg per hour) for 14 days; controls received placebo. Four days after surgery, one MK329 and one control group were fed a high-fat semi-synthetic diet (35% fat); the other groups were given a similar composition with low-fat content (5%). Four days after these diets were started, all animals received a single injection of N-nitrosobis(2-oxopropyl)amine (BOP, 20 mg/kg body weight). Dietary intake and body weight were recorded for 55 weeks; surviving animals were killed and autopsied at this time. Histology was performed blind by an experienced pathologist on three step sections through the entire pancreas.

The total incidence of malignant tumors was higher in high-fat diet (49%) than low-fat (17%, $p < 0.01$) animals. Importantly, advanced lesion (adenocarcinoma) incidence was higher in the high-fat (26%) than the low-fat group (5%, $p < 0.01$). No significant differences in total malignant lesions or incidence of advanced tumors was seen between MK329-treated animals and controls.

These findings confirm an increased incidence of malignant tumors in animals receiving a high-fat diet. The lack of effect of MK329 on tumor incidence provides no evidence for an important role for endogenous CCK during tumor initiation. Further studies are required to investigate the role of CCK during tumor promotion by high-fat diet.

Selenite-Induced Inhibition of Colony Formation by Buthionine Sulfoximine-Sensitive and -Resistant Cell Lines

P.B. CAFFREY and G.D. FRENKEL

Department of Biological Sciences,
Rutgers University, Newark, NJ

We previously demonstrated that treatment of HeLa cells with buthionine sulfoximine (BSO), which decreases the level of cellular glutathione, resulted in a decrease in the potency of selenite in inhibiting cell colony formation. We have now examined the effect of selenite on normal human lung fibroblast (CCL-210) cells, which resemble HeLa cells in their sensitivity to BSO and on human lung adenocarcinoma (A549) cells, which are relatively insensitive to BSO. We have found that BSO treatment caused an approximately four-fold decrease in selenite potency in the CCL-210 cells but had no significant effect on its potency in A549 cells. In contrast, BSO treatment of the CCL-210 cells did not decrease the potency of selenodiglutathione, the product of the reaction of selenite with glutathione. These results support the hypothesis that for selenite to exert its cytotoxic effect it must undergo the first step in its metabolism, reaction with an SH compound to form the selenotrisulfide. These results also demonstrate that a large differential sensitivity to the cytotoxic effect of selenite can be achieved as a result of the lower sensitivity of the tumor cells to BSO.

Supported by the American Institute for Cancer Research grant 91A40 and a grant from the National Institutes of Health.

The Role of Lipids in the Regulation of Ras-GTPase Activating Proteins

M. GOLUBIC,[1] P. HOMAYOUN,[1] K. TANAKA,[2]
S. DOBROWOLSKI,[1] D. WOOD,[2] M.-H. TSAI,[1]
F. TAMANOI[2] and D.W. STACEY[1]

[1]The Department of Molecular Biology, The Cleveland Clinic
Foundation, Cleveland, OH; [2]The Department of Biochemistry and
Molecular Biology, The University of Chicago, Chicago, IL

Lipids may influence the carcinogenic process by modulating the functions of onco-genes, tumor suppressor genes and signal transduction pathways. We have shown earlier that lipids, such as arachidonic acid, phosphatidic acid and phosphatidylinositol phosphates are able to influence the activity of mammalian Ras proto-oncogenic protein by inhibiting its regulatory molecule — the GTPase activating protein (GAP). GAP normally down-regulates the Ras function by stimulating the GTPase activity of Ras protein, thus converting the active Ras-GTP form to the inactive Ras-GDP form. The inhibition of GAP activity by lipids could, therefore, increase Ras biological activity and thus promote cellular proliferation.

In addition to GAP, neurofibromatosis type 1 (NF1) and yeast IRA2 proteins are able to stimulate the GTPase activity of Ras proteins. We wanted to determine if lipids might also have an effect upon the activity of NF1 and IRA2. The catalytic fragment of NF1 was expressed in bacteria and compared to the catalytic fragment of GAP. We found that the NF1 protein was indeed inhibited by lipids in its ability to stimulate the GTPase activity of H-Ras. Linoleic acid and arachidonic acid inhibited the GTPase stimulatory activity of NF1 even more efficiently than that of GAP. Phosphatidic acid (containing arachidonic and stearic acid) was unable to inhibit GTPase stimulation by the catalytic fragment of GAP, but did inhibit such a fragment of NF1. Similar studies were carried out with the catalytic fragment of yeast IRA2 protein. This protein was also inhibited quite efficiently by arachidonic acid, but not by phosphatidic acid.

The fact that all three GTPase stimulatory proteins are similarly inhibited by mitogenic-ally produced lipids supports the notion that lipids might be important in their biologic control. The apparent role of lipids in the control of cellular Ras activity raises the possibili-ty that dietary fats could play a role in regulating the activity of normal Ras protein and therefore cellular proliferation.

Assessment of Exercise-Related Changes in Fat Distribution Using Ultrasound Images

M.E. RAMIREZ

*Cardiovascular Genetics, University of Utah,
Salt Lake City, UT*

Recent studies have shown that regional fat deposits play important roles in hormone production and lipolytic activity. Exercise appears to have different effects on the body composition and weight maintenance of men and women. The importance of physical activity has been discussed in studies showing that weight fluctuation can have serious health implications. The measurements often used in assessing body composition are body circumferences and skinfolds, which have proven to be excellent screening tools. Unfortunately, they lack precision in measuring fat distribution changes.

Methods: To measure changes in subcutaneous fat thickness and fat distribution resulting from intense physical activity, we measured body composition and fat distribution in college gymnasts using anthropometry and ultrasound. Three sets of measurements were obtained: at the beginning of the training season, at peak training, and post-season.

Results: Intense training resulted in a reduction in most of the body measurements. The changes in body circumferences and total body fat were not statistically significant. The skinfold measurements at the upper arm and calf decreased significantly, but the trunk and anterior thigh skinfolds did not. Subcutaneous fat thickness measured using ultrasound decreased significantly on the trunk, arm, calf, and anterior thigh. However, the lateral and medial thigh deposits did not decrease significantly.

Measurements obtained after a marked decrease in activity level showed that subcutaneous fat deposits had been replenished to original levels without significant increases in weight, circumferences, or percent fat.

Effect of Corn Oil and Omega-3 Fatty Acid Diet on Human Breast Cancer Cells (MCF-7) Growth in Nude Mice

G. FERNANDES and J. VENKATRAMAN

Department of Medicine, The University of Texas
Health Science Center, San Antonio, TX

Several recent observations have described the beneficial effects of omega-3 fatty acid diet on reducing the incidence of carcinogen-induced tumors in small animal models. The present study was undertaken to compare the growth of MCF-7, human breast cancer origin tumor cells, in nude mice maintained on semi-purified diets containing 20% polyunsaturated (corn oil), and omega-3 fatty acids (menhaden oil). After maintaining the weanling animals on each dietary regimen for 8 weeks, each mouse was injected subcutaneously with 5×10^6 MCF-7 tumor cells. The transplanted tumor incidence after 90 days was as follows: corn oil (71%) - 17/24; fish oil (23%) - 5/22.

The rate of tumor growth and the tumor volume was significantly higher in corn oil-fed mice and was significantly lower in fish oil-fed mice. There was no significant difference in body weight between the groups. High levels of 18:2 (ω-6) and 20:4 (ω-6) fatty acids were present in tumor tissues of corn oil-fed mice whereas tumor tissue from fish oil-fed mice showed higher levels of 20:5 (ω-3) and 22:6 (ω-3) fatty acids which are known to regulate decreased PGE_2 production. Serum and tumor tissue sample analysis indicated decreased serum estrogen and prolactin levels as well as less tissue content of PGE_2 and reduced c-*myc* oncogene mRNA levels in the tumor tissues of fish oil-fed mice. Further, when SDS-PAGE-separated polypeptides were electrophoretically transferred onto immobilon P and immunoblotted with P21 antibodies, the level of P21 proteins was also found lower in tumor tissues of fish oil-fed animals and was much higher in corn oil-fed mice. In summary, our pilot studies suggest that both reduction of PGE_2 and endocrine hormones by fish oil diet appear to act on reducing the expression of oncogene and possibly several other growth factor mRNA levels that may facilitate in reducing human breast cancer cell growth in nude mice. However, new experiments are required to elucidate a more precise molecular mechanism involved in the reduction of breast cancer cell growth by suitable diet and anti-estrogen therapy in nude mice.

Supported by the Kleberg Foundation, San Antonio.

International FOODBASE™ Consumption Database

Y.S. CYPEL, N. BENELL, J.S. DOUGLASS,
S.K. EGAN, K.H. FLEMING and B.J. PETERSEN

Technical Assessment Systems, Inc., 1000 Potomac Street, N.W., Washington, DC

Technical Assessment Systems, Inc. (TAS) is collaborating with the U.S. National Cancer Institute (NCI) on a 3-year project to develop a data management and analysis system based on international food consumption surveys. FOODBASE™ will be a powerful tool for nutritionists, epidemiologists, medical researchers, and other health professionals to use in assessing the intake of foods and food constituents for individuals from all parts of the world. The FOODBASE™ IBM-PC compatible data retrieval system is designed for users with little or no computer experience and allows for the sorting of dietary intake information to meet user needs. Future application of the FOODBASE™ system has been directed towards greater investigation of diet-disease associations, mainly via supplementation of FOODBASE™-generated data with other data sets (e.g., cancer incidence).

FOODBASE™ has three linked components: (1) descriptive data for each dietary survey, (2) food and nutrient intake summary data for selected surveys, and a (3) bibliography of related documents. The descriptive component allows users to select those surveys that best answer their research questions. Once the appropriate surveys are selected, food and nutrient intake data from component two are available on line. The bibliographic citations, or component three, provide further background information and documentation for those surveys specified.

The Effect of Diet and Exercise on Incidence of 7,12-Dimethylbenz(a)anthracene-Induced Mammary Tumors in Virgin BALB/c Mice

H.W. LANE,[1] M.T. WHITE,[2] P. TEER,[3]
R.E. KEITH[2] and S. STRAHAN[2]

[1]NASA Medical Sciences Division, Houston, TX;
[2]Department of Nutrition & Foods; and [3]College of
Veterinary Medicine, Auburn University, AL

The effects of rotating-drum treadmill exercise and diet on 7,12-dimethylbenz(a)anthracene (DMBA)-induced mammary tumors were investigated in virgin female BALB/c mice. The animals were fed one of three diets: AIN 76 (SD), high-fat diet (HFD), or a restricted-calorie diet (RCD). All diets were begun at 6 weeks of age and fed *ad libitum* except for the restricted diet, which was fed at 70% of the SD. At 8 weeks of age all animals received the first of 6 consecutive DMBA doses (1 mg/2 ml corn oil) via gastric tube. Each diet had an exercise and no-exercise subgroup. Exercise began at 10 weeks of age (6 m/min for 60 min, 5 d/wd) and continued throughout the 9.5-month study. Exercise reduced feed consumption in SD and HFD groups. Body weight was similar in all groups with HFDEx having the lowest body weight. Calorie restriction had no effect on body weight but reduced mammary tumor incidence. Exercise had no effect on mammary tumor incidence in the SD groups (47% SD and 45% SDEx); however, exercise did affect mammary tumor incidence in the other groups as follows: RCD=82%, RCDEx+13%, HFD+31%, HFDEx+19%. Caloric consumption appeared to be related to mammary tumor incidence rather than body weight or dietary fat.

Supported by the American Institute for Cancer Research grant 87A33.

Protection against Skin Tumor Promotion in SENCAR Mice by Green Tea Polyphenols

H. MUKHTAR, S.K. KATIYAR and R. AGARWAL

Department of Dermatology, University Hospitals of Cleveland,
Case Western Reserve University, and Department of
Veterans Affairs Medical Center, Cleveland, OH

Green tea, next to water, is the most popular and commonly consumed beverage in the world especially in Eastern countries. In prior studies we have shown that the polyphenol-enriched fraction of green tea (GTP) inhibits the mutagenicity of several promutagens in *Salmonella typhimurium* (*Mutation Res*, 223:273-285, 1989), and protects against polycyclic aromatic hydrocarbon-induced tumor initiation (*Cancer Lett*, 42:7-12, 1988; *Carcinogenesis*, 10:441-415, 1989) and ultraviolet B radiation-induced carcinogenesis in murine skin (*Carcinogenesis*, 12(8), 1991 in press). In the present study the effect of skin application of GTP to SENCAR mice on 12-O-tetradecanoylphorbol-13-acetate (TPA)-caused induction of epidermal ornithine decarboxylase (ODC) activity and skin tumor promotion was assessed. Topical application of GTP to mouse skin in a dose-dependent manner inhibited TPA-caused induction of epidermal ODC activity. The inhibitory effect of GTP was also dependent on the time of its application relative to TPA treatment. GTP application to animals also inhibited the induction of epidermal ODC activity caused by several structurally different mouse skin tumor promoters including benzoyl peroxide; however, maximal inhibitory effect was observed with TPA. When assessed in anti-tumor promotion protocol in 7,12-dimethyl-benz[a]anthracene-initiated SENCAR mouse skin, pre-treatment of animals with GTP before each application of TPA resulted in significant protection in total number of tumors per mouse and percent of mice with tumors when compared to non-GTP pre-treated animals. These protective effects of GTP were also dose-dependent; at doses of 1 and 24 mg GTP per animal per application, greater than 30% and nearly 100% protection, respectively, against tumor formation occurred. These results, in conjunction with our prior publications, suggest that GTP may prove to be a useful chemopreventive agent against some forms of human cancers induced by environmental agents.

Supported by the American Institute for Cancer Research grant 90A47.

Energy Expenditure in Patients with Breast Cancer: A Preliminary Report

R.W. IAFELICE, W.L. SIMONICH,
D.K. LEWIS and J.F. BAUTISTA

American International Hospital–Cancer Treatment
Centers of America, Zion, IL

The object of this study is to characterize resting energy expenditure (REE) in breast cancer patients and identify its possible determinants. We measured resting energy expenditure by indirect calorimetry in 55 breast cancer patients. We then compared the findings with predicted energy expenditure (PEE) from the Harris-Benedict formula. Each patient was classified as normometabolic (REE = PEE ± 10%), hypometabolic (REE < 0.90 PEE), or hypermetabolic (REE > 1.10 PEE). Because of the danger of cancer cachexia, we treat these statuses as forming the ordered variable of "metabolic status," from desirable (normometabolic) to less desirable (hypometabolic) to least desirable (hypermetabolic). Based on the prior work of Knox and Dempsey, in nonbreast cancer, we predict that about 43% will be normometabolic, 33% hypometabolic, and 24% hypermetabolic. We also predict that duration of disease, duration of metastatic disease, and liver metastases each worsen metabolic status (MS). Actual MS percentages (36/22/42) do not differ from predicted (p>0.05). However, neither duration of disease, duration of metastatic disease, nor liver metastases are associated with MS (p>0.05, one-tailed). Breast cancer patients show the same pattern of energy expenditure as other cancer patients. Resting energy expenditure does not correlate with age, weight, surgery, chemotherapy, TPN, percent ideal weight, percent usual weight, or albumin. However, a significant negative association was found between height and MS, despite normalization of REE.

Enhancement of Pancreatic Carcinogenesis by Dehydroepiandrosterone

B.D. ROEBUCK, A.R. TAGLIAFERRO, A.M. RONAN and L.D. MEEKER

Dartmouth Medical School, Hanover, NH, and University of New Hampshire, Durham, NH

The effects of the anti-obesity steroid, dehydroepiandrosterone (DHEA) on energy balance and azaserine-induced pancreatic pre-neoplastic lesions were examined. Twenty-four-male Lewis weanling rat pups were randomly assigned to three groups: DHEA (n=8), pair-fed (PF; n=6), and *ad libitum* controls (n=10) and were fed a 20% high-fat diet containing either 0.6% DHEA or no DHEA, respectively, for 4 months. Daily food intake of DHEA, PF, and *ad libitum* groups were 12.0, 12.6, and 15.0 g, respectively. Fasted and post-prandial energy expenditure (kcal/kg body weight) of DHEA rats was significantly higher than that of PF. DHEA rats were 12% shorter in length and 59% smaller in body mass (p<0.001) than PF. Percentages of total body mass as fat and fat-free mass were significantly lower and higher, respectively, than PF or *ad libitum* controls. Light microscopic analysis showed that the DHEA rats had a greater number (602/cm^3) and volume percent of pancreas (2.6%) occupied by pre-neoplastic foci than PF (338/cm^3; 1.6%), and *ad libitum* controls (372/cm^3; 2.2%). Evidence suggests that DHEA promotes pancreatic carcinogenesis directly or indirectly via a substrate-dependent mechanism.

Supported by NH AES 285 (ART) and (BDR) and by the American Institute for Cancer Research grant 88A29.

Retinoid Regulation of Gene Expression in Human Papilloma Virus Immortalized Human Cervical Epithelial Cells

C. AGARWAL,[1] E.A. RORKE[2] and R.L. ECKERT[3]

[1,2,3]*Departments of Physiology and Biophysics,*
[2]*Environmental Health Sciences,* [2,3]*Reproductive Biology,*
[3]*Dermatology, and Biochemistry, Case Western Reserve*
University, School of Medicine, Cleveland, OH

Human papilloma virus type 16 (HPV16) is an important etiologic agent in the development of cervical cancer. As a model system for the study of HPV effects on cervical cell function we immortalized human cervical epithelial cells with molecularly cloned HPV16. Retinoids are nutritional constituents that are important regulators of epithelial cell differentiation and may be therapeutically useful in treating various types of cancer. We therefore examined the effects of various retinoids on the differentiation of a clonal line of HPV16 immortalized cervical cells, ECE16-1. Keratin expression is cell type specific and keratin profile can be utilized as an index of cell differentiation. Treatment of ECE16-1 cells with *trans*-retinoic acid results in a marked change in the keratin structural protein profile. In retinoid-free medium ECE16-1 cells synthesize keratins K5, K6, K7, K8, K13, K14, K16/17, and K19; a pattern identical to that of normal cervical cells. Retinoid addition reduces K5, K6, and K16/17 to nearly undetectable levels, while the level of K7, K8, and K19 increase. K13, a specific marker of cervical epithelial cells, is not regulated. These changes are mediated by retinoid-dependent changes in keratin mRNA levels. This is in contrast to normal cells where retinoids do not regulate keratin gene expression. Other markers of differentiation [superficial cell (squame) formation, involucrin level, involucrin crosslinking and transglutaminase activity] respond to retinoids in a manner similar to that of normal cervical cells. These results indicate that (1) HPV16 immortalized cells possess a heightened sensitivity to retinoids, (2) that HPV16 transformation renders normally unresponsive cytokeratin genes retinoid responsive and, (3) only part of the cervical cell differentiation program is altered by immortalization.

Effects of Caloric Restriction on Colon Cellularity, DNA Synthesis, and Chemically Induced Tumorigenesis in the Rat

D. ALBANES,[1] C. LEWIS,[2] M. ANVER[3] and P.R. TAYLOR[1]

[1]National Cancer Institute, Bethesda, MD;
[2]U.S. Department of Agriculture, Beltsville MD;
[3]PRI/DynCorp, Frederick, MD

The mechanism(s) by which caloric restriction (CR) inhibits tumorigenesis is (are) unknown. One active hypothesis is that CR affects absolute cell number and the rate of cell proliferation. This study in rats correlates the incidence of colon cancer induced by 1,2-dimethylhydrazine (DMH) with changes in colon cellularity and DNA synthesis in response to CR during two periods in life: (1) a 9-week post-weaning period of hyperplastic colon growth; and, (2) a 48-week post-growth period. A group of 220 weanling Fischer 344 female rats were randomized to one of two dietary regimens for the early period: *ad libitum* feeding (AL) or restriction to 50% of the *ad libitum* caloric intake (R). After 9 weeks on these regimens, each group was further divided into 2 groups that were fed the AL or R diet during the second period. The four final study groups were AL/AL, AL/R, R/AL, R/R. Two weeks into the second period, all animals received DMH (30 mg/kg body weight) by gavage once weekly for 6 consecutive weeks. Subgroups of animals were randomly chosen for determination of colon DNA, RNA, protein, and ^{3}H-thymidine incorporation into DNA after 1, 2, 3, and 12 weeks in period two. At the end of the experiment (age 60 weeks), average body weights for the 4 groups were 305, 168, 265, and 174 g. Colon weight paralleled these group differences, as did total colon DNA (301, 278, 323, and 281 µg/l), RNA, and protein. ^{3}H-thymidine incorporation was highest in the two groups fed *ad libitum* in the second period: 362 and 350 cpm for AL/AL and R/AL, compared with 176 and 125 cpm for groups AL/R and R/R. Total tumor incidence in the colon (adenoma or adenocarcinoma) was 47%, 20%, 58%, and 22% in the AL/AL, AL/R, R/AL, R/R groups, respectively. Colon adenocarcinoma incidence was 33%, 0%, 32%, and 11%, respectively. These results indicate that CR and the concomitant reductions in colon cellularity and cell proliferation, when they occur during a carcinogenic exposure, can reduce colon cancer incidence.

Selenium and Immune Cell Function

L. KIREMIDJIAN-SCHUMACHER, M. ROY,
H.I. WISHE, M.W. COHEN and G. STOTZKY

*New York University, College of Dentistry and
Graduate School of Arts and Science, New York, NY*

Selenium (Se) is an essential nutritional factor that affects the development and expression of cell-mediated immune responses directed toward malignant cells. These studies have shown that dietary (2 ppm for 8 weeks) or *in vitro* (1 x 10^{-7}M) supplementation with Se (as sodium selenite) results in a significant enhancement of the proliferative responses of spleen lymphocytes from C57B1/6J mice in response to stimulation with mitogen or antigen. Se deficiency (0.02 ppm for 8 weeks) had the opposite effect. The alterations in the ability of the cells to proliferate, which occurred in the absence of changes in the endogenous levels of interleukin-2 (Il_2) or interleukin-1, were apparently related to the ability of Se to alter the kinetics of expression of high-affinity Il_2 receptors on the surface of activated lymphocytes. This resulted in an enhanced or delayed clonal expansion of the cells and in an increased or decreased frequency of cytotoxic cells within a given cell population. The changes in tumor cytotoxicity were paralleled by changes in the amounts of lymphotoxin produced by the activated cells. The results also suggested that Se exerts its effect 8 to 24 hours after stimulation, and that it most likely affects processes in the cytoplasmic and/or nuclear compartments of activated lymphocytes. Dietary Se modulations had a comparable effect on macrophage-mediated tumor cytodestruction. Supplementation with Se enhanced tumor cytodestruction and tumor necrosis factor-α production by peritoneal macrophages elicited by allogenic stimulation *in vivo*, while Se deficiency inhibited tumor cytodestruction. It appears that modulation of Se levels in the diet significantly affects the development and magnitude of immune responses.

Supported by the American Institute for Cancer Research grant 86A08R87B.

A Community-Based Exercise and Nutrition Intervention Targeting African Americans and Latinos

A.K. YANCY

*UCLA School of Public Health, Cancer Prevention
Research Unit, Division of Cancer Control,
UCLA Jonsson Comprehensive Cancer Center, Los Angeles, CA*

Cancer and cardiovascular disease are the predominant sources of morbidity and mortality in the U.S. The convergence of their primary prevention approaches is an active area of research, particularly in exploring the interface between nutrition and exercise. Individuals from socially devalued racial and ethnic groups are at greater risk of developing many chronic diseases, including cancer, linked both to poverty and to newly acquired affluence. The *malnutrition of affluence* and sedentary lifestyles have been increasingly implicated in cancer epidemiology.

Little applied research, however, has been done in extending primary prevention interventions successful in Anglo populations to African-American and Latino communities. For example, none of the classic recent studies on nutrition and fitness, including Miller, Gordon, Marston, Tucker and Friedman, Gortmaker, Dietz and Cheung, Blair, Wood, and Paffenbarger, reported inclusion of significant numbers of African Americans or Latinos in their samples. Similarly, few patient education materials, especially in audiovisual modalities more likely to be attended to by those with less formal education, are specifically targeted to them (in the manner that tobacco and alcohol marketing and promotion have perfected). As health behaviors are culture-bound, attention and resources should be directed at developing interventions that are culturally relevant and linguistically appropriate.

The research proposed here seeks to develop, implement and evaluate a primary prevention intervention utilizing identification with ethnically relevant role models in emotionally significant contexts, available both inter-personally and electronically, to impart knowledge; influence self-concept, attitudes, values and beliefs; and thereby, increase cancer-protective health behaviors. It is anticipated that, with incremental behavioral change, the synergy between optimal nutrition and exercise will also favorably alter the individual's physiologic and neuroendocrine milieu. Thus, a biopsychosocial model is represented.

A randomized, prospective, community-based, cohort, nutrition-exercise-smoking cessation study targeting a large, majority African-American and Latino sample is planned. The intervention includes group nutrition instruction incorporating video modalities, individual exercise prescriptions, supervised group exercise, personal training PRN, group process stress-management sessions, and *healthy cuisine* juice bar/cafe offerings. The proposed intervention site is a an African-American-owned, urban Los Angeles health club in the ethnically and socioeconomically diverse mid-Wilshire district. The current clientele is observably heterogeneous with respect to age, SES, and corpulence, with a predominance of lower-middle class individuals. A *teachable moment* exists when an individual seeks a gym membership. Motivation is heightened by personal appearance concerns, as well as health-related ones. Capitalizing on the price elasticity of a free membership offer, in exchange for study participation, others might be encouraged to join, especially those in the lowest quintile of fitness. While after-work socializing among many Anglos has shifted from neighborhood bar to gym, this transition has not been as successfully effected among people of color.

A national multi-disciplinary medical advisory board has been recruited. It functions to lend viewpoints representing a broad range of community providers of care to these populations, as well as providing a starting point for culturally targeting messages. A majority are African American and Latino, representing a range of body types, and all are behaviorally health conscious. As it has been demonstrated that adoption of good health behaviors by physicians has a *multiplier effect*, these providers will serve as role models for clients attempting to make similar changes.

This poster presentation will outline the proposed pilot study and detail the scientific core of the intervention. These nutritional recommendations and exercise guidelines are based upon extensive literature review and nearly 10 years of the author's experience as an international fashion model and physician to a collective of entertainers and artists critical of allopathic medicine and actively taking control of their own life-styles to protect and enhance their health. The structure of the intervention is an adaptation of the Better Choices Nutrition Program designed for the American Cancer Society as a training program for nutritionists by William McCarthy, Ph.D., Adjunct Assistant Professor of Psychology, UCLA School of Public Health and co-principal investigator of this project.

American-Blend Fiber Lowers Serum Cholesterol without Stimulating Colonic Cell Proliferation

J.R. LUPTON, S.W. SHARP and T.K. ROONEY

Human Nutrition, Texas A&M University, College Station, TX

Single fiber sources that lower serum cholesterol stimulate colonic cell proliferation and may enhance experimentally induced colon tumorigenesis. We designed a mixed-fiber source to mimic that found in the American diet and fed it to rats at levels that could be extrapolated to current human recommendations. Serum and tissue cholesterols were measured enzymatically as were daily cholesterol and bile acid excretions. Colonic cell proliferation was measured by *in vivo* uptake of bromodeoxyuridine. Results from the mixed fiber (MF) were compared to a fiber-free control (FF) or diets supplemented with 6% fiber from cellulose (C), oat bran (OB), or pectin (P). Both P and MF significantly lowered serum cholesterol as compared to C (P=111 $\pm$ 13 mg/dl; MF=119 $\pm$ 5 mg/dl; C=157 $\pm$ 13 mg/dl; $P<0.05$). However, MF resulted in a more quiescent proliferative pattern in the colon than did P. For example, in the cecum P had a greater number of proliferating cells/crypt column and a greater zone of proliferating cells than FF whereas MF was not different from FF. Similarly, in the distal colon P resulted in a higher proliferative index than controls, whereas MF did not. These data suggest positive physiologic effects of the mixture of fibers currently ingested by Americans if this mixture is consumed at recommended levels.

Supported by the American Institute for Cancer Research grant 91A19.

Inhibitory Effects of Diallyl Sulfide on Metabolism and Tumorigenicity of the Tobacco-Specific Carcinogen 4-(methylnitrosamino)-1-(3-pyridyl)-1-butanone (NNK) in A/J Mouse Lung

J.-Y. HONG, Z.-Y. WANG, T. SMITH, S. ZHOU, S.T. SHI and C.S. YANG

Laboratory for Cancer Research, College of Pharmacy, Rutgers University, Piscataway, NJ

Diallyl sulfide (DAS), a component of garlic oil, has been shown to inhibit tumorigenesis by several chemical carcinogens. Our previous work demonstrated that DAS inhibited the metabolic activation of carcinogenic nitrosamines, including the tobacco-specific nitrosamine NNK, in rat lung and nasal mucosa. In the present study, the effects of DAS on the tumorigenicity and the metabolism of NNK in A/J mouse lung were examined. Female A/J mice at 7 weeks of age were pretreated with DAS (200 mg/kg bw in corn oil, po daily) for 3 days. Two hours after the final DAS treatment, the mice were either given a single dose of NNK (2 mg/mouse, ip) and kept for an additional 16 weeks for determining the production of pulmonary adenomas, or sacrificed immediately for measuring the microsomal activity in metabolizing NNK. In comparison to the control group, DAS pre-treatment significantly decreased the incidence of NNK-induced lung adenomas (37.9 vs. 97.8%) and the tumor multiplicity (0.6 vs. 8.4 tumors/mouse). In pulmonary metabolism of NNK, DAS pre-treatment reduced the formation of keto-aldehyde, keto-alcohol, NNAL-N-oxide, and NNK-N-oxide by 70 to 90%. In addition, the hepatic formation of NNK oxidative metabolites from DAS-pre-treated mice was remarkably reduced. DAS also inhibited the metabolism of NNK *in vitro* in mouse lung microsomes. These results demonstrate that DAS is an effective chemopreventive agent against NNK-induced lung tumorigenesis, possibly by inhibiting the metabolic activation of NNK.

Supported by the American Institute for Cancer Research grant 90B49.

Retinoic Acid, 1,25-Dihydroxy Vitamin D$_2$: Coordinated Down-Regulation of c-*myc* and RB Gene Expression in HL-60 Differentiation

A. YEN and M. FORBES

Cornell University, Ithaca, NY

Retinoic acid and 1,25-dihydroxy vitamin D$_2$ each induce down-regulation of RB retinoblastoma (tumor suppressor) and c-*myc* gene expression prior to onset of terminal myeloid or monocytic differentiation. Dose-response relations for RA and VD induced down-regulation of RB and c-*myc* expression were compared with each other and with induced cell differentiation. A low concentration (10^{-8} M) of RA induced down-regulation of RB expression associated with down-regulation of c-*myc* expression but without cell differentiation. Higher concentrations caused progressively greater corresponding reductions in RB and c-*myc* expression with an attendant progressively increasing fraction of cells terminally differentiating. VD caused analogous effects on gene expression with monocytic instead of myeloid differentiation. The down-regulation of these two genes may be coupled during cell differentiation. This is consistent with a hypothesized role for RB as a "Status Quo" gene whose expression is needed to sustain a developmentally ordained state of differentiation with down-regulation ergo needed to allow change from that state.

Supported by the American Institute for Cancer Research grant 87A59R9.

Effect of the Phytoestrogen Zearalenone on Human Breast Cancer Cells

F. LEONESSA, W.-Y. LIM, V. BOULAY,
J. LIPPMAN and R. CLARKE

*V.T. Lombardi Cancer Research Center, Georgetown
University Medical Center, Washington, DC*

Zearalenone is a resorcylic acid lactone that can be found in several major food grains infected with the mold *Fusarium roseum*. Because of its estrogenic properties, zearalenone and its metabolites have been held responsible for impaired fertility and genital tract diseases in livestock. Zearalenone binds to the estrogen receptor (ER) with an affinity approaching 5% that of 17-beta-estradiol. Subsequent interactions with DNA estrogen-responsive elements stimulate the expression of estrogen-specific proteins and proliferation in target cells, such as breast cancer cells. It is well known that a high percentage of breast cancers are responsive to estrogens. Treatments aimed to decrease the availability or prevent the stimulation by physiologic estrogens represent a common form of treatment. Consequently, dietary phytoestrogens, such as zearalenone, are likely to have a potential impact on breast cancer natural history and the outcome of treatment.

We have characterized the ability of zearalenone to regulate cell growth and the synthesis of an estrogen-specific protein, pS2, in human breast cancer cells. In our hands, zearalenone maximally stimulated growth and ^{3}H-thymidine incorporation by estrogen-responsive MCF-7 human breast cancer cells already at concentration 10^{-10} M. This maximal stimulation was comparable to that achievable by estradiol stimulation and was maintained through concentrations up to 10^{-6} M without any sign of aspecific inhibition. Cell kinetic recruitment by zearalenone at concentrations from 10^{-8} M to 5×10^{-6} M for 48 hours was confirmed by flow cytometric techniques. Moreover, zearalenone stimulated the expression of pS2, as assessed by Northern blotting.

Supported in part by the American Institute for Cancer Research grant 90BW65.

Inhibition of Nitrosamine-Induced Tumorigenesis in A/J Mice by Green Tea and Black Tea

Z.-Y. WANG, J.-Y. HONG, S.T. SHI, M.-T. HUANG, K. REUHL, A.H. CONNEY and C.S. YANG

Laboratory for Cancer, Research, College of Pharmacy, Rutgers University, Piscataway, NJ

The effects of oral administration of tea on nitrosamine-induced carcinogenesis were investigated. Female A/J mice were given N-nitrosodiethylamine (NDEA) (10 mg/kg) orally once a week for 8 weeks and were killed 16 weeks later. More than 90% of the mice had forestomach and lung tumors. The mice had an average of 8.3 forestomach and 2.5 lung tumors per mouse. Administration of 0.63% or 1.25% green tea extract as the sole source of drinking water for the entire experimental period decreased the forestomach tumor multiplicity by 59 or 63%, respectively, and the pulmonary adenoma multiplicity by 36 or 60%, respectively. Administration of 0.63 or 1.25% of green tea extract, during the NDEA treatment period only, decreased the forestomach tumor multiplicity by 31 or 58%, respectively, and the pulmonary adenoma multiplicity by 36 or 56%, respectively. Administration of 0.63 or 1.25% green tea extract for 16 weeks, starting 1 week after the completion of NDEA treatment, decreased the forestomach tumor multiplicity by 35 or 47%, respectively, and the pulmonary adenoma multiplicity by 52 or 44%, respectively. The tea extracts were prepared by extracting 12.5 g of green tea leaves with 1 l of boiling water (1.25% extract) and by 1 to 2 dilution to make the 0.63% extract. Treatment of female A/J mice with a single dose (103 mg/kg) of 4-(methylnitrosamino)-1-(3-pridyl)-1-butanone (NNK) resulted in the formation of pulmonary adenomas in almost all the animals after 16 weeks. When 0.6% decaffeinated green tea or black tea extract was given during the NNK treatment period, tumor incidence was reduced by 18 or 15% and multiplicity by 63 or 61%, respectively. When the tea extract was given after the NNK treatment period until the end of the experiment, 0.6% green tea extract inhibited the tumor incidence and multiplicity by 32 and 84%, respectively. In this protocol, a 0.6% of black tea extract inhibited tumor multiplicity by about 60%, but did not inhibit the tumor incidence. The results clearly demonstrated the inhibitory action of green tea and black tea on NDEA- and NNK-induced tumorigenesis.

Supported in part by the American Institute for Cancer Research grant 90B49.

Cancer Prevention Trials Using Micronutrients: Design Issues

B.H. PATTERSON,[1] L.C. CLARK,[2]
D.L. WEED[1] and B.W. TURNBULL[3]

[1]*National Cancer Institute, Bethesda, MD;*
[2]*University of Arizona, Tucson, AZ;*
[3]*Cornell University, Ithaca, NY*

Cancer chemoprevention trials are more than just an extension of therapeutic trials; they pose special design problems. In trials that use micronutrients, deficiency is hypothesized to be related to increased cancer risk, and supplementation to a reduction in risk. An initial issue is whether to supplement to levels associated with good nutrition, or to higher, pharmacologic levels. Unlike in therapeutic trials, subjects are already exposed to the intervention because vitamins and trace elements are already present, in varying degrees, in the daily diet. Micronutrient status, a measure of an individual's body stores (e.g., blood or tissue levels), depends both on an individual's diet and his metabolism.

"High-risk" subjects, defined both with respect to micronutrient status and to other risk factors, may be sought to enchance study power. Study duration depends in part on lag time to treatment efficacy, which may be a function of micronutrient half-life. If treatment efficacy is achieved when subjects are close to steady-state levels (possibly several years for some micronutiients), the study must be sufffciently long to provide a true test of the null hypothesis. Within-subject variability in blood levels must be considered in the design because it complicates compliance monitoring as well as determination of levels associated with either efficacy or toxicity. Examples will be provided from a selenium skin-cancer trial and from a selenium pharmacokinetics study.

Supported in part by the American Institute for Cancer Research grant 84B0188B.

Effects of RRR-α-Tocopheryl Succinate on Human Promyelocytic (HL-60) Cells

J.M. TURLEY, B.G. SANDERS and K. KLINE

Divison of Nutritional Science and Department of Zoology, University of Texas, Austin, TX

HL-60 human promyelocytic leukemia cells are capable of being induced to undergo terminal differentiation to mature granulocytes or monocytes/macrophages by various inducing agents. Dimethyl sulfoxide and retinoic acid (a biologically active form of vitamin A) induce differentiation of HL-60 cells along the granulocytic pathway, whereas phorbol esters and 1-25-dihydroxy vitamin D_3 (the active hormonal form of vitamin D) induce monocytic differentiation. In this study, vitamin E in the form of RRR-α-tocopheryl succinate has been shown to inhibit cellular proliferation by producing a soluble anti-proliferative factor and by blocking cells in the cell cycle. RRR-α-tocopheryl succinate has also been found to induce the expression of cell surface adhesion proteins which are members of the leukocyte integrin family.

HL-60 cells when treated with 20 μg/ml RRR-α-tocopheryl succinate exhibit a 26% and 62%, inhibition of cellular proliferation following 24 and 48 hours of culture, respectively. The conditioned media from HL-60 cells cultured with 20 μg/ml RRR-α-tocopheryl succinate for 24 hours has been found to contain a soluble anti-proliferative factor capable of suppressing the growth of C4#1 tumor cells by 51% and FACS analysis of RRR-α-tocopheryl succinate treated HL-60 cells revealed that the cells were blocked in the G2 stage of the cell cycle. Both the RRR-α-tocopheryl succinate elicited production of an anti-proliferative factor and blockage of the cell cycle may function to inhibit HL-60 cell proliferation. In addition to effecting HL-60 cell proliferation, when HL-60 cells are treated with 15 or 20 μg/ml vitamin E succinate for 24 or 48 hours they exhibit dramatic homotypic aggregation. Preliminary studies to immunochemically characterize the molecules involved in the homotypic aggregration employed monoclonal antibodies specific for CD18 (the common β subunit of the intregrin adhesion proteins) and showed RRR-α-tocopheryl succinate to induce the expression of CD11a (LFA-1; α subunit) and CD18. The results of these studies suggest a role for RRR-α-tocopheryl succinate in the modulation of tumor cell proliferation and differentiation, and a novel role for RRR-α-tocopheryl succinate in regulating cell-cell adhesion protein expression.

Supported by Public Health Service grant CA45422, Awarded by the National Cancer Institute, Department of Health and Human Services.

Macrophage Tumoricidal Activity Is Inhibited by Docosahexaenoic Acid (DHA), an Omega-3 Fatty Acid

C.Y. LU, L.B. DUSTIN and M.A. VAZQUEZ

University of Texas, Southwestern Medical Center, Dallas, TX

Fish oils rich in docosahexaenoic acid (C22:6, n-3) exert significant effects on tumor growth in experimental animals—inhibiting some, but not all cancers. Tumor growth *in vivo* depends upon the effect of fish oils on the tumor itself and also upon the anti-tumor immune response. Our studies were focused upon the effect of DHA on macrophage-mediated tumor killing, one important component of the anti-tumor response. P815 mastocytoma cells were used as targets. Killing of this tumor requires macrophage priming by interferon gamma and triggering by endotoxin. DHA, but not arachidonic acid (C20:4 n-4), inhibited macrophage-mediated tumor killing in a dose-dependent fashion between 20-160µM. The inhibition was reversed by increasing the interferon gamma/endotoxin signal. When the interferon gamma and endotoxin signals were separated in time, DHA was far more inhibitory if delivered with the triggering signal than if delivered with interferon gamma. Although DHA inhibits cyclooxygenase activity, its inhibition of macrophage-mediated tumor killing was not reversed with the following cyclooxygenase products: PGE2, a stable TXA2 analog (U46,619) or a stable PGI2 analog (Iloprost). Although DHA is metabolized by lipoxygenases, the inhibition was not reversed by the lipoxygenase inhibitors 5,8,11,14-eicosatetraenoic acid and nordihydroguaiaretic acid.

Caloric Restriction (CR) Enhances the Effective Activity of Rat Liver Catalase

R.J. FEUERS, R. WEINDRUCH[1] and J.E.A. LEAKEY

National Center for Toxicological Research,
Jefferson, AR; [1]University of Wisconsin,
Department of Medicine, Madison, WI

CR is the only intervention known to increase maximum lifespan in mammals but little is known about its mode of action. CR may act by reducing free radical levels either by decreasing their production or increasing detoxification. Prior work indicates that liver and kidney catalase activity decline in rats and mice with aging. Also, CR increases liver catalase activity in old rats when assayed at very high $[H_2O_2]$, which is nonphysiologic and quickly inactivates the enzyme. We investigated the influence on cytosolic catalase of a 40% CR started at 14 weeks of age in 12-month-old male (BN X F344)F_1 rats. Also, the effect of time of day was evaluated as rats were killed for study at 0600, 1200, 1800, and 2400 hours. At high, nonphysiologic $[H_2O_2]$ (e.g., >26 mM) no significant effects on enzyme activity (U/l or U/mg protein) of CR or time of day were observed. We next analyzed the samples across a broad range of $[H_2O_2]$. The length of time through which the reaction remained linear was determined and multiplied by enzyme activity. This value is viewed as the effective catalase activity. At high $[H_2O_2]$ no significant effects of CR or time of day were observed. However, at 15.6 or 19.8 mM H_2O_2 significant circadian rhythms with maximums at 1200 hours (after feeding) were seen in both diet groups. At 15.6 mM, CR rats had significantly higher (40%) effective levels of catalase at 1800 and 0600 hours. Similar results were observed at 7.8 mM H_2O_2. Current work suggests that the impact of CR on effective catalase activity is even larger at very low $[H_2O_2]$ (<1 mM). These data suggest that CR leads to important changes in the mechanism for the regulation of catalase activity.

Caloric Restriction (CR) Enhances the Effective Activity of Rat Liver Catalase

R.J. Feuers

National Center for Toxicological Research,
Jefferson, AR 72079
Department of Biometry

Index

CPSIA information can be obtained at www.ICGtesting.com
Printed in the USA
LVOW021318070413

327971LV00005B/144/P